P9-DTV-354

WITHDRAWN
UTSA LIBRARIES

4574

A

DI

COGNITIVE VULNERABILITY TO DEPRESSION

Cognitive Vulnerability to Depression

RICK E. INGRAM
JEANNE MIRANDA
ZINDEL V. SEGAL

Foreword by Aaron T. Beck

THE GUILFORD PRESS
New York   London

© 1998 The Guilford Press
A Division of Guilford Publications, Inc.
72 Spring Street, New York, NY 10012
http://www.guilford.com

All rights reserved

No part of this book may be reproduced, translated, stored in a
retrieval system, or transmitted, in any form or by any means,
electronic, mechanical, photocopying, microfilming, recording, or
otherwise, without written permission from the Publisher.

Printed in the United States of America

This book is printed on acid-free paper.

Last digit is print number: 9 8 7 6 5 4 3 2 1

Library of Congress Cataloging-in-Publication Data

Ingram, Rick E. / Rick E. Ingram, Jeanne Miranda, and Zindel
V. Segal.
    p.   cm.
  Includes bibliographical references and index.
  ISBN 1-57230-304-2
  1. Depression, Mental—Risk factors.
  2. Emotions and cognition. 3. Cognitive styles.
  I. Miranda, Jeanne, 1950– . II. Segal, Zindel V., 1956– .
III.Title.
  RC537.I54 1998
  616.85 27—dc21   97–48997
                                                        CIP

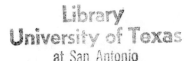
Library
University of Texas
at San Antonio

To Nancy—R. E. I.

To Ed and Cecilia—J. M.

To Ariel, Shira, and Solomon—Z. V. S.

Acknowledgments

It goes without saying that any book authored by more than one person requires extensive deliberation, discussion, and sometimes compromise. A book written by authors who live across three time zones, who work in not only different places, but also in very different kinds of institutional settings, requires these discussions to occur via e-mail, over the phone, and, on delightful but unfortunately rare occasions, in person. Our discussions were always interesting, thought-provoking, and sometimes quite spirited. This book represents the end result of our thinking and conversations.

Several people deserve our thanks—Seymour Weingarten, Editor-in-Chief at The Guilford Press, in particular for his patience in seeing this project through, and Jeannie Tang, Senior Production Editor at Guilford, for guiding the book through the production process. We would also like to specifically acknowledge Tim Beck for not only valuable discussions, but for the inspiration he has provided through the years, which has played such a fundamental role in shaping our views on depression. Additionally, Nancy Hamilton, Vanessa Malcarne, Joseph Price, John Teasdale, and Mark Williams deserve thanks for ongoing discussions and for provoking our thinking about cognitive functioning in depression. Finally, we owe a debt of gratitude to our families who provided the supportive atmosphere necessary to write this book.

Foreword

As our understanding of the nature of depression increases, many of the earlier assumptions about this disorder have been replaced by more accurate descriptions of both its course and the toll that the illness takes on patients' lives. It had been thought, for example, that since episodes of major depression responded well to short-term therapy, this condition was self-limiting in nature and associated with a favorable prognostic picture. There is now a growing recognition, however, that relapse and recurrence following successful treatment are common and debilitating outcomes.

In order to respond effectively to these newer conceptions of depression, we need to have models of risk and vulnerability that will allow us to develop strategies for reducing the risk of recurrence post-recovery. This knowledge would go a long way toward helping to shorten the span of depression, which is potentially lifelong in duration, and help to reduce the social and familial costs of depression, which have been estimated as comparable to or worse than major chronic medical conditions. The authors have seized on this premise and provide intriguing leads to the question of what variables place patients at cognitive risk to develop depression or experience a relapse following their recovery. The ultimate insights into this problem are likely to be informed by future work integrating findings from a number of fields, including neuroscience, cognitive science, and social theory. However, the contours of a model describing psychological factors are now at hand.

Ever since my early efforts to document the characteristic reasoning and thinking styles of depressed patients, I have been struck by how well these features also lead to a vulnerability model. In the early 1960s, I suggested that cognitive vulnerability to depression lay at the level of dysfunctional beliefs and attitudes that were hypothesized to reflect enduring negative self-views: "If I am not successful then others will reject me" or "Making a mistake is a sign of weakness." Clinically, these attitudes and assumptions remained important because they were largely unspoken, abstract regulators of behavior and could be maladaptive by disrupting more constructive responses in the patient's repertoire.

This book addresses itself to this clinical verity. The authors draw on basic research in cognitive science to document the relationship between negative mood and negative cognitions. They then go on to explain how depressed mood is maintained by these cognitions and how adverse life events can trigger these self-perpetuating mood–thought cycles into operation. The diathesis in this model is the person's cognitive reactivity in the face of mild dysphoria. Vulnerability to depression is based on tacit patterns of thinking that become activated once an individual is in a mildly depressed mood. These patterns or styles of thinking are the result of prior negative experiences and, when activated by a mildly depressed mood, promote further negative thoughts and feelings. This mechanism thus produces a downward spiral of depression, magnifying the initial mild state of dysphoria into a full-blown depressive episode. It is heartening that in their review of the empirical literature on cognitive models of vulnerability, the authors demonstrate that there is good support for a number of core premises. Cognitive reactivity following a mood induction, for example, predicts depressive relapse as late as 2 1/2 years following recovery. How robust and replicable this find will prove to be is hard to say at this point. What is more important, perhaps, is that the problem of vulnerability to depression is receiving the attention it deserves and that a focus on the cognitive aspects of this problem may contribute to its eventual understanding. This volume presents a refreshing perspective on the psychology of depression that should be a spur to a good deal of productive research.

AARON T. BECK, MD
University Professor of Psychiatry
University of Pennsylvania
Philadelphia

Preface

> By some persons, madness has been considered as a state of mind analogous to dreaming: but an inference of this kind supposes us fully acquainted with the actual state, or condition of the mind in dreaming, and in madness. The whole question hinges on a knowledge of this *state of mind*, which I fear is still involved in obscurity.
>
> HALSAM (1809, p. 75)

Writing nearly 200 years ago, John Halsam, the Apothecary to Bethlehem Hospital, London, suggested that to apprehend the nature of insanity one must understand the states of mind of the afflicted. Indeed, a consistent feature among many of the early case histories of patients suffering from "nervous conditions" is the careful tracing of the thoughts and beliefs endorsed by these individuals. In describing the thinking of patients with "religious melancholia" or "intense vanity," for example, the deviation from normal patterns of thinking could be more acutely appreciated and the use of labels such as mad or deranged became self-evident.

This view does not differ greatly from current cognitive perspectives on psychopathology, which are concerned with human mental activity as it relates to emotional disorder. Then, as now, cognition was generally thought to encompass the mental processes of perceiving, recognizing, conceiving, judging, and reasoning. Likewise, both then and now, these cognitive variables were thought to have significant causal implications for the onset, maintenance, and remission of disordered states. Indeed, numerous similarities can be found between historical and contemporary perspectives on cognition and psychopathology.

Important differences do exist, however. One critical difference is that, while Halsam's (1809) study of his patients' thoughts entailed only prudent observation and phenomenological description, contemporary cognitive psychopathologists can add the paradigms of cognitive science to assist in the conceptualization of maladaptive cognitive processes. These paradigms encompass rigorous experimental methods developed within the context of cognitive psychology, which allow psychopathologists to study the human cognitive system as it interacts with psychological dysfunction. Have these contemporary approaches aided psychopathologists in their ability to understand the deviations in thinking so carefully recorded by Halsam close to two centuries ago? Based on numerous research reports, we believe so. We also believe that the paradigms and methods of cognitive science afford the opportunity to attempt an understanding of an aspect of psychological dysfunction that has been relatively neglected by many psychopathologists: vulnerability to depression.

Depression is a problem that afflicts millions of individuals worldwide. Indeed, some estimates suggest that as many as 17% of all individuals will experience a major depressive episode at some point in their lives. Although the incidence of depression can vary somewhat across different groups, no group is exempt. For instance, depression cuts across diverse ethnic and cultural groups, familial structures, age differences, geographical and national boundaries, occupational and educational levels, and socioeconomic status. As anyone who has experienced this disorder knows, depression is an intensely aversive emotional state that is characterized by a wide range of symptoms. Equally aversive are the correlates and consequences of depression. Epidemiological data show that depression can be associated with impaired interpersonal relationships and divorce, impaired psychological and social competence, vastly diminished work capacity, poor parenting, and significant health problems. Indeed, in some cases depression is a deadly disorder. Affective disorder, for example, is a common precipitant of suicide. In sum, depression has a profound negative impact on the lives of numerous individuals. Understanding the factors that render some individuals vulnerable to this disorder is both tremendously important and immensely challenging.

Our aim in this volume is to describe and document a cognitive approach to the study of vulnerability to depression. This perspective does not suggest that all important vulnerability factors are cognitive in nature, but it does suggest that a consideration of mental activities such as perceiving, encoding, thinking, retrieving, and reasoning is vitally important in determining what factors put individuals at risk for developing depression. One must also understand the learning processes that affect the cognitive variables linked to depression vulnerability. Additionally, we hold the view that vulnerability extends across the lifespan. Finally, we emphasize that sound experimental methods must be applied to the empirical study of cognition and depression before any genuine progress can be made in understanding the critical determinants and effects of cognitive vulnerability to depression.

To begin our exploration of cognitive vulnerability to depression, in Chapter 1 we provide an overview of recent developments in cognitive psychology so that readers will be familiar with some of the central concepts in this area. We also examine the historical background of cognitive approaches and then discuss several major cognitive paradigms that may have applicability to depression vulnerability.

We do not believe that it is possible to understand vulnerability to a disorder without reflecting on the disorder itself. Therefore, in Chapter 2 we turn to a discussion of the syndrome of depression as defined by the standard psychiatric nosology of the fourth edition of the *Diagnostic and Statistical Manual of Mental Disorders* (DSM-IV), and then in Chapter 5, we present a related but slightly different operational definition of the depression construct that guides our discussion about the nature of cognitive vulnerability.

In Chapter 3 we provide an overview of the major cognitive models of depression. While some of these theories include specific statements about vulnerability, most focus on a description of the cognitive variables that operate after the onset of the depressed state. Nevertheless, understanding these theories is crucial for understanding vulnerability because many cognitive vulnerability notions are intrinsically embedded within these theories.

Equally crucial to understanding vulnerability to a specific disorder such as depression is an adequate understanding of the concept of vulnerability in general. The ideas of vulnerability and risk are introduced and their role in the study of psychopathology is described in Chapter 4. In particular, we discuss the origins of the vulnerability to psychopathology approach; we then assess what appear to constitute the core features of vulnerability paradigms, and we distinguish between the concepts of vulnerability and risk. In Chapter 5 we build on these general vulnerability features to focus on the definitional and conceptual issues that are specific to cognitive vulnerability to depression. As noted, we outline a working definition of the depression construct to guide our examination of vulnerability. We examine important distinctions in conceptions of causality—specifically those that differentiate between the onset and maintenance of depression—and also distinctions between distal and proximal vulnerability. In brief, proximal vulnerability refers to those factors operating close to the onset of a disorder while distal factors precede the disorder by a longer time span.

In Chapters 6 and 7, respectively, we discuss the methodological issues and strategies for the study of, and then examine theory and data on, proximal cognitive vulnerability. We follow a similar outline in Chapters 8 and 9 for distal vulnerability. Our goals in these four chapters are twofold. The first is to present a view of the cognitive factors that place persons at risk for depression by reviewing and evaluating data that bear on cognitive models. Our second goal is to distinguish risk factors whose effects may be relatively close in time to the development of an episode of depression from those variables whose effects may be somewhat removed in time from the episode.

In the final chapter of the book we present a model that integrates the theory and data previously presented into a comprehensive view of cognitive risk for depression. We seek here not to offer startlingly new insights or to cover all possible vulnerability to depression, but rather to integrate and explore the existing body of literature to arrive at a unifying conceptualization of cognitive vulnerability spanning the earliest origins up into adulthood. Our greatest hope is that these views will not only inform future experimental work on the questions of vulnerability to depression in general, and cognitive vulnerability to depression in particular, but will also stimulate new thinking and theorizing and perhaps prevention and treatment strategies for a problem that affects the lives of countless individuals.

Contents

CHAPTER 1

The Cognitive Approach to Psychopathology

To begin our exploration of cognitive factors in psychopathology, specifically those that may predispose some individuals toward depression, we assess the foundations of the cognitive approach to psychological disorder. To do so we illustrate some basic cognitive constructs and show how they have been applied to the investigation of psychopathology. In some places we touch upon the application of these constructs to the understanding of depression, but in this chapter we focus on the interrelationship between cognition and psychopathology in general.

Our exploration of the cognitive foundations of psychopathology leads us initially to an examination of the guiding assumptions of the cognitive approach to psychological science. We then examine the historical background of the cognitive approach to dysfunction and the progress toward current conceptualizations of the role of cognition in emotional disorders. After briefly exploring questions concerning the basic nature of the cognition construct, we examine the information-processing view of psychopathology and note the importance of considering cognition within an overall context of the underlying dysfunctional processes that give rise to abnormal behavior. Following this discussion we turn to the antecedents of current cognitive approaches and discuss an organizational framework for categorizing cognitive variables. Finally, we examine some cognitive variables, many of which are derived from cognitive experimental psychology and cognitive science. These constructs have formed much of the core of current cognitive approaches to psychopathology, which will serve as the foundation from which we explore cognitive vulnerability to depression.

GUIDING ASSUMPTIONS
OF COGNITIVE APPROACHES

Models of psychopathology that feature the role of cognitive variables in producing psychological dysfunction are often built on findings in cognitive psychology and information processing that describe how these variables behave in normal populations. For example, depressed patients often show a selectivity in their memories for certain types of material over others, which is often explained by referring to the work on mood congruence effects in normal memory function (Teasdale, 1983). It is, therefore, important to understand the rationale developed by cognitive psychologists for guiding their study of the mind, because it permeates many of the methods used in experimental psychopathology.

A critical guiding assumption in the study of cognition is that the objective features of a stimulus alone are insufficient to predict human cognitive performance. Rather, mental functions, such as representation and computation, play important mediating roles in determining a response to any particular stimulus. Put more simply, individuals do not all see objects, let alone more complex behavior, in the same way. This is an elaboration of the basic stimulus–response model of behavior, which, simply put, includes mental operations as an intermediary step in the chain of events. These mental operations are what we find when we look inside the "black box" of the mind.

Some cognitive psychologists studying the mental processes that produce reactions to stimuli have identified the subcomponents that perform different mental operations on a stimulus. It is the unique combination of these elementary mental processes or operations that produce complex responses (Posner & McLeod, 1982; J. M. G. Williams, Watts, MacLeod, & Matthews, 1997). As an illustration of this principle, consider the commonly accepted view that the time between a stimulus and a response is occupied by a series of processes or stages, some of which are mental operations, and many of which are arranged in such a fashion that one process does not begin until the preceding one has ended (Sternberg, 1969). Using this framework, psychologists studying reaction time have developed methods in which the difference between average response times for two tasks is used to estimate the duration of each process (Donders, 1868–1869/1969). This has enabled a more accurate study of basic mental operations and how they combine to produce complex performance. Understanding these basic mental operations thus forms the basis of the key assumptions and principles that underlie the cognitive approach to human behavior.

HISTORICAL AND CONTEMPORARY CONSIDERATIONS

Theoretical paradigms do not develop in a vacuum, and cognitive theories are certainly no exception to this rule. To appreciate fully contemporary developments in cognitive psychology it is important to consider the historical context from which they have arisen. Thus, prior to assessing contemporary aspects of the study of cognition, we address several important historical constructs and milestones in the study of cognition.

Historical Background

Many of the early experimental studies of mental processes were conducted in Wilhelm Wundt's (1899) psychology laboratory in Leipzig, Germany as the introspectionists were beginning to pursue their cognitive agenda at the turn of the century. They were interested in mapping the contents of consciousness, but to do so, they relied on markedly different methods than those used today. The introspectionists' guiding belief was that a theory of cognition could be developed by examining the contents of introspective reports and that these reports could be obtained through self-observation (Gardner, 1985). Although subsequent work in cognitive psychology has demonstrated the shortcomings of this position due to the lack of an isomorphic correspondence between those contents accessible to self-report and the underlying processes responsible for these contents, the notion that the mind can be studied through the examination of its products continues to fascinate psychopathologists.

One technique commonly employed by the introspectionists was free association. An experimenter would read a list of words to a subject and measure the amount of time it would take the person to generate responses to these words. This methodology was guided by the underlying belief that time differences reflected the operation of different cognitive processes. This idea still holds sway in the current cognitive arena, as evidenced by the plethora of methodologies that rely on reaction time, rating time, or decision time measures. Thus, while the basic ideas behind the concept of introspection remain important, the methodologies for studying these ideas have improved substantially.

Experimental psychologists, however, were not the only ones studying the mind at the turn of the century. Practitioners concerned with the treatment of "nervous disorders" also contributed to the burgeoning field of cognitive inquiry, setting a precedent for a complementary exploration of cognition that is often overlooked today. Jung (1910), for example, employed a word association technique to uncover complexes (e.g., areas of emotional conflict), which he assumed existed in patients with neurotic disorders. Words were presented to individuals who were instructed to respond by naming the first word that came to mind. Time to respond was recorded, along with other physical measures such as pneumography, used to record breathing changes. Jung believed that indications of emotional reactions to these words such as flushing or longer reaction times revealed the emotional valence of the stimulus item which allowed therapists to hypothesize about their significance to the patient. The number of associations or amount of emotion elicited by stimulus words would indicate the presence of complexes, or clusters of information that attracted greater amounts of psychic energy than did neutral words or clusters of information. The conceptual resemblance between this work and current models of spreading activation and semantic network models (Bower & Clapper, 1989) is considerable. Ironically, although Jung's experimental studies had little effect on psychoanalytic thinking at the time, they have withstood some degree of empirical scrutiny (see Carlson & Levy, 1973). It is certainly interesting and possibly important to note that, even in the formative stages of cognitive analyses of emotional disorders, experimental methods were sometimes closely tied to the clinical bases of the disorder under investigation.

Contemporary Developments

The dominance of behaviorism in the early decades of this century temporarily impeded the development of methods for the study of the mind. The reemergence of interest in cognitive psychology has been traced by J. R. Anderson (1985) to developments in three distinct areas. First, human factors research received a boost in World War II when practical information about human cognitive skills was in great need to help improve responses to potentially lethal situations. The second development stemmed from advances in computer science, especially work that demonstrated the ability of computer programs to problem solve, thus provoking new interest and analogies regarding the nature of intelligence. This work helped to establish the mind-as-computer metaphor that is still prominent today. Third, advances in the study of linguistics portrayed language acquisition and fluency as inherently complex abilities that could not be explained by prevailing behavioral theories. This pushed the agenda of cognitive psychology to the forefront of psychological science and helped to eclipse the previously dominant behavioral emphasis in these areas.

In many respects, the emergence of cognitive and information-processing approaches to emotional disorders can also be traced to a commitment of many theorists and researchers to the integration of clinical and experimental psychological science. Few would argue the point that clinical research efforts have profited immensely from examination and adaptation of the theories and methods of basic psychological science (Ingram & Kendall, 1986). This is not the first time, however, that clinical theory and research has looked explicitly to the ideas, concepts, and methods of basic psychological science. The principles of learning theory developed in experimental laboratories in the 1930s (e.g., Guhtrie, 1935; Tolman, 1932), for example, provided enormously fertile ground for generating a diversity of applied and clinical research applications (Kanfer & Hagerman, 1985). These principles, of course, constituted the antecedents of clinical behaviorism. Once again, there are substantial benefits for theory, research, and clinical applications that draw upon work in the experimental analysis of cognition. The utilization of such basic experimental principles and empirical work situates clinical science in general, and the analysis of cognition in depression in particular, squarely within the category of an applied specialization of basic experimental psychological science (Ingram, 1991a).

The waxing and waning of the influence of purely behavioral accounts of learning had a profound impact on clinical psychology. Through the 1960s, the behavioral model predominated in the field. But, beginning in the late 1960s and early 1970s, theories of emotional disorder, which had been dominated by animal conditioning studies and models, and which assumed the acquisition of maladaptive behavioral repertoires to be due to simplistic stimulus–response pairings, were gradually being challenged by a framework that admitted the possibility of cognitive mediation. This led to a renewed interest in the role of thinking and reasoning in psychopathology. Bandura's (1969) influential work, for example, legitimized the study of cognitive variables such as expectancies, self-verbalizations, predictions, and other covert processes that had previously been excluded from accounts of human behavior and learning.

As the interest in cognitive accounts of disordered behavior grew, therapies began to be developed that capitalized on the idea that cognition might be an important clinical target. Although some of these were straightforward extensions of behavioristic learning principles that went largely unverified (e.g., covert reinforcement; Cautela, 1970), at the very least this applied interest stimulated further interest in the clinical utility of cognitive constructs. Yet, few guiding paradigms were available with which to conceptualize the role and functioning of cognition in clinical problems; what existed instead were both a broad area of interest and inquiry that recognized that maladaptive cognitions were part of emotional disorders, and the development of strategies to modify these cognitions (Ingram & Kendall, 1986).

Fortunately from a conceptual standpoint, the growing recognition of the role of cognitive mediation in learning was soon accompanied by an influx of information from the neurosciences and computer sciences that focused the study of behavior change on questions of representation, the role of memory in learning, and constructive processes in perception (Pribram, 1986). Loosely termed the *information-processing perspective*, the clinical extensions of this viewpoint emphasized that humans are not merely passive recipients of information, but are instead active and selective seekers, creators, and users of information (Ingram & Kendall, 1986; Mahoney, 1990). Accounts of how people learn, which had previously only accepted stimuli, responses, and contingencies, started to consider deliberate cognitive activity as consequential; a wealth of meaningful activity occurring in the "black box," which behavioristic approaches had conceptually been unable to explore was now available for exploration.

Attempts to define the basic principles of cognitive functioning, both in general, and as they relate to clinical concerns, have been made by a number of theorists. According to a compelling definition offered by Mahoney (1990), the basic tenets of a cognitive mediation perspective in clinical psychology are that (1) humans respond primarily to cognitive representations of the environment rather than to the environments per se; (2) these cognitive representations are related to the principles of learning; (3) most learning is cognitively mediated; and (4) thoughts, feelings, and behaviors influence one another.

The applied aspects of cognitive assumptions stemming from the recognition that thoughts, feelings, and behaviors influence one another can be seen further in the premises of cognitive-behavioral treatment approaches. As noted by a number of writers (Dobson & Block, 1988; Ingram, Kendall, & Chen, 1991; Ingram & Scott, 1990; Kendall & Bemis, 1983; Kendall & Hollon, 1979; Mahoney & Arnkoff, 1978), the assumption that thoughts, feelings, and behaviors influence each other leads to the postulates that (1) modifying cognition can lead to the corollary modification of maladaptive patterns of emotion and behavior, and (2) cognitive and behavioral change methods can be integrated for effective intervention of emotional distress. These assumptions have received support as evidenced by the data demonstrating the efficacy of a number of cognitive-behavioral treatment approaches (Ingram et al., 1991; Ingram & Scott, 1990).

One key theme that occurs throughout the discussion of cognition is an emphasis on mental representation. This focus on representation is crucial in information-processing models as it implicates the mind in learning and allows for behavioral sequences to be explained by referring to cognitive operations. This principle forms a bridge, enabling links to be made between already established accounts of thinking and reasoning in normal human performance and models of abnormal psychology where the mental representation serves as the guiding idea for the study of cognitive and affective dysfunction. Likewise, clinical efforts to conceptualize cognition and relate it to the principal domain of cognitive sciences, that is, "normal" functioning, stand similarly to profit from an examination of cognition that has gone awry.

WHAT IS COGNITION?

Discussion of both the historical and contemporary aspects of the cognitive approach to clinical psychology begs one important question. Specifically, any discussion of cognitive vulnerability must, by necessity, devote some attention to examining the basic nature and meaning of the construct of cognition. Examination of this topic may seem unnecessary to many who study or understand psychological problems from a cognitive viewpoint. Yet, psychological conceptions of cognition may vary considerably. Historically, for example, cognition has been defined as the conscious contents of the mind as explored by introspection (Wundt, 1899) or the various associations between mental elements (Ebbinghaus, 1885). From a more contemporary perspective, a divergence of viewpoints is illustrated in a well-known exchange on the primacy of cognition versus affect. In arguing that affect is not postcognitive, Zajonc (1980) views cognition as constituting "considerable processing of information" (p. 151) or "extensive perceptual and cognitive encoding" (p. 151). For Lazarus (1982), however, such extensive analysis is not a defining feature of cognition, which "does not imply anything about deliberate reflection, rationality, or awareness" (p. 1,022). Lazarus (1982) instead argues that cognition can consist of activating the individual's belief and meaning systems, which he and others refer to as "appraisal" (for an early description of this process, see Arnold, 1960). Thus, cognition need not be extensive and lengthy, but can instead be considered a global evaluation of the significance of events as they pertain to the individual's well-being. At the same time, Lazarus argues against a view of cognition that he ascribes to cognitive psychology:

> . . . [that] decision and action as built up from essentially meaningless stimulus display elements or bits and that systematic scanning of

this display generates information. Thus, human cognition, like the operations of a computer, proceeds by serially receiving, registering, encoding, storing for the short or long run, and retrieving meaningless bits—a transformation to meaning that is called information processing. (pp. 1020–1021)

Views similar to this have been expressed by other investigators. Arnkoff (1980) has argued that definitions of cognition from an "information processing model are inadequate from a clinical perspective because clients are active creators, not passive receivers or automatic transformers of stimuli" (p. 342). Yet, many would disagree that these views accurately reflect experimental cognitive psychology's view of cognition. As noted by Ingram and Kendall (1986), for instance, another view of cognition is the "information processing perspective which . . . conceptualizes and empirically examines [how cognitive] structures work to allow for the 'active' construction of perception and experience" (pp. 20–21). Information-processing views are thus not confined to passive views of cognition, nor do they require the sequential flow of "meaningless" information through various processes and stores before meaning for the organism can be derived.

As is evidenced by these views, there are differing views on what constitutes a satisfactory conceptualization of cognition. We do not intend to resolve this issue so much as to offer a definition that will guide our discussion of cognitive vulnerability to depression. Our working definition of the construct of cognition is quite broad and adheres closely to the views offered by many experimental cognitive psychologists. In general, we subscribe to the view offered by Juola (1986): "Humans are viewed as active processors of information in that every behavior, from recognition of common objects to participation in a conversation, involves the operation of a number of different systems acting in concert" (p. 51). Our concern in this volume is thus the mental structures and processes that are involved in perception, memory, decision making, thinking, and behavior. Following many investigators, we do not view these processes as necessarily synonymous with conscious awareness, nor do we think that these processes need to reflect intensive processing for them to qualify as cognitive. Indeed, although we can hopefully develop valid inferences as to the structure and function of cognition in vulnerability to depression, many cognitive variables as we have defined them may operate outside of awareness and with limited processing. Having defined cognition is such a broad manner, we now turn to a description of a particular approach to cognition: specifically, a general examination of information processing and psychopathology.

INFORMATION PROCESSING AND A COGNITIVE VIEW OF PSYCHOPATHOLOGY

Information-processing models attempt to describe the nature of very elementary mental processes or operations that are thought to contribute to the production of complex behavior (Gardner, 1985). As Juola (1986) describes this, an information-processing perspective views behavior as being "modeled as a flow of information through a system in which different processing stages receive inputs from the environment, from memory, or from other stages" (p. 51). Some of these processing operations perform changes of code, enabling one form of information to be transformed into another (Posner, 1978). For example, recall of a string of numbers increases if the string can be condensed or recoded into a smaller number of chunks of digits (Mandler, 1967). In this case the transformation involves changing the task from one of memorizing digits individually to considering a smaller number of chunks of digits grouped according to some type of subjective organization. Others involve the use of strategies in which a combination of basic computations is assembled for a particular task (Posner & McLeod, 1982). For example, verbal protocol analysis reveals that efficient problem solving entails asking a series of questions about the problem, gathering information about the outcome of the inquiry, and then using the feedback to refine the questions asked on the next pass-through. This can be contrasted with less efficient approaches based on guesswork or intuitive leaps (Newell & Simon, 1972).

As shown in Figure 1.1, mental operations can also be characterized by their specificity and duration (Posner & McLeod, 1982). Accordingly, cognitive operations that involve the performance of a specific computation and that are enduring are referred to as structures (e.g., grammar structures). Operations that are combined for a given task are considered to be strategies (e.g., rehearsal of material to be recalled). Other influences on performance may be time-sensitive and variable in which case they are called states (e.g., mood), while others may be relatively enduring and are labeled traits (e.g., reactance, hypervigilance). The cognitive approach to psychopathology, and ultimately to vulnerability to psychopathology, is rooted in an understanding of the role played by these basic building blocks in normative information processing, and uses this understanding as a point of departure for studying aberrant mental activity. But this is a point of departure only. Clinical scientists are unlikely to further understanding by adopting wholesale the theories and methods of cognitive science. What is more likely to be productive is an examination of the conceptual paradigms utilized in cognitive

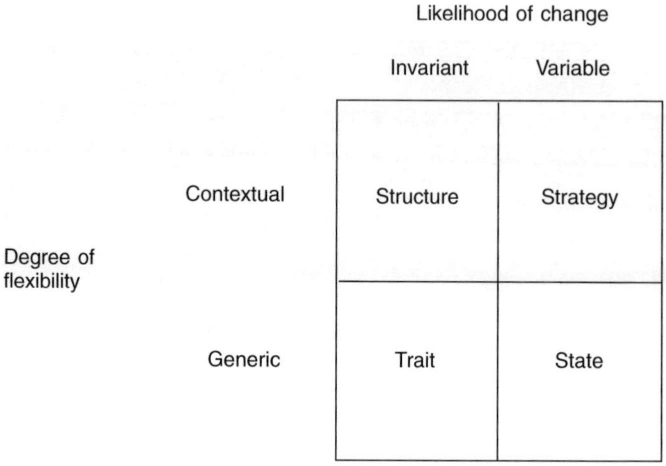

Likelihood of change

Invariant   Variable

	Invariant	Variable
Contextual	Structure	Strategy
Generic	Trait	State

Degree of
flexibility

FIGURE 1.1. Mental operations categorized according to their generality and variability.

science and their adaptation in cognitive theories and methods as they apply to specific clinical problems (Lachman & Lachman, 1986).

An Applied Science Approach

Cognitive psychopathology is essentially an exercise in applied psychological science (Ingram & Kendall, 1986). According to Teasdale and Barnard (1993) this involves choosing an ecologically valid clinical problem (e.g., catastrophic interpretation of bodily sensations in panic disorder) as a starting point and as a continuing reference point against which the relevance of subsequent experimentation and theorizing can be evaluated. Researchers would then employ existing experimental cognitive tasks, adapt existing tasks, or develop new ones to help capture in the laboratory the essential aspects of the applied problem (e.g., a dichotic listening task with anxiety words in the unattended channel, the Stroop color naming of threat words, a visual dot probe task with threat word distracters, etc.). Theoretical accounts can then be developed that take advantage of the precision and power offered by these experimental methods. These theories can then be tested and refined by referring back to the clinical problem and to ongoing laboratory studies intended to test key premises of the theory (e.g., hypervigilance and attentional bias). In continually cycling between experiment, theory, and problem solving, more detailed information is accumulated and our theoretical models are improved. With time, this may enhance our ability to deal with the original clinical concern through the development of methods based on a better understanding of related aspects of psychological function, derived from empirical study.

Cognition as One Piece of the Psychopathological Puzzle

To appreciate the role of cognitive variables in psychopathology, we need to remember that mental events are only one of a number of relevant levels of analysis in psychopathology. A variety of alternative approaches have made numerous and significant contributions to understanding normal as well as psychopathological functioning. Despite these contributions, no single approach can account for all facets of behavior, and cognitive approaches are no exception. Hence, cognitive factors represent one aspect of a confluence of forces that shape and determine behavior. Likewise, Braff (1985) reminds us that psychopathology comprises the domains of neuroanatomic, neurotransmitter, and hormonal; psycho- and neurophysiological; attentional and information processing, cognitive and neuropsychological; symptom-based state markers; and trait-based clinical outcome markers. To this we would add interpersonal and sociological levels of analysis. Among the difficulties faced by the psychopathologist is the need to weave these levels of analysis into a comprehensive account of the disorder, along with demonstrating whatever deficit or finding is pathognomic for the disorder and also establishing that such findings are not due to generalized, nonspecific factors (e.g., low motivation, medication side effects, chronicity of illness).

In view of the complex clinical phenomena comprising numerous levels of functioning that are being studied, it becomes extremely important to articulate the construct system and causal and vulnerability model from which one is operating. Articulation of construct, causality, and vulnerability assumptions potentially helps to clarify which of a disorder's multiple dysfunctions are most clinically significant, the expected relationships among them, and their possible determinants (Haynes, 1992). Further, understanding the nature of these relationships and determinants offers the potential for recognizing the steps required for remediation of the disorder.

With respect to depression, both thoughts and biology seem to influence onset (Gabbard, 1992; Kandel, 1983; Shelton, Hollon, Purdon, & Loosen, 1991). Accounts of disorder that restrict themselves to a single level of analysis deemed sufficient for explanation may thus be limited because they tend to describe the role of depressive cognition and biology in unidirectional terms. Indeed, recent depression research indicates that changing the conditions maintaining one dysfunctional subsystem of the disorder can have consequences on other, untargeted subsystems. For instance, the depression literature shows clear evidence of interaction between cognitive and biological systems. Studies have shown that changes in depressive cognition—such as automatic thinking, dysfunctional attitudes or attributional style—can be produced by somatic treatments (DeRubeis, Evans, & Hollon, 1990; Simons, Garfield, & Murphy, 1984). Similarly, cognitive treatment is associated with alterations of biological markers such as normalization of posttreatment dexamethasone suppression test response (Blackburn, Whalley, & Christie, 1987; McKnight, Nelson-Gray, & Barnhill, 1992), increases in sleep efficiency (Beutler, Scogin, Kirkish, & Schretlen, 1987), or increases in thyroid hormone levels (Joffe, Segal, & Singer, 1996). Patients with biological markers of depression (electroencephalographic sleep disturbance, endogenous symptom profiles) have also shown good outcome with cognitive behavior therapy in two recently reported trials (Simons & Thase, 1992; Thase, Simons, & Cahalane, 1991). The effects of psychological interventions are not just limited to alterations of biological markers of disorder, but can impact at the level of brain structures. Baxter, Schwartz, and Bergman (1992) used positron emission tomography (PET) to study local cerebral metabolic rates for glucose in patients with obsessive–compulsive disorder. Patients were tested before and after treatment with either fluoxetine hydrochloride or behavior therapy and results indicated that glucose metabolic rates in the right head of the caudate nucleus changed with successful treatment, regardless of the modality used. Pardo, Pardo, and Raichle (1993) report a study along similar lines in which PET was utilized to detect changes in cerebral blood flow associated with two self-induced states of mind (restfulness, dysphoria).

Clearly, the determinants of vulnerability to affective disorder are multiple and complex. In our view, cognition is but one of a series of systems that may be in dysfunction, and not merely a byproduct of a more fundamental somatic process. Recognizing the reciprocal influence of different subsystems in depression may allow the link between its cognitive features and other aspects of the disorder to be understood more clearly.

ANTECEDENTS OF COGNITIVE CONSTRUCTS AND ORGANIZING MODELS OF PSYCHOPATHOLOGY

Having considered the relation of cognition to other causal or contributory variables that may ultimately affect vulnerability to depression, we now turn our attention to those variables featured within cognitively based models. Specifically, in this section we examine the theoretical antecedents of contemporary cognitive models of psychopathology. We also consider a set of organizing principles for different cognitive constructs. We start with an examination of theoretical antecedents of current cognitive models and briefly examine several specific models of depression to illustrate these antecedents. We then turn to a discussion of one framework for organizing cognitive constructs.

Antecedents of Cognitive Models of Psychopathology

There are many possible ways to conceptualize and group the antecedents of cognitive models of mental disorder. One way that we think is particularly useful is to categorize the primary variables comprising these models into three broad domains (see Ingram & Wisnicki, 1991). These domains include (1) information-processing models, (2) social-cognitive models, and (3) behavioral-cognitive models.

Information-Processing-Based Models

Information-processing models are derived directly from theory and research in experimental cognitive psychology. For example, Ingram (1984) has described an information-processing model of depression based on the relationships between mood and cognition described in Bower's (1981) associative network theory. In this model, certain cognitive associative networks are connected to the affective structures responsible for the initiation of each emotion. When the structure for sadness or depression is activated through the individual's appraisal processes, depression-linked networks are then activated and become an increasingly intrusive influence on the individual's cognitive functioning. In another example, H. C. Ellis and Ashbrook's (1988) resource allocation model of depression is derived from more general models of attention. This view proposes that there is a limited amount of attentional capacity to be allocated to given tasks and that affective states, such as depression, compete for this processing capacity. Depressed patients' impaired performance on effortful tasks is explained by the diversion of attentional resources, due to mood state, away from task demands. Consequently, these competing task demands extend the duration of depression by their interference with the performance of adaptive behaviors (e.g., distraction or problem solving).

Social-Cognitive Models

Social cognition features prominently in the hopelessness theory of depression (Abramson, Metalsky, & Alloy, 1989), which posits that certain types of causal attributions contribute to the development of hopelessness and that hopelessness is a sufficient cause of the symptoms of hopelessness depression. This view offers a different level of analysis than information processing approaches. Variables in the social-cognitive tradition—such as negative expectations about the occurrence of highly valued outcomes and expectations of helplessness about changing the likelihood of their occurrence—are featured in this approach. The social-cognitive approach also suggests some differences in methodology. For instance, variables such as expectations can be measured with self-report instruments and are available to subjective awareness, whereas activation of the semantic networks that are prominent in information-processing approaches cannot be directly assessed.

Behavioral-Cognitive Models

Behavioral-cognitive models derive primarily from social learning analyses of depressive behavior that emphasize the role of cognitive activity in modulating availability of environmental reinforcement. Rehm's (1977) self-control model of depression represents an example of this approach. Rehm's model targets depressed patients' deficits in self-regulation. Through selective monitoring of negative events, biased predictions based on the immediate as opposed to the delayed consequences of behavior, and excessive standards for self-evaluation, depressed patients increase the probability that self-punishment will follow performance initiatives and that response contingent positive reinforcement will be further reduced (see also Lewinsohn, Hoberman, Teri, & Hautzinger, 1985).

Cognitive Organizing Frameworks

In considering conceptual antecedents, it is clear that a number of different cognitive variables are being studied by depression researchers. Despite the impressive gains of this research, a framework is missing for specifying the important theoretical links among these various levels of cognitive activity and how these factors interact with affective and behavioral variables in a given psychopathology. In the absence of such links, cognitive models have been criticized for suggesting relatively simple and linear causal relationships between cognition (e.g., self-critical automatic thoughts or appraisals of danger) and affective or behavioral dysfunction, such as "more distorted thinking means more depression" or that "negative thinking causes depression" (Coyne, 1992). Ingram and Kendall (1986) have described one possible framework, the "meta-construct model," for organizing the multitude of variables currently employed in a number of cognitive models. This framework adds to the distinctions suggested by Posner and McLeod (1982) by showing how an information-processing perspective may be integrated with clinically relevant theory and research (see Figure 1.2). The meta-construct model incorporates both a cognitive taxonomy and a components analysis of psychopathological variables. We now examine this organizational framework in greater detail.

The Meta-Construct Model: A Cognitive Taxonomy

The variety of different cognitive constructs that have been proposed by researchers argues for the development of taxonomic efforts to help classify and organize these different aspects of cognition. The cognitive taxonomy depicted here is one way to classify these constructs. It is but one possible construct system or operational definition, whose ultimate value will depend on its utility in furthering understanding of cognition and behavioral dysfunction. Development of this particular taxonomic structure for cognitive variables is based on the conceptual and empirical distinctions between cognitive structures and processes that have been proposed by researchers such as Goldfried and Robins (1983), Hollon and Kriss (1984), Kihlstrom and Nasby (1981), and Nasby and Kihlstrom (1986). In particular, this taxonomy suggests that important distinctions can be made among cognitive variables and measures; for example, selective attention processes and attributions, although both clearly cognitive and related at some level, are relevant to different kinds or conceptualizations of cognition. Thus, these variables can be classified according to specified cognitive categories; selective attention and causal attributions would fall into fundamentally different cognitive categories.

Before describing this framework, an important caveat is necessary. What we refer to as cognition in this framework represents an integrated series of mechanisms; it is not possible to isolate pure cognitive variables in either theoretical conceptualizations or empirical methodologies. Thus, cognitive classification represents a matter of emphasis rather than of mutual exclusion. There are four categories, as follows (see Table 1.1):

1. *Cognitive structural constructs.* Structural variables refer generally to the "architecture" of the system; that is, the aspect of information processing encompassing how information is stored and organized within some type of structure. Concepts such as short- and long-term memory as well as implicit and explicit memory are prominent examples of variables that focus primarily on the structural aspects of information processing.

2. *Cognitive propositional constructs.* In contrast to structural mechanisms, which by definition do not emphasize content, propositions refer to the content of information that is stored and organized within some structure. Episodic and semantic knowledge are examples of propositional variables. Propositions are thus variables that point to the meaning that has been encoded within the system. Schemas are typically conceptualized as combined structures and propositions (see Table 1.1).

3. *Cognitive operational constructs.* Operations refer to the processes by which the system operates. Some examples of cognitive operations variables include information encoding, retrieval, and attentional allocation. This category could be termed cognitive processes (e.g., Goldfried & Robins, 1983; Kihlstrom & Nasby, 1981; Hollon & Kriss, 1984; Nasby & Kihlstrom, 1986), but to avoid confusion with other cognitive uses of the term "process," these variables were labeled operations.

4. *Cognitive product constructs.* Products are defined as the end result of the cognitive system's information-processing operation; these are the cognitions or thoughts that the individual experiences as a result of the interaction of incoming information with cognitive structures, propositions, and operations. Examples include constructs such as self-statements, images, and attributions. Of note is that this is the only category of variables where there is awareness of cognition, although this does not imply that all cognitive products are inevitably within awareness; some recent work has suggested that some cognitive products may function outside of awareness (e.g., the work of Mogg, Bradley, Williams, & Mathews, 1993).

TABLE 1.1. Examples of Cognitive Constructs Categorized According to a Provisional Cognitive Taxonomic System

Schema		Operations	Products
Structures	Propositions		
Short-term memory	Episodic knowledge	Spreading activation	Attributions
Long-term memory	Semantic knowledge	Cognitive elaboration	Decisions
Iconic/sensory storage	Internally generated information	Encoding	Images
Neural networks	Beliefs (stored)	Retrieval	Thoughts
Memory nodes		Speed of information transfer	Beliefs (accessed)
Associative linkages		Attention	Recognition/ detection of stimuli

The Meta-Construct Model: Components Analysis
of Psychopathological Variables

A second aspect of this conceptual framework focuses on partitioning the components that comprise psychopathological functioning. Given the numerous cognitive variables proposed to operate in a multitude of disordered states, it is unrealistic to assume that all or even most of these variables, even if adequately conceptualized and flawlessly measured, are unique to a particular disorder. We propose that a useful conceptual metaphor for understanding the relationship between these variables and the variety of different disorders is to employ a model that views the variance in psychopathology analogously to the manner in which variance in experimental research is conceptualized (Ingram & Kendall, 1986, 1987; Ingram & Wisnicki, 1991). Specifically, the variance in psychopathology can be conceptually "partitioned" in much the same way that experimental variance is partitioned by an analysis of variance or virtually any other statistical procedure. In an experimental outcome, for example, several presumably identifiable sources of variance converge to contribute to a score on a given measure; variance uniquely due to an experimental manipulation or treatment (main effects), variance that is common to more than one experimental procedure (interaction), and error variance, typically due to individual differences that are not assessed in the experiment. Similarly, the ultimate symptomatic expression of a particular disorder can be conceptualized as the convergence of what we have called unique or "critical psychopathological features," "common psychopathological features," and error variance that is unpredictable.

1. *Critical features.* These features reflect variance that is uniquely characteristic of a particular disorder and thus describe variables specific to a given psychopathology. Hence, these features are defined as those that not only differentiate disorder from nondisorder, but that also differentiate one disorder from another. Critical features can thus be represented as cognitive "main effects."

2. *Common features.* In contrast to critical psychopathological features, common features are generally characteristic of all or most disorders and are therefore conceptualized as common or shared psychopathological variance. Although these features do not differentiate particular disorders, they do differentiate disorder from nondisorder. That is, whereas common features are not unique to a given disorder, they are "unique" to psychopathology in general, and thus they broadly separate adaptive from maladaptive functioning.

3. *Error variance.* Finally, error variance represents the unpredictable variance in psychopathology that is due to nonsystematic factors

such as individual differences. Although the majority of variance in the expression of psychopathology can most likely be accounted for by critical and common features, the precise symptoms and characteristics of the disorder will also be influenced to some degree by factors unique to the particular person involved.

As noted, the cognitive taxonomy and components frameworks together form the meta-construct model, a theoretical structure for organizing various constructs into broad conceptual categories encompassing both critical and common psychopathological features. Hence, cognition in disordered functioning can be theoretically and empirically viewed in terms of whether it is a critical feature or a common feature and whether it fits primarily into structural, propositional, operational, or product elements of cognition. The components of the meta-construct model are represented in Figure 1.2. Depending on the conceptual question being asked, the task is empirically to fill in the framework's spaces as they pertain to specified disorders.

META-CONSTRUCT MODEL

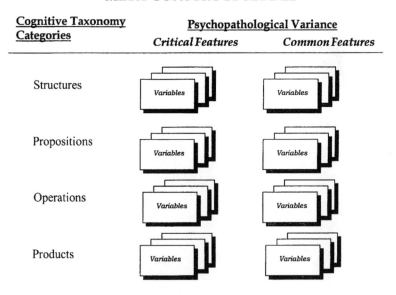

FIGURE 1.2. Components of the meta-construct model encompassing construct categories and partition of variance. One task of empirical research is to categorize the taxonomic level of the variable, and to assess which variables are critical to the disorder under consideration, or common across different disorders.

Having examined the rationale for the specific components that comprise the Meta-construct model, we now turn to a discussion of some common factors that cut across this framework.

CENTRAL CONCEPTS SUGGESTED BY A COGNITIVE APPROACH TO PSYCHOPATHOLOGY

Experimental studies of cognition are increasingly informing theories of psychopathology (Ingram, 1986; Magaro, 1991; Teasdale & Barnard, 1993; J. M. G. Williams et al., 1997). What is potentially informative about this approach is the opportunity to bring a large body of theory and research in cognitive psychology to bear on the investigation of vulnerability to emotional disorders, which would not have been possible even at the halfway point of the century. In addition, some of the processes investigated by cognitive psychologists (e.g., selective attention) bear a close resemblance to prominent features of certain emotional disorders (e.g., panic disorder) and suggest the value of calibrating a model of disorder to findings from the cognitive science literature. We now examine those concepts and process distinctions upon which many cognitive accounts of emotional disorder are founded. In doing so we recognize that the information-processing framework we are exploring, although established, is best described as a paradigm in transition. Our goal is not to encourage the wholesale transfer of ways of thinking about psychological processes from the realm of the experimental to the clinical, but, rather, to examine what may be gained by adopting a perspective on abnormal behavior that implicates possibly flawed perceiving, thinking, or reasoning in the development and maintenance of such behavior. There is also value in describing the clinical manifestations consistent with taking this position on the nature of dysfunction. To illustrate the relevance of basic cognitive concepts for informing clinical theorizing, research, and practice, in what follows we describe how several well-established cognitive approaches and findings have been used in the study of emotional disorder.

Neural Networks

Cognitive science approaches, particularly connectionist models intended to model neural networks, tend to emphasize the importance of distributed representations of multiple processing units. Units are conceptualized as the psychological depiction of neurons, or groups of neurons, that serve the same function, which are organized around connections to other units. Units can be represented as "input units" or "output units," or if units are hypothesized to exist between input and output, these are typically referred to as "hidden units." Networks developed to include hidden units are conceptualized as "multilayer" networks (see Stein & Young, 1992) and are intended to correspond to the internal or cognitive representation of knowledge that affects how information is processed.

There are a variety of constructs suggested by cognitive science, but among the most common are those that focus on the creation of networks comprised of interconnected units. As we just noted, these constructs are typically referred to as neural networks, a label designed to connote their organizational analogy to the neural organization of the brain (Caspar, Rothenfluh, & Segal, 1992). Such networks are conceptualized as complex organizational entities that enable cognition through large-scale fluctuations of activity within the network (Stinson & Palmer, 1991). Computational models of hypothesized networks are usually assessed by employing computer simulations.

Computational models of neural networks have been recently applied to clinical concerns, including depression. For example, Siegle and Ingram (1997) have attempted to explain some of the attentional disturbances in depression by developing a computational model of how negative information interferes with information processing in depression. In brief, Siegle and Ingram (1997) suggest that depressed individuals have active cognitive networks that focus on the emotional parameters of information to be processed rather than on the more functional semantic content of the information. Regardless of whether this particular hypothesis is supported, connectionist-based neural network approaches are apt to become increasingly important cognitive constructs in the study of psychopathology.

Capacity Limitations in the Cognitive System

Capacity limitation concepts have figured significantly in a number of models of psychopathology. The basic finding that people can only pay attention to so many things at any one time suggests that they have a limited capacity to process information (J. M. G. Williams et al., 1997). This implies that performance may be determined, in part, by the number of concurrent demands on the individual. One explanation for this has been to think of tasks as utilizing "resources" or "effort" and to study the ways in which different tasks may tax the capacity of the cognitive system (Norman, 1969; Shiffrin & Schneider, 1977). Within psychopathology, the notion of capacity limitation has been expressed in H. C. Ellis and Ashbrook's (1988) resource allocation model of depression, in which the finite cognitive resources available in the system are divided between task demands and the demands associated with chronic mood states.

Automatic and Effortful Processing

Most people would agree that the acquisition of new skills or abilities takes a good deal of effort and concentration. For example, it is difficult when first learning how to drive a car to be able to turn on the radio with one hand while balancing a donut and steering with the other. Yet, with practice this becomes easier to manage and can occur even while the driver is engaged in conversation with a passenger. One way to understand this is that those behaviors that had previously been so taxing of the cognitive system have become automatic or "overlearned" and are now able to be performed with very little effort, leaving resources for other behaviors to be performed concurrently. Whereas the acquisition of the driving skills is initially effortful, it becomes automatic with increasing practice (Hasher & Zacks, 1979; Kahneman, 1973; Shiffrin & Schneider, 1977).

In general, depression seems to interfere more with highly effortful tasks that require attentional resources and does not tend to interfere with automatic processes (Hartlage, Alloy, Vazquez, & Dykman, 1993). This notion has been invoked in psychopathology to explain depressed patients' performance on tasks that measure both implicit and explicit memorial processes (Danion et al., 1991; Elliot & Greene, 1992). Depressed patients tend to perform more poorly on tasks that tap recognition or recall functions, but tend to do as well as controls on measures of implicit memory. This is also seen in studies where depressed patients are asked to perform a task under two conditions, once with and once without a memory load (such as counting backwards while memorizing a list of words). Although performance under conditions of a memory load is generally poorer for both depressed and control subjects, depressed individuals are especially impaired.

Selective Processing of Information

Given the enormous amount of information each of us encounters on a moment-by-moment basis, it seems sensible that our cognitive systems have been developed to allow for a filtering of this input into categories that are more or less deserving of our immediate attention (Posner & McLeod, 1982). There are number of bases on which this selectivity operates and these can reflect characteristics of the stimulus, such as intensity, or can be guided by expectations of what to anticipate in the data stream.

Psychopathologists have used this concept to examine biases in the judgmental processes of individuals with a number of different disorders. For example, Mathews and MacLeod (1985) found that patients with phobia and panic disorder were more likely to perceive or be distracted by stimulus content that was threat- or danger-related than were non-disordered controls. In a task that required patients to respond to target words presented at a central fixation point on a computer screen, they found that anxious patients were more likely than controls to have their attention pulled away by irrelevant words related to fear presented on the periphery of the screen. Consequently, the response times to the target words for anxious patients were significantly slower than for controls. Using a similar paradigm in the case of patients with an eating disorder, Labarge, Cash, and Brown (1995) found that those who were asked to name the color of different words took longer to do so if the words were related to body shape or size concerns (e.g., fat, thin) than if the content of the words was neutral. The relevance of the body shape information interfered with the task of suppressing the meaning of the word in order to name the color as quickly as possible.

Levels of Processing

Although selection serves the important function of narrowing down the sheer volume of information confronting the individual, the type of processing this material receives is by no means homogeneous. There are a number of hierarchical encoding operations that can be performed on new information, each of which has consequences for how well this material is later retrieved or remembered. The notion that the initial organization of information can affect the memory for this stored material has been referred to as the "levels-of-processing model" (Craik & Lockhart, 1972). Craik and Lockhart distinguish between encoding strategies that focus on perceptual aspects of the stimulus, regularities, or pattern recognition that inform meaning; or the semantic/conceptual relationship of the stimulus to other material. Greater depth of processing is associated with greater elaboration in the cognitive system and leaves a more enduring trace in memory.

A direct application of the levels-of-processing model to the study of depression is in work with the self-referent encoding task (SRET; Kuiper & Olinger, 1986). Although there are several variations, in the basic SRET, subjects are serially presented a number of personal adjectives (positive and negative) and asked to make a number of decisions about the material. If perceptual encoding is being studied, subjects might be asked whether the word is spelled in upper case or lower case letters; if patterns or stimulus regularities are being studied, subjects would examine whether the work contains a specific letter string such as 't' following 's'. Finally, and most importantly, if a self-referent level of organization is being studied, subjects might be asked to decide whether an adjective is self-descriptive. After all the stimulus words have been rated, an incidental recall test is administered.

Empirical findings with this task suggest that depressed people endorse more negative adjectives as self-descriptive than do nondepressed controls, who tend to rate more positive adjectives as self-descriptive (MacDonald & Kuiper, 1982). Depressed people have also been shown to recall more negative self-referent adjectives following the SRET, whereas nondepressed controls recall more positive ones (Derry & Kuiper, 1981), presumably indicating the presence of depressive self-relevant cognitive structures. Analogous findings have been reported for anxious individuals (Ingram, Kendall, Smith, Donnell, & Ronan, 1987; Smith, Ingram, & Brehm, 1983).

Top-Down or Bottom-Up Processing

The idea that accurate perception or successful problem solving reflects the operation of a series of independent stages of processing, starting from simple and proceeding to complex, is misleading. There is good evidence, for example, to suggest that higher order representations related to the information at hand can influence the manner in which current input is analyzed (Neisser, 1976). J. M. G. Williams et al. (1997) have pointed out that "most aspects of cognitive functioning are . . . less accurately characterized as simple linear chains of processing stages, linking input to output, than as non-linear processing loops in which information is transferred in both directions. Those models which concentrate upon the way in which low-level basic processes lead to higher-order representations are often termed 'bottom up' models. Those which emphasize how higher-order representations influence basic low-level operations are termed 'top down' models" (p. 23).

Lang's (1977) work is a good example of a "top-down" model of information processing applied to the study of anxiety disorders. He posits that a highly coherent "fear network" or "fear schema" contains information about the feared stimulus situation, as well as about fear responses and their meanings. This fear network is an enduring system that develops based on past experience and is represented in propositional form in semantic memory. According to this theory, the network can be activated by objective threat stimuli and by symbolic stimuli, such as ambiguous stimuli or threat-related words. Such activation is thought to lead to intrusive thoughts, hypervigilance to threat, or other manifestations of anxiety.

Evidence consistent with this view comes from Burgess, Jones, Robertson, Radcliffe, and Emerson (1981), who used a "dichotic listening" paradigm. In this paradigm, threat words and neutral words were embedded in prose passages presented to the unattended channel. Individuals with agoraphobia, social phobia, and normal control subjects were asked to shadow aloud the passage presented in the attended channel, and to press a button whenever they detected a phobia-related or neutral target word. The patients evidenced an attentional bias for threat stimuli as shown by higher detection rates for phobic words, relative to neutral words; in contrast, the normal control subjects evidenced no difference in detection rates. Similar results have been obtained with other anxious populations such as those who have generalized anxiety disorder (Mathews & MacLeod, 1985) or obsessive–compulsive disorder (Foa & McNally, 1986).

Processing of Information outside of Focal Awareness

Cognition can operate and produce effects on mood and behavior without a person knowing that this is occurring. For instance, in the volume that ushered in much of contemporary cognitive psychology, Neisser (1967) points out that by far the majority of cognitive processing responsible for encoding, information transformation, and retrieval occurs well beyond the conscious awareness of people. In a now classic paper, Nisbett and Wilson (1977) also argued persuasively for the influence and importance of cognitive processes occurring outside of awareness. In the more specific arena of depression, Beck (1976) and others (Ingram, 1984; Teasdale, 1983) have maintained that a preconscious process, "automatic thinking," operates at the periphery of awareness and plays a central role in determining emotional responses to events. Brewin (1988) has expanded on this notion by positing the existence of separate processing pathways for conscious and nonconscious emotional stimuli. At a conscious level, verbally accessible rules can be modified through novel experiences in the person's life that disconfirm the content of these rules. So, for example, a man who believes that he is not attractive to members of the opposite sex may modify this belief if he asks a woman out and she accepts. At a nonconscious level, however, such rules cannot be directly modified, but they can be made to come to mind less easily by creating new nonconscious memories through novel experiences that share many contextual features with the old memories.

Schemas

One construct operating outside the realm of focal awareness that may be particularly relevant to an understanding of depression is the schema. Although definitions vary somewhat, in general, a schema can be thought of as a stored body of knowledge that interacts with incoming information to influence selective attention and memory search (J. M. G.

Williams et al., 1997). Schemas tend to be self-perpetuating because the information available to the person over time becomes increasingly congruent with the knowledge structures directing the search. As a result, input that may disconfirm or contradict what is already known is not attended to as easily. For example, evidence suggests that depressed persons have schemas of the self that are negatively biased, filtering out positive self-knowledge and exaggerating negative self-referent information. Evidence regarding cognitive mechanisms in depression covers a wide range of constructs and will be discussed in more detail in Chapter 7, and but for now we can note that depressed patients have been shown to endorse and recall adjectives with more negative than positive content (Derry & Kuiper, 1981), to perceive and recall social feedback as being more negative than is actually the case (Gotlib, 1983), and to personalize failure events while dismissing instances of successful performance (De-Monbreun & Craighead, 1977). All of these findings have been attributed to the operation of a depressotypic schema.

Availability and Accessibility

Several of the information-processing constructs we have discussed have incorporated the notion of activation (e.g., the activation of cognitive networks). One way that the theoretical and methodological implications of the idea of activation can be more fully understood is through the concepts of accessibility and availability. *Accessibility* can be thought of as the activation of cognitive structures while *availability* refers to whether or not these structures exist (see Higgins & King, 1981).[1]

As will become apparent later in this volume, this distinction is quite significant. If these concepts are valid, then research that seeks to examine the presence of hypothesized structures must take steps to ensure that they are adequately accessed. Likewise, even if these structures are found to exist, they must be accessed before their parameters can be mapped. Thus, for example, if the negative schemas hypothesized to characterize depression are further hypothesized to be latent until activated, then theoretical ideas about the functioning of schemas must take into account both accessibility and availability parameters.

---

[1]The idea of availability as we have described it should not be confused with the "availability heuristic." While an important cognitive concept in its own right, the availability heuristic (Tversky & Kahneman, 1973) refers not to whether structures are available but rather to probability judgments that are affected by the ease of which information comes to mind.

Cognition in Interpersonal Context: Internal Working Models

The concept of an internal working model was first articulated by Bowlby (1980), although similar conceptualizations have emerged from this construct, such as relational schemas (Baldwin, 1992; M. J. Horowitz, 1988) and interpersonal schemas (Safran, 1990; Safran & Segal, 1990). We will return to this idea in Chapters 9 and 10 when we discuss developmentally based constructs that shape current thinking about cognitive vulnerability to depression. For now, we note that internal working models serve as cognitive–interpersonal blueprints that form the basis of how interpersonal interactions are processed and interpreted. These models encompass implicit beliefs about the self and others along with procedural rules and knowledge for processing information and determining affective, behavioral, and verbal responses to interpersonal situations. This knowledge includes internal representations of the self and others, expectations for self and others in potential as well as actual interactions, rules for assigning meaning to the behavior of self and others, and propensities for the selection of information and how information is encoded, stored, and retrieved. In theory, such models are developed through generalizations that are abstracted from real or perceived regularities in past experience, frequently from past experience with key attachment figures (Bowlby, 1969). Internal working models thus form the link between current interactional patterns and past interpersonal experiences.

As Westen (1991) notes, such internal working models function outside conscious awareness and constitute a powerful basis for determining numerous facets of interactional patterns (see also Chapter 9). These models shape with whom, and how, new relationships are entered into, as well as how one interprets information and interacts within these relationships. The man who has learned that any expression of weakness leads to rejection from others enters into, perceives, and attempts to structure business, companionship, and romantic relationships in ways that will differ substantially from those of a man who has not experienced rejection from others over perceived weakness. Similarly, the woman who has experienced a sexually inappropriate stepfather and uncle will likely interpret and act accordingly with other men, particularly those with whom she might potentially grow close. On the other hand, a woman with a loving and appropriate father will interpret an interaction with a man in a very different fashion. Perhaps the most important aspect of these working models, at least for the sake of the current discussion, is that although people can certainly articulate some of the processes behind these behaviors, the internal representations of social interaction that guide these relationships are not typically accessible to the person at a conscious level. In a light-hearted explication of this idea, we are reminded of a line from the movie *Sleepless in Seattle*: Anne, not sure of her attraction to her fiancé, asks her brother Dennis if in some cosmic, magical way people know who is "right" for them. Dennis replies, "When you're attracted to someone it just means that your subconscious is attracted to their subconscious . . . subconsciously. So what we think of as fate is just two neuroses knowing they're a perfect match."

Of course, such models lead to reciprocal interpersonal interactions and, particularly in the case of "unhealthy" models, create self-fulfilling prophecies. The man with a cognitive schema that leads to the perception and prediction of hostility from others will not only perceive hostility in messages where there is none, but will respond "accordingly" with his own anger and hostility. Repeated interactions with a person with such paranoid ideation ultimately elicit hostility from others, which reinforces and strengthens the working model and leads to a dysfunctional and reciprocal interpersonal cycle of perceived and actual hostility. Such cognitive–interpersonal cycles will be repeated with many people who enter the person's life, regardless of the context of the interaction (academic, business, interpersonal). The concept of internal working models suggests that these cycles are due to powerful cognitive maps that operate beyond ordinary awareness. As will be discussed later in this volume, internal working models may prove among the most powerful of psychological concepts for understanding cognitive vulnerability to depression.

SUMMARY AND CONCLUSIONS

To summarize, the cognitive approach to psychopathology has roots in experimental investigations of cognitive functioning conducted at the turn of the century. Although relatively recent in comparison to the longer history of interest in abnormal behavior and mental illness, the cognitive approach has contributed a number of potentially important paradigms for investigating these phenomena. These paradigms draw heavily from work in selective attention, memory, and representational systems, all of which are embedded within the larger field of information processing. Important information constructs are capacity limitations, automatic and effortful processing, neural networks, levels of processing and self-referent encoding, top-down and bottom-up processing, and accessibility and availability.

Of noteworthy significance among the cognitive variables we have examined are the roles of specific representations such as schemas and working models, which contain depressive information and can bias cognitive operations against the encoding of information that is adaptive or potentially disconfirming of negative sets. These constructs will prove to be especially important in the accounts of cognitive vulnerability we discuss later in this volume.

Overall, the sampling of constructs we have reviewed, and the methods developed to test them will, we believe, continue to inform research aimed at elucidating the unique cognitive contributions to this costly, socially impairing, and multidetermined mental disorder. With these basic cognitive concepts in mind, we now turn to an examination of affective disorder as a category of psychopathology.

CHAPTER 2

Depression: An Overview

In this book we attempt to understand how cognition might predispose individuals to depression. Prior to delving into vulnerability, we will present a general overview of our current understanding of depression. In Chapter 5, as part of a larger discussion of conceptual issues, we discuss questions concerning the definition and meaning of the depression construct. In this chapter, we provide a brief summary of the prevalence and correlates of depression as defined by standard psychiatric nomenclature, that is, by definition of DSM-IV of the American Psychiatric Association (1994). Because the epidemiology, genetics, morbidity, correlates, and treatment of depression have been examined extensively in a variety of excellent studies, we will briefly review these important topics, which shed light on the nature of depression. We begin by discussing the epidemiology of depression. Next, we provide an overview of the genetics of depression. We then turn to the morbidity associated with depression, as well as other related features, such as stressful life events. Finally, we discuss current trends in treating depression.

EPIDEMIOLOGY OF DEPRESSION

As defined by DSM-IV, depression is a common, yet serious and debilitating disorder. Although a variety of different types of depression are officially recognized, two major subtypes are included in psychiatric diagnoses. The first, major depressive disorder, can present as a single episode or as a recurrent disorder; about 50% of those who have one episode will go on to have another. Current formal diagnostic systems, such as the *International Classification of Diseases* (ICD-10; World Health Organization, 1992) and DSM-IV, include criteria for sad mood or anhedonia, as well as a checklist of various symptoms. An episode of major depression is defined as a period of at least 2 weeks during which there is either depressed mood or a loss of interest or pleasure in nearly all activities. Because nearly everyone has periods of sad mood, at least four additional symptoms must be present to meet criteria for major depression. These four symptoms are drawn from a list that includes changes in appetite, weight, sleep, and psychomotor activities; decreased energy; feelings of worthlessness or guilt; difficulty thinking, concentrating, or making decisions; or recurrent thoughts of death or suicidal ideation, plans, or attempts.

The second subtype of depression, dysthymia, is a less intense but more chronic form of depression. According to DSM-IV, dysthymia involves a pervasive negative mood or lack of interest or pleasure in most activities that occurs most of the day, for more days than not. These symptoms are coupled with two or more additional symptoms such as sleep or appetite disturbance, and problems with concentration, libido, and energy. To qualify for a diagnosis of dysthymia, DSM-IV criteria specify that during a 2-year period, the person should not be symptom free for more than 2 months at a time.

Considerable data support the distinction between depression and other diagnoses; that is, depression can be clearly distinguished from disorders such as panic disorder or schizophrenia. Similarly, persons with major depression or dysthymia differ in many ways from those without such a diagnosis. Yet, there is no explicit rationale for why some symptoms but not others are officially recognized as characteristic of depression. For example, social withdrawal is a frequent concomitant of depression but is not a symptom listed in the diagnostic category. Similarly, a clear rationale for the time requirement for symptoms or the exact number of symptoms necessary for diagnosis does not exist. Some researchers have argued that the existing depression criteria are too stringent. Wells et al. (1989) found that medical patients with significant depressive symptoms who did not reach criteria for major depression incurred as much disability as a result of their depression as did those who met criteria for major depression. Clearly, the diagnostic criteria for depression are likely to evolve further in the future (see Chapter 5).

Prevalence

Relative to other psychiatric conditions, depressive disorders as defined by DSM-IV are extremely common. Various lifetime estimates have ranged from as high as 20% for women and 12% for men (Sturt, Kumakura, & Der, 1989). To assess prevalence comprehensively, two major epidemiological studies have been conducted that determine the rates of psychiatric disorders, including depression, in the United States. The first, the National Institute of Mental Health Epidemiologic Catchment Area (ECA) study, interviewed more than 20,000 community and institutionalized adults in five sites: New Haven, Connecticut; Baltimore, Maryland; St. Louis, Missouri; Durham, North Carolina; and Los Angeles, California (Eaton & Kessler, 1985; Eaton, Holzer, & Von Kortt, 1984; Regier, Myers, & Kramer, 1984). The Diagnostic Interview Schedule (Robins, Helzer, Croughan, & Ratcliff, 1981) was used to determine the presence of symptoms of sufficient severity and duration to warrant diagnosis of major depression or dysthymia. Data from all five sites were merged and standardized to the 1980 U.S. population to provide a best estimate of national prevalence rates of mental disorders (Regier et al., 1988). According to those results, approximately 2.2% of the population experienced a major depressive episode over a 1-month period. Furthermore, 5.8% of the population had experienced an episode of major depression at sometime during his or her life. Dysthymic disorder, which in DSM-III required a 2-year duration of symptoms, was diagnosed on a lifetime basis only. Approximately 3.3% of the population had experienced dysthymia. About one-quarter of those with a diagnosis of dysthymia had suffered from major depression within the past 6 months; almost half had a lifetime diagnosis of major depression.

The second major study to address rates of psychiatric disorders in the United States is the National Comorbidity Survey (NCS; Kessler et al., 1994). The NCS is the first survey to administer a psychiatric interview to a representative national sample in the United States. This study found generally higher rates of disorder than previously documented. Specifically, lifetime rates of depression were found to be 17.1% and dysthymia, 6.4%, quite significantly higher than rates found in the ECA studies. This may be because of the population difference (i.e., the national probability sample for the NCS study vs. community samples for the ECA study) or measurement differences (the NCS study revised the interview used by the ECA study). Regardless of these specific differences, both the ECA and the NCS studies suggest that depression is one of the most common mental disorders found in the general public.

Diagnostic, Descriptive, and Demographic Issues

Even though epidemiological studies show the extent of depression, they do not tell the complete story of the problems associated with depression. To provide a foundation for examining these problems, in this section we provide an overview of the correlates and features of depressive disorder.

Course of Depression

Although some estimates have suggested that untreated depression lasts between 6 months to 1 year (Dorzab, Baker, Winokur, & Cadoret, 1971; Keller, Shapiro, Lavori, & Wolfe, 1982), other estimates have suggested that patients with an untreated major depressive episode can remain symptomatic for up to 24 months (see Goodwin & Jamison, 1990). For two-thirds of cases, symptoms remit completely and functioning returns to the premorbid level. In the remaining cases, the full episode may persist for more than 2 years (5–10%) or recovery between episodes may be partial (20–25%). Approximately one-fourth of patients who have had recurrent depression develop chronic dysthymia. In addition, relapse rates are quite high and some estimates have suggested that for those who do relapse, there is a 20% chance of encountering chronic depression (Lavori, Keller, & Klerman, 1984).

Bipolar versus Unipolar Depression

One of the most common distinctions between different types of depression is the bipolar versus unipolar distinction. Depressive disorders that occur with and without manic periods should be viewed as two distinct disorders. Manic periods involve elation or excessive irritability, heightened activity and energy level, increased self-esteem, racing thoughts, distractibility, impulsive behavior, and a decreased need for sleep. For some individuals, depression is intermittent with periods of mania and is then classified as bipolar disorder. Bipolar disorder appears to be strongly determined by genetics (Winokur, Clayton, & Reich, 1969; Winokur, Coryell, Endicott, & Akiskal, 1993). Hence, bipolar disorder is clearly distinguishable from major depression and should be considered an altogether different disorder.

Subtypes of Depression

Historically there have been a variety of subtypes of depression (e.g., neurotic depression). Although there may be some validity to these subtypes, our focus here is on those that have been recognized by current psychiatric nosology. In particular, several subtypes of depression have been recognized within the formal diagnostic (i.e., DSM-IV) category of major depression. First, *atypical depression* is a subtype of depression that is characterized by two atypical symptoms, overeating and oversleeping, as well as a long-standing pattern of interpersonal rejection sensitivity. *Melancholia* is a subtype of depression that requires three or more of the following symptoms: (1) a distinct quality of negative mood that differs from intense sadness, (2) symptoms that worsen in the morning as compared with evening, (3) early morning awakenings, (4) marked psychomotor retardation or agitation, (5) significant anorexia or weight loss, and (6) excessive or inappropriate guilt. The *psychotic* subtype of depression requires accompanying psychotic symptomatology. The *seasonal pattern* is a subtype of depression with a regular temporal relationship with a particular time of year, typically during the winter months. These subtypes generally show different response patterns to treatment.

Gender Differences

Women are at a much higher risk for depression than are men. Although female-to-male ratios vary across studies, the average ratio is close to 2:1 (Culbertson, 1997; Goldman & Ravid, 1980; Nolen-Hoeksema, 1987; Strickland, 1988; M. M. Weissman & Klerman, 1977, 1985; M. M. Weissman, Leaf, Holzer, Myers, & Tischler, 1984). The difference holds for white, African American, and Latina women and persists when income, education, and occupation are controlled (Ensel, 1982; Radloff, 1975). Kessler, McGonagle, Swartz, Blazer, and Nelson (1993) explored this gender difference in results from the NCS study. According to these data, men and women develop first episodes of depression at about the same age. Similarly, rates of chronicity and recurrence are approximately equivalent for men and women. However, women are much more likely than men to incur a first episode of depression. The two-fold increase in rates of depression in women as compared to men appears first in adolescence; interestingly, rates are similar between girls and boys in childhood (Garrison, Addy, Jackson, McKeown, & Waller, 1992; D. B. Kandel & Davies, 1982; Lewinsohn, Hops, Roberts, Seeley, & Andrews, 1993).

Although the existence of gender differences is remarkably consistent and well documented in numerous epidemiological studies of depression, the processes underlying these pervasive differences are poorly understood. Clearly, understanding the increased incidence of depression in women might help in our overall understanding of vulnerability to depression. Several broad and sometimes interrelated hypotheses have been offered to account for findings that women are more likely than men to be diagnosed as depressed. An early idea was that men and women actually experience depression in roughly equal proportions, but that women are more likely to acknowledge and seek help for their depression, and clinicians more likely to overdiagnose depression in women than in men (Phillips & Segal, 1969). This *artifact* hypothesis has not received much support in epidemiological research in the community. This research, which helps to avoid the problems of self-identification and referral, continues to document gender differences in symptomatology and rates of depression in the population as a whole.

Another hypothesis advanced to explain the differences in rates of depression in men and women considers the role of precipitating events in onset of depression. The *precipitating factors* hypothesis proposes that women are more likely than men to encounter the critical factors that initiate depressive episodes (Radloff & Rae, 1979). Clear evidence demonstrates that women do, in fact, encounter more life change events than do men, but probably not sufficiently different to account for the large differential rates of depression in women as compared with men. Alternatively, *biological* hypotheses maintain that depression is linked to neurotransmitter dysregulation and that women are more vulnerable to depression because of endocrinological differences (Akiskal, 1987). Variants to the biological hypotheses suggest that changes associated with hormones, including the menstrual cycle (Schmidt et al., 1991), menopause (Greene, 1980), and the postpartum period (Pitt, 1982), predispose women to depression. However, available evidence does not support the view that hormones play a role in predisposing women to depression. In fact, the commonly held belief that postpartum depression is biologically based is being clearly challenged with evidence showing that rates of depression for postpartum women compared with matched nonchildbearing women are not significantly different (O'Hara, Zekoski, Phillips, & Wright, 1990). In sum, at the current time, biological differences have not received support as vulnerability factors for depression.

Along with biological factors, *psychosocial* factors have been examined to account for the differential rates of depression in men and women. Specifically, cognitive factors have been implicated in sex differences. Several investigators have found that women are more likely to ruminate (Nolen-Hoeksema, 1987) and focus their attention on themselves (Ingram, Cruet, Johnson, & Wisnicki, 1988) than are men. Such cognitive processes have been linked to a variety of disordered states, including depression (Ingram, 1990). Clearly, these cognitive differences may result from social background or biological differences themselves, but they appear to account for a portion of the differential rates of depression between men and women.

Although many of these hypotheses regarding sex differences in depression are plausible, and some combination of them may eventually account for sex differences in depression, none has yet received unambiguous support (Amenson & Lewinsohn, 1981; Ingram et al., 1988; Nolen-Hoeksema, 1987). As the field progresses in understanding vulnerability to depression, a clearer understanding of sex differences should also emerge.

Age and Cohort Effects

Depression tends to occur early in life, sometimes quite early; although reliable epidemiological data are unavailable, depression does occur in children and adolescents (Nurcombe, 1992). With regard to ages for which epidemiological data are available, the ECA study showed that most cases of major depressive disorder have their onset in young adulthood. In fact, 20% of cases met criteria for diagnosis for the first time before the age of 25 years, and 50% before the age 39 (Dryman & Eaton, 1991). Certainly, depression is a problem that tends to afflict young people.

This early onset may be a relatively new phenomena in that there appears to be a cohort effect for depressive disorder. That is, cohorts born in this century show higher prevalence of depression for each decade (Hagnell, Lanke, Rorsman, & Ojesjo, 1982; Klerman et al., 1985; Klerman & Weissman, 1992). More recent birth cohorts seem to be at increased risk for depression, a risk that can be dramatically illustrated by comparing prevalence rate for people born early in versus in the middle of the 20th century. For example, people born early in the 20th century demonstrate a prevalence rate of approximately 1%. Conversely, individuals born around the middle of the century have approximately an 8–9% risk, despite having less time available to experience the onset of depression. Although artifact explanations for these differences are possible, few appear plausible (Seligman, 1990). For example, Seligman (1990) notes that although when surveyed older individuals may be more hesitant to report the experience of depressive symptoms, they did not appear more hesitant to report symptoms of psychotic disorders or substance abuse. Therefore, whatever combination of factors create vulnerability to depression, those factors are increasingly prevalent with each decade of this century.

Cross-Cultural Aspects of Depression

Depression seems to be ubiquitous. That is, struggling with negative mood and associated symptoms is common across cultures. Many clinical studies of depressive symptomatology in non-Western cultures have been reported and all document high rates of depressive disorders. In some non-Western cultures, there is a reduced frequency or absence of psychological components of depression and a dominance of somatic aspects (Marsella, Sartorius, Jablensky, & Fenton, 1985). For example, two international surveys (Murphy, Wittkower, & Chance, 1964) completed in 30 countries found a cluster of symptoms, including depressed mood, diurnal variations, insomnia, and loss of interest, to be common in Western cultures whereas fatigue, anorexia, weight loss, and loss of libido were primary symptoms in non-Western cultures. The World Health Organization Collaborative Study of Depression (Sartorius, Jablensky, Gulbinat, & Ernberg, 1980) examined patients from five countries (Canada, India, Iran, Japan, and Switzerland). They found similar patterns of depressive disorder in all settings; however, cultural variations in frequency of symptoms did exist. For example, suicidal ideation was present in 70% of the depressed Canadian sample as compared with only 40% of the depressed Japanese sample.

In sum, cross-cultural research has identified a core experience and expression of depressive disorders that exist in varying degrees across cultures. However, symptomatology tends to be more "psychological" in Western societies and more "somatized" in non-Western societies.

GENETICS OF DEPRESSION

Over the past decade, several family studies have found that major depression is influenced by family of origin. The lifetime rate of major depression in the first-degree relatives ranges from 8.6% to 34.9% (Baron, Gruen, Asnis, & Kane, 1982; Bland, Newman, & Orn, 1986; Gershon & Nurnberger, 1982; Giles, Biggs, Rush, & Roffworg, 1988; McGuffin, Katz, Aldrich, & Bebbington, 1988; Stancer, Persad, Wagener, & Jorna, 1987; M. M. Weissman, Gershon, Kidd, Prusoff, & Lekman, 1984; Winokur, Tsuang, & Crowe, 1982). This rate is two to three times higher than in relatives of matched comparison groups.

Although the family studies of risk for depression are impressive, they do confound genetic and environmental factors in understanding the etiology of depression. Several twin studies have examined the relationship of genetics to depression. Since 1990, four twin studies have been published. G. Andrews, Nelson, Hunt, and Stewart (1990) found that concordance rates for major depression were low but somewhat greater in dizygotic than in monozygotic twins. McGuffin, Katz, and Rutherford (1991) found concordance rates of 58% in monozygotic twins as compared with 28% in dizygotic twins. Kendler, Neale, Kessler, and Heath (1992) found rates of 44% in monozygotic twins and 19% in dizygotic twins. In a 1-year follow-up to their twin study, Kendler, Kessler, and Neale (1993) found that genetic factors play a moderate etiological role in 1-year prevalence of major depression. In addition, they found that environmental factors play a significant role in onset of major depression, but that their effects are generally transitory. That is, genetic factors predispose to depression across a lifetime, whereas environmental stressors lead to current major depression, but do not appear to predispose to depression beyond a 1-year period of time. Without a doubt, there is some genetic component to depression; however, the way in which genetics renders individuals vulnerable to depression is not at all clear.

MORBIDITY, COMORBIDITY, AND CORRELATES OF DEPRESSION

Depressive disorders are associated with substantial impairment. Patients having a major depressive episode report substantially poorer intimate relationships and less satisfying social interactions than do members of the general population who have previously suffered from depression or who currently have other psychiatric disorders (Fredman, Weissman, Leaf, & Bruce, 1988). Patients with untreated depression also suffer severe health- and work-related disability. In one study, 23% of depressed patients reported some days in which they were in bed all or most of the day in the previous 2 weeks, compared to 5% of the general population (Wells, Golding, & Burnam, 1988). Similarly, 48% of depressed community respondents described their health as either fair or poor, compared to only 29% of those without depression (Wells et al., 1988). In addition, those with major depressive disorder reported 11 disability days per 90-day interval versus 2.2 disability days for the general population (Broadhead, Blazer, & George, 1990). Finally, 38% of persons with major depressive disorder had some chronic activity restriction compared with 9% of persons without psychiatric disorders, and 29% of those with depression reported decreased activity days in the previous 2 weeks compared to 9% of those without psychiatric disorder (Wells et al., 1988).

Many studies have also linked depression with suicide. More than half of suicides occur in persons suffering from depression (Barraclough, Bunch, Nelson, & Sainsbury, 1974). Persons who are depressed are 30 times more likely to commit suicide than the general population (Guze & Robins, 1970). Thus, depression can result in loss of life as well as loss of functioning.

Depression is costly to society as well as to individuals. In one recent study, the economic burden of depression in the United States was estimated to be $43.7 billion dollars annually. Of this total, $12.4 billion, or 28%, can be attributed to direct costs, such as inpatient and outpatient treatment, as well as pharmacological costs. An additional $7.5 billion, or 17%, are comprised by mortality costs associated with suicides, such as loss of lifetime earnings. The final category includes $23.8 billion, or 55%, that can be attributed to the decrements in functioning associated with depression. Clearly, depression is costly at the societal as well as the individual level (Greenberg, Stiglin, Finkelstein, & Berndt, 1993).

Depression can be costly to future generations as well. Maternal depression has been extensively studied as a risk factor for child psychopathology. Children of mothers with depression are at high risk for a range of problems including psychopathology (Beardslee, Bemporad, Keller, & Klerman, 1983; Billings & Moos, 1983; Burbach & Borduin, 1986; Hammen et al., 1987). The results of several studies suggest that children of depressed parents show deficits in academic performance, school behavior, and social competence relative to children of psychiatrically normal parents (Rolf & Garmezy, 1974; Weintraub, Winters, & Neale, 1986; Worland, Weeks, Janes, & Strock, 1984). Furthermore, children of depressed mothers do more poorly in social and academic spheres than do children of bipolar, medically ill, or psychiatrically normal women (C. A. Anderson & Hammen, 1993). We will discuss additional research on the effect of maternal depression in Chapter 9.

Comorbidity

Conceptual issues of comorbidity and depression are examined in greater detail in Chapter 5. For now, we briefly discuss some of the major issues of comorbidity and psychiatric disorders, substance abuse disorders, medical disorders, and personality disorders. Overall, the lifetime risk for comorbidity with depression is as high as 43% (Sargeant, Bruce, Florio, & Weissman, 1990). The 1-month comorbidity for depression is 8%; that is, 8% of those with current major depression have a comorbid psychiatric disorder.

Anxiety

Anxiety is one of the most common psychiatric correlates of depression. Some, although certainly not all, of this co-occurrence may be accounted for by an overlap in diagnostic criteria. For example, difficulty concentrating, sleep disturbances, and fatigue appear in the diagnostic criteria for both major depressive disorder and generalized anxiety disorder. However, even when factors such as diagnostic criteria overlap are taken into account, there is still substantial comorbidity between depressive and anxious states; a number of studies have found either significant correlations between measures of depressive and anxious states, or the occurrence of a significant degree of anxiety in depressed individuals (and vice versa) (see L. A. Clark & Watson, 1991; Watson & Clark, 1984).

Psychiatric Disorders

Schizophrenia is often associated with depression. In fact, people diagnosed with schizophrenia have 28.5 times greater odds of being depressed than do nonschizophrenic individuals (Boyd et al., 1984). Similarly, those with anxiety disorder frequently get depressed. For example, the odds of individuals with panic disorder becoming depressed are 18.8 times greater than for those without panic. Likewise, many patients with eating disorders also have symptoms of depression. Major depression may be found in as high as 56% of anorexics (Hendren, 1983). Similarly, current major depression occurs in approximately 24–33% of people with bulimia (Walsh, Roose, Glassman, Gladis, & Sadik, 1985). Although the directionality of the disorders is not clear, significant psychopathology is often linked with depression.

Substance Abuse Disorders

Depression and substance abuse disorders are also highly related. Among those with major depression, 14.5% have substance abuse or dependence problems. For people with dysthymia, 20.9% concurrently have a substance abuse or dependence disorder. Two opposing theories have explained this link. Winokur and Clayton (1967) propose that there is a gene for depressive-spectrum disease that is likely to eventuate in depression for females and alcoholism for males. In opposition, Khantzian (1985) argues that addictive substances are used by those with depression in order to "self-medicate." Specifically, depressed people become addicted to psychoactive substances, such as alcohol or cocaine, in an attempt to treat their depression. Although neither theory has been completely supported or negated, both have found some support. Clearly, the interrelationship of substance abuse and depression is likely to be complex and vulnerability factors for one may be tightly linked to vulnerability factors for the other.

Medical Disorders

Depression is also prevalent among patients with medical disorders. For instance, approximately 4.8–9.2% of ambulatory medical patients have major depression (Agency for Health Care Policy and Research Clinical Practice Guidelines, 1993). Depression also appears to be particularly associated with chronic disorders. For example, 18.2% of diabetic patients have been found to have concurrent depression (Marcus, Wing, Guare, Blair, & Jawad, 1992; Mayou, Peveler, Davies, Beverley, & Fairburn, 1991). Even higher rates of depression have been found among hospitalized medical patients, with 22–33% reporting depression (for a review, see Katon & Sullivan, 1990). Data have also shown a high degree of comorbidity between depression and both rheumatoid arthritis and osteoarthritis (Banks & Kerns, 1996; Romano & Turner, 1985; Smith, Wallston, & Dwyer, 1995).

Although common in chronic disorders, the co-occurrence of depression and medical illness is not limited to these conditions; depression is also a frequent concomitant of acute, severe medical problems. For example, 20–30% of oncology patients report depression, with pancreatic cancer patients having the highest rates (Massie & Holland, 1987). Similarly, 18% of patients report major depression following myocardial infarction (Schleifer et al., 1989). Thus, both chronic and acute medical illnesses are linked with depression.

The frequent link between depression and medical illnesses raises problematic situations both for the clinical recognition of depression in medical patients and for studies seeking to examine depressive symptomatology in the context of medical illness. This problem pertains primarily to symptom overlap. For example, if a patient with cancer complains of loss of appetite, should this symptom be ascribed to the malignancy or depression? Symptoms of depression that can easily be correlates of medical illness include appetite/weight disturbance, psychomotor agitation/retardation, insomnia/hypersomnia, decreased libido, and fatigue. This is particularly (although not exclusively) true for chronic illness, and can substantially affect research results. For instance, Peck, Smith, Ward, and Milano (1989) and Calfas, Ingram, and Kaplan (1997) have shown that the cognitive correlates of depression in chronic pain conditions are different when "depressive" symptoms that are somatic in nature, and thus possibly the result of pain (e.g., difficulty sleeping, diminished enjoyment of activities), are removed from diagnostic consideration. Hence, it appears certain that studies measuring only symptoms of depression and using cutoff scores established in healthy populations probably overdiagnose psychiatric distress in medically ill patients and possibly confound research findings.

The use of explicit diagnostic criteria based on structured interviews for major depressive disorder is more likely to be accurate in determining depression in medical populations. For example, meeting diagnostic criteria for major depression requires severe, persistent low mood, as well as other symptoms, only some of which are likely to stem from a physical ailment. Therefore, studies relating diagnostic criteria for depression to medical illness are likely to be more accurate, although caution is still needed in dealing with somatic symptoms.

Personality Disorders

Two recent studies have carefully examined the co-occurrence of personality disorders and depression. In the first, Shea, Glass, Pilkonis, Watkins, and Docherty (1987) found that 75% of a sample of 249 persons with major depression had a definite or probable diagnosis of personality disorder. Pilkonis and Frank (1988) found that 48% of a sample of recurrent unipolar depressed patients who had responded to treatment had concurrent probable or definite personality disorders. Rates of co-occurrence are even higher for inpatients. Friedman, Aronoff, Clarkin, Corn, and Hurt (1983) reported that 81% of 53 consecutive inpatients with depression had concurrent personality disorders.

Concurrent personality disorder is related to decreased responsiveness to treatment of depression. Many studies have found that those depressed persons with personality disorders tend to do more poorly in psychotherapy and pharmacotherapy interventions (e.g., Frank, Kupfer, Jacob, & Jarrett, 1987; Pilkonis & Frank, 1988). Furthermore, depressed individuals with personality disorders are at greater risk for psychiatric hospitalizations (Zimmerman, Coryell, Pfohl, Corenthal, & Stangl, 1986). Clearly, the presence of a personality disorder complicates depression.

Impact of Life Events, Social Support, and Coping on Depression

Life Events

The impact of negative life events on onset and course of depression has been well established. Life events, or experiences that are disruptive and require readjustment on the part of the individual, relate positively to both onset and maintenance of psychiatric distress (B. S. Dohrenwend & Dohrenwend, 1974). Events that involve significant loss, such as loss of a spouse or job, are particularly likely to result in significant psychological distress (Aneshensel, 1985; Billings, Cronkite, & Moos, 1983). Clearly, negative life events, as opposed to positive change events, are most powerful in predicting subsequent distress. When negative events occur, those that are uncontrollable are most strongly related to depression (McFarlane, Norman, Streiner, Roy, & Scott, 1980; Paykel, 1974, 1979).

Acute stressors have long been identified as precipitants for depression. More recently, the role of chronic stressors in inducing and maintaining depression has been evaluated. Chronic stressors including problems with finances, work, spouse, children, and physical health, are all related to subsequent distress (Moos & Moos, 1992). For example, marital and parenting stressors are associated with depression (Andrews & Brewing, 1990; Moos, Fenn, Billings, & Moos, 1989; Pearlin & Schooler, 1978) as are work stressors (Billings & Moos, 1982b; Revicki, Whitley, Gallery, & Allison, 1993). Those stressors that endure are associated with both depressive symptoms, as well as recurrence of depression (Aneshensel, 1985; Moos et al., 1989).

Minor stressors, or stressors that are not drastic but are ongoing, have also been found to be predictive of depression. Kanner, Coyne, Schaefer, and Lazarus (1981) found that ongoing minor stressors or daily hassles were better predictors of depressive symptoms than were major life events. Unfortunately, at this time it is not possible to untangle the occurrence of minor stressors from a larger context. For example, one minor stressor that is predictive of depression is constant interruptions. This is likely to be highly associated with having young children. Past research has clearly indicated that the presence of young children in the home is a predictor of depression, if there is inadequate social support (Brown & Harris, 1978). The role of minor stressors in precipitating depression needs to be more thoroughly examined.

An important question regarding life stressors and depression is whether life stress causes depression or depression-prone persons incur more life stress. Recent studies have found that chronically depressed people tend to experience more negative events as part of the social environment that they create and maintain (Hammen, 1991, 1992; Monroe, Kupfer, & Frank, 1992). Depression may generate stressful life events that in turn lead to continued depression (Coyne et al., 1987; Hammen, 1991). Further work is needed to understand the impact of daily life stressors, as well as major life stressors, in the onset and maintenance of depression.

Social Support

Many theorists have hypothesized that social support may serve as a buffer between stressful life events and depression. A consistent relationship between social support and depression has been found (Aneshensel & Frerichs, 1982; Barnett & Gotlib, 1988; Barerra, 1985; Billings et al., 1983; Schaefer, Coyne, & Lazarus, 1981). Clearly, low levels of social integration, or connection to one's community, characterize persons who are depressed or prone to depression (Aneshensel, 1985; Barnett & Gotlib, 1988; Billings & Moos, 1985). How this lack of connection to community is related to vulnerability is currently unknown; for example, does disconnection from community cause vulnerability to depression or do factors associated with vulnerability to depression lead to disconnection from the community? Unfortunately, what is known is that the symptoms of depression mitigate against gaining and maintaining a social network.

Intimate relationships or confidants are particularly important to maintaining positive mental health. Depression is associated with lack of an intimate relationship (Brown & Harris, 1978), as well as with marital conflict (Billings & Moos, 1982a, 1982b). Marital distress is likely to play an etiological role in depression, as well as be the result of depression. Again, although intimacy tends to protect against depression, the causal role of this factor in the onset and maintenance of depression is not clear.

Coping

Coping skills may also help to prevent depression following stressful life events. Depressed persons use more avoidance-type coping, such as emotional discharge, wishful thinking, or distraction, whereas nondepressed people use more active, problem-solving styles of coping (Billings et al., 1983; Coyne, Aldwin, & Lazarus, 1981). Coping skills also interact with treatments. Those who use an avoidant style of coping at the beginning of treatment for depression are more likely to remain depressed that those who use more active styles of coping (Krantz & Moos, 1988). Similarly, depressed avoiders have poorer relationships with their therapists (Gaston, Marmar, Thompson, & Gallagher, 1988). Overall, active coping is more effective in dealing with depression than is avoidant or passive coping. In addition, active coping style probably is effective in reducing onset of depression as compared with more avoidant or passive coping.

Overall, the impact of negative life events on producing and maintaining depression is well established. Furthermore, those prone to depression may "cause" more negative life events based on the environments that they choose and build for themselves. Similarly, social support and active coping style are hypothesized to mitigate against the effects of negative life events in producing depression. Although this relationship has not been well supported, partially because of the difficulties in studying these complex interactions over time, both lack of social support and passive, avoidant coping are related to depression onset, maintenance, and therapy outcome.

TREATMENT OF DEPRESSION

Effective treatments for depression are available. Both medications and psychotherapies have been found to be effective in treating depression.

Prior to the 1970s, electroconvulsive treatment was the major intervention for depression. Since that time, both tricyclic antidepressants and monoamine oxidase inhibitors have been used extensively for treatment of depression, as have newer psychopharmacological treatments such as serotonin reuptake inhibitors.

Many medications have been found to be effective for treating acute phases of major depression. Controlled randomized trials have been conducted to evaluate the effectiveness of tricyclic antidepressants, heterocyclic antidepressants, selective serotonin reuptake inhibitors, and monoamine oxidase inhibitors. Most antidepressant medications have comparable efficacy. Most reports find that over a 3- to 4-week period, 65–70% of those taking medications improve (AHCPR Clinical Practice Guidelines, 1993). However, when you consider those who are unable to take medication because of side effects or who decide to discontinue treatment, closer to 50% achieve substantial improvement (Depression Guideline Panel, 1993).

Numerous psychotherapies have been used to treat depression. The oldest is the psychodynamic approach. Interpersonal psychotherapy (IPT; Klerman, Weissman, Rounsaville, & Chevron, 1984) is a psychodynamic approach to the treatment of depression that emphasizes the importance of the person's interpersonal relationships. Interpersonal therapy was developed by Klerman and colleagues as part of a clinical trial to test the efficacy of maintenance psychotherapy for outpatients with major depression (Klerman et al., 1984). The success of this therapy has been tested in a series of controlled comparative treatment trials (see Markowitz & Weissman, 1995, for review). The treatment usually lasts 12–20 weeks and explicitly targets depressive symptoms. The therapy is conducted with a directive, active stance that identifies an interpersonal problem area and deals with the problem in treatment. The problem may be struggling with others, making a change in role, or showing a deficit in interpersonal interactions. The treatment encourages appropriate social interactions, with a consolidation of interpersonal gains at the end. IPT was found to be effective in a 16-week trial with depressed outpatients (DiMascio et al., 1979). This study compared IPT, amitriptyline, and their combination, with a nonstructured psychotherapy program. Both active treatments were more effective than the control; the combination was superior to either alone. At 1-year follow-up, patients who received IPT with or without medication demonstrated better psychosocial functioning than those who had received either amitriptyline alone or the control (M. M. Weissman, Klerman, Prusoff, Sholomskas, & Padian, 1981).

Cognitive-behavioral therapy (CBT) has also been shown to be effective for treating the acute phase of depression. Beck and colleagues

(Beck, Rush, Shaw, & Emery, 1979) treat depression by leading patients to think more rationally about their lives and problems. The theory underlying this treatment is that dysfunctional thinking actually predisposes one to depression. For example, if a student believes that she is worthwhile only if she makes straight As, she is vulnerable to depression if she receives a B. The treatment helps the patient to believe that she is worthwhile even if she receives a B by reminding her, for example, that she is valuable for many reasons other than grades, and that a B grade is very acceptable. At this time, overwhelming evidence exists to document that CBT is effective for treatment of an episode of major depression. Meta-analyses indicate that CBT reduces symptoms substantially faster than would occur without treatment (e.g., Dobson, 1989), and CBT compares favorably with other treatments for depression.

Therapies focused on other cognitive deficits, such as interpersonal skills (D'Zurilla, 1986) or self-control skills (Rehm, 1977), have also been used to treat depression. In addition, behavioral approaches that invite patients to participate in more pleasant activities (Lewinsohn, 1985; Lewinsohn, Hoberman, Teri, & Hautzinger, 1985) have been used to treat depression. Although all of the above-mentioned psychotherapies have been shown to be effective in treating depression, the specific effect intended by the therapy has not been as easy to detect. That is, cognitive therapy has not been found to change cognitions, interpersonal therapy to improve relationships, and so forth. In addition, as with pharmacotherapy, dropout rates are relatively high (20–47%).

Unfortunately, the lack of specificity of treatment to outcome precludes treatment outcome studies from helping us to elucidate vulnerability to depression. These treatments tend to suggest that there is some common final pathway to depression that results in decrements in thinking, acting, and relating to others. By changing any of these systems, patients tend to improve. Understanding which decrements may lead to depression in which patients is still an unanswered question.

SUMMARY AND CONCLUSIONS

As is apparent from our preceding discussion, much is known about the symptoms, characteristics, and features of depression as it is defined by current psychiatric nomenclature. Depending on different estimates, somewhere between 6% and 17% of the population has experienced a clinically severe episode of depression at some point in their lives, with women reporting roughly twice the rate as men. Depression in some form exists in all cultures and subcultures, and, at least in North America, the rate of depression is increasing with each new decade.

Although much needs to be learned about the precipitants of depression, it is clear that both genetic and environmental factors contribute to the causes of at least some forms of the disorder. Finally, both pharmacological and psychological interventions have been found to be effective in the treatment of depression; unfortunately, the effectiveness of these treatments sheds little light on proposed causal or vulnerability factors. Although there are numerous theories of depression, among the most well-documented theories are those that employ a cognitive approach, an approach to which we will turn in the following chapter.

CHAPTER 3

Cognitive Theories of Depression

Our ultimate interest in this book is, of course, cognitive vulnerability. To set the stage for our consideration of the factors related to such vulnerability, in this chapter we review a number of the prominent theories of depression. Our goal is not to review these theories in depth or to provide a critical analysis, but rather to provide an overview of the variables that are conceptually central to these theories. After this review, we will also briefly discuss some of the empirical evidence concerning these theories. Finally, although some of these theories make specific statements about vulnerability, our focus will be on describing the basic cognitive principles of the theory rather than focusing on vulnerability.

We begin our examination of cognitive theories of depression with a brief statement that sums up the relevance of these theories with the context of current conceptualizing about psychopathology. We then respectively review those theories that emphasize cognitive products, cognitive structures and propositions, and cognitive operations. We conclude this chapter with a discussion of several issues that pertain to all models of depression that focus on cognition.

THE INFLUENCE OF COGNITIVE APPROACHES TO DEPRESSION

Cognitive approaches to the conceptualization, assessment, and treatment of psychopathological conditions have expanded rapidly over the past two decades. This extensive development of cognitive approaches to psychopathology is evidenced by the numerous research reports and volumes examining the conceptual foundations, empirical research, and practical applications of these approaches (e.g., Beck & Emery, 1985; Brewin, 1988; Dobson & Kendall, 1993; Ingram, 1986; Kendall & Hollon, 1979, 1981; Magaro, 1991; Matthews, in press; Stein & Young, 1992).

Paralleling, and in many cases fueling, this rapid growth are the numerous cognitive theories of depression that have been developed during this time period. As with cognitive approaches to psychopathology in general, the vitality of the cognitive view of depression is evidenced by a number of sources, most notably the number of major reviews and commentaries that have appeared over the last 15 or so years (e.g., Blaney, 1986; Coyne, 1982; Coyne & Gotlib, 1983, 1986; Ingram & Holle, 1992; Ingram & Reed, 1986; Segal & Dobson, 1992). Although some have predicted the demise of the cognitive approach to psychopathological states such as depression (Averil, 1983; Coyne, 1992), the cognitive perspective has continued to thrive.

That cognitive models of depression have proliferated is clear, but the nature of what constitutes a cognitive model of depression cannot merely be assumed (Pyszczynski & Greenberg, 1992b). At the most general level, the primary assumption underlying cognitive models of depression is that certain cognitive processes (such as those noted in Chapter 1) are related in a nontrivial fashion to the onset, course, and/or alleviation of the disorder. Within the context of this general definition, the degree of "cognitiveness" of a model can vary substantially. Some models that can be considered cognitive contain only some cognitive elements among a much larger network of constructs. For example, the theory proposed by Lewinsohn et al. (1985) accords a central role to a cognitive construct, self-focused attention, but this is virtually the only such construct in this model. Alternatively, for other cognitive models the majority of conceptual variance is accounted for by cognitive constructs. For our purposes, we will operationally define as a cognitive model any framework that includes a major cognitive component within its conceptual framework.

COGNITIVE THEORIES OF DEPRESSION

In Chapter 1 we noted that there are many ways to conceptualize and group the principles that underlie cognitive approaches to psychopathology. For instance, we noted that cognitive models could be categorized according to their theoretical antecedents (i.e., information-processing models, social-cognitive models, and cognitive-behavioral models). We also noted an organizational framework for conceptualizing the differing levels of cognitive analysis that have been examined in the literature (the meta-construct model). Although we could examine cognitive models in this chapter according to their historical antecedents, we will focus instead on the cognitive variables featured by these models. We therefore employ the meta-construct framework to help organize our discussion of cognitive models (see Figure 3.1). Although this structure is by no means perfect, and significant overlap may occur in the models that we place in different categories, this framework nonetheless helps us to differentiate models according to the cognitive variables they emphasize. Thus, models can be categorized according to those emphasizing cognitive products (or the thoughts and cognitions that are characteristic of depression), cognitive structures and propositions that underlie cognition (such as schemas), or those underscoring the primacy of cognitive operations in the depressed state. We begin with an examination of theories that highlight cognitive products.

Theories Focusing on Cognitive Products

Theories focusing on cognitive products place primary emphasis on those kinds of cognitions individuals experience that are linked to depression. In this section we concentrate on perhaps the original cognitive theory,

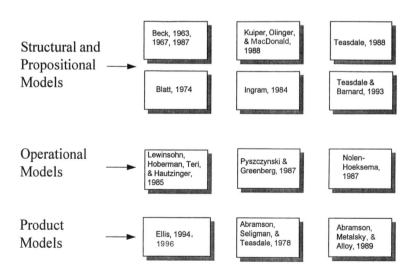

Structural and Propositional Models

| Beck, 1963, 1967, 1987 | Kuiper, Olinger, & MacDonald, 1988 | Teasdale, 1988 |
| Blatt, 1974 | Ingram, 1984 | Teasdale & Barnard, 1993 |

Operational Models

| Lewinsohn, Hoberman, Teri, & Hautzinger, 1985 | Pyszczynski & Greenberg, 1987 | Nolen-Hoeksema, 1987 |

Product Models

| Ellis, 1994, 1996 | Abramson, Seligman, & Teasdale, 1978 | Abramson, Metalsky, & Alloy, 1989 |

FIGURE 3.1. Cognitive models of depression categorized according to the cognitive constructs featured in the model.

Albert Ellis's irrational beliefs model (1962), and discuss its place in contemporary cognitive theorizing about depression. In contrast, we also examine perhaps the most recent theory to emphasize cognitive products as critical elements in the depression process (the hopelessness model; Abramson et al., 1989).

Cognitive Errors

A hallmark of cognitive theories of depression has been linking errors in thinking to onset of depression. The earliest theories tended to emphasize a relatively simple linear association between thinking errors and the consequent onset of emotional distress (Ellis, 1962). Such theoretical approaches can be traced to the development of the pioneering cognitive-behavioral interventions that focused on the treatment of psychological dysfunction through procedures designed to correct errors in thinking. The emphasis of these approaches was clearly on the development of effective therapeutic interventions and much less on specifying and elaborating the underlying theoretical mechanisms. Consequently, the theoretical articulation of cognitive processes tended to be fairly limited and relied on straightforward linear assumptions about errors in thinking leading to the onset of depression.

As the effectiveness of these cognitive interventions was increasingly empirically demonstrated, researchers began to focus on more sophisticated and elaborate specifications of the cognitive mechanisms of disorder. No longer was the emphasis on these mechanisms as they pertained to treatment considerations (although this has always been and remains important), but rather on a better understanding of the cognitive processes involved in the onset and perpetuation of dysfunctional psychological states. Thus, recent theories have tended to reject the more simplistic view that simple errors in thinking cause depression in favor of focusing more on principles of complex information-processing errors as the causal factors for depression.

In this section we will briefly review the linear cognitive model proposed by A. Ellis (1962) and comment on its research support. Although a number of more complex models of cognition in depression have been developed, Ellis's model is relevant because of its historical status as the forerunner of more contemporary cognitive models of depression. Ellis's model has been revised somewhat, but it still incorporates the critical elements of its predecessor (1994, 1996). Moreover, even though Ellis's approach was not specific to the causes of depression, but was rather aimed at emotional disorders in general, it is easily applied to depressive disorders.

Rational-emotive behavioral theory (REBT; A. Ellis, 1994, 1996) is the most recent revision of Ellis's theory. Stated simply, Ellis postulates that irrational beliefs lead to psychological disorders such as depression. According to REBT, depression-prone individuals are typified as holding overly rigid standards by which life is judged. These standards are applied to one's own performance, the performance of others, and life happenings in general. As a consequence of these inappropriately high standards, the individual who expects too much of him- or herself, others, or life in general is likely to be disappointed and, ultimately, to become depressed.

Although research has tended to support A. Ellis's theory (1994), a number of serious problems have been noted in these studies. Perhaps the most important problem in terms of methodology has been measurement of irrational beliefs (Hagga & Davison, 1993). In a series of reviews and empirical studies, Smith and colleagues (Smith, 1989; Zurawski & Smith, 1987) found that the most commonly used measures of irrational beliefs, the Rational Behavior Inventory (Shorkey & Whiteman, 1977) and the Rational Beliefs Test (Jones, 1968) are highly confounded with negative mood. That is, these measures are strongly related to depressive symptomatology in that depressed individuals score high on them but only when they are depressed. This may undermine interpretability of studies evaluating irrational beliefs as a factor in the onset for depression; A. Ellis does not distinguish conditions when such rigid beliefs become accessed and thus, theoretically, they should be constant and always available to precipitate depression. However, because these rigidly held beliefs proposed by Ellis as the causal factor in depression appear to be present only during episodes of depression, they may constitute symptoms of depression rather than causal factors.

The criticism that cognitive factors proposed to be linked to depression may only be detected when the person is depressed is not limited to A. Ellis's theory. In Chapter 6 we discuss the problems with this interpretation in more detail. In brief, such findings are a more serious problem for a cognitive model if it specifies that the critical cognitive features should continually be present. As noted by the distinction between accessibility and availability (see Chapter 1), however, the lack of continually detectable cognitive factors is only fatal for a model that, implicitly at least, specifies that the cognitive causal factors are always available and accessed. The fact that Ellis's approach does not draw a clear distinction between accessibility and availability is a limitation.

Learned Helplessness/Hopelessness Theory

A major theory of vulnerability to depression has been the helplessness theory of depression. This theory began with work by Martin Seligman (see Seligman, 1975) who observed that animals who were unable to control negative stimuli often developed behavior consistent with depression. Specifically, dogs who were unable to control intermittent electrical shocks to their feet eventually became helpless and did not escape this aversive situation even when a pathway to escape became available. While not originally intended as a theory of depression, Seligman noted the apparent similarity between animals exposed to helplessness conditions and people with depressive symptoms. Seligman's theory of depression focused on how depression-prone individuals have expectations that they are helpless to control aversive outcomes and, therefore, behave in ways that are consistent with these expectations.

Learned helplessness theory, perhaps because of its intuitive appeal and apparent simplicity, generated an enormous amount of research (Abramson, Seligman, & Teasdale, 1978). Although much of this research was supportive of the basic tenets of the theory, other research highlighted the theory's shortcomings. Recognizing these shortcomings, in 1978 the theory was reformulated as the theory of helplessness and depression and focused on individuals' attributions about the causes of events (Abramson et al., 1978). In this revised theory, attributional style was hypothesized as the key causal factor in depression. Specifically, making global, stable, internal attributions for negative events, and conversely, making specific, unstable, external attributions for positive events, was proposed to lead to depression.

Support for the various iterations of the learned helplessness/hopelessness theory of depression has been similar to that of other cognitive approaches. That is, when individuals are depressed, cross-sectional research shows that they do indeed make the kinds of attributions suggested by the theory. Moreover, there are some data that suggest that the tendency to make these kinds of attributions precedes negative mood reactions by college students in response to negative events. In particular, two prospective studies found that college students who tend to attribute negative achievement events to stable, global causes experienced more enduring depressive mood to low midterm grades than did students without this attributional style (Metalsky, Halberstadt, & Abramson, 1987; Metalsky, Joiner, Hardin, & Abramson, 1993). The broader causal implications of this theory (i.e., that these kinds of thinking processes cause depression), however, have yet to be confirmed.

More recently, Abramson et al. (1989) have presented a new iteration of the attributional theories, which they have referred to as the hopelessness theory of depression. More than just a theory, however, they have also proposed that this represents a subtype of depressive disorders; in particular, they describe a subtype of depression that is characterized by hopelessness. The cause of hopelessness depression is the expectation that highly desired outcomes will not occur or that highly aversive outcomes will occur and that no response in one's repertoire will change the likelihood of the occurrence of these outcomes (hence the concept of hopelessness).

By definition, the hopelessness-prone individual has a depressogenic attributional style; that is, he or she sees the factors causing catalytic, negative life events as stable and global, with a high degree of importance attached to these events. As with several cognitive models of depression, the hopelessness hypothesis requires a match between the content area of an individual's depressogenic attributional style (i.e., areas of specific sensitivity) and the negative life events encountered before the attributional diathesis–stress interaction is proposed to lead to depression.

Because the hopelessness theory of depression is relatively new, fewer data are available to evaluate it, although early studies examining the association between attributions and negative affect in college students have been largely positive. For example, many cross-sectional and longitudinal studies have examined the relationship between attributional style and depression (for reviews see Barnett & Gotlib, 1988; Brewin, 1985b; Coyne & Gotlib, 1983; Peterson & Seligman, 1984; Sweeney, Anderson, & Bailey, 1986). Although these findings have not always been strong, they do point to evidence for some association between depression and the tendency to make internal, stable, and global attributions for negative events. Nonetheless, as with the earlier theories, this theory has failed to demonstrate clearly that attributional style, the putative causal factor, is present in those vulnerable to depression *prior* to an episode of depression. Recently, however, Alloy and Abramson (1990) undertook a large prospective, longitudinal study to determine whether hopelessness-prone individuals (those with the proposed negative attributional style) become depressed over the course of the longitudinal study. This well-designed prospective study will follow college students over time after they have been classified as at high or low risk for hopelessness depression and will provide valuable data in regards to the vulnerability factors proposed by the hopelessness theory to predispose individuals to depression.

Theories Focusing on Cognitive Structures and Propositions

In contrast to those theories placing primary emphasis on some aspect of thinking (cognitive products), theories focusing on cognitive structures place the key emphasis on putative depressogenic cognitive structures and the content that is represented within these structures. Although these theories incorporate other cognitive elements such as thoughts or cognitions and various cognitive processes, the central organizing principle of these approaches is the structure.

Dysfunctional Cognitive Schemas

Several cognitive approaches focus on some conceptualization of dysfunctional cognitive structures as the critical causal elements in depression. By virtually any measure, the most widely known and well-accepted cognitive model that focuses on dysfunctional structures has been proposed by Beck (1963, 1967, 1987). Beck's cognitive theory argues that dysfunctional cognitions are the causal elements for depression. This theory goes beyond simple cognitive errors and argues that "deeper" structures related to thinking are also involved in precipitating depression. Specifically, this theory contends that there are three "layers" of cognitions that are involved in precipitating depression. First, automatic thoughts are the negative thoughts that occur in depressed individuals throughout the day. Underlying the automatic thoughts are irrational cognitions or beliefs that are in turn a product of even deeper depressive schemas. According to Beck, dysfunctional thinking is activated by stress to which the individual has been previously sensitized. For example, a student may think, "I'm really stupid and useless," every time she gets a poor grade on a test. Then, if this student does poorly at the end of a semester, this stress may result in activation of the student's negative schema. She would become aware of believing, "If I do poorly in school, I am a failure." Underlying this dysfunctional belief may be a set of negative beliefs represented within schemas about being worthwhile only insofar as one is productive. According to Beck, once the depressogenic schema is activated by stress, the student will become depressed.

A key postulate of Beck's theory is that depressogenic schemas are latent until activated by certain stresses, a notion that until relatively recently has been difficult to assess. We will discuss this idea more fully in Chapters 6, 7, and 10. For now, we simply note that when he first discussed cognitive structures over 30 years ago (Beck, 1963, 1967), Beck proposed that depression-prone individuals possess dysfunctional schemas that are latent until they are activated by key stressful life events. When activated, such schemas are thought to provide access to a complex system of negative themes and give rise to a corresponding pattern of negative self-referent information processing that precipitates depression (Segal & Shaw, 1986).

Although numerous studies have found that those who are currently depressed report more evidence of dysfunctional cognitive structures than do those who are not currently depressed (Blaney, Behar, & Head, 1980; Hamilton & Abramson, 1983; Hollon & Kendall, 1980; Ingram & Holle, 1992; Krantz & Hammen, 1979; Lefebve, 1981), such dysfunctional structures become undetectable as an episode of depression remits (Eaves & Rush, 1984; Hamilton & Abramson, 1983; Hammen,

Miklowitz, & Dyck, 1986; Persons & Rao, 1985; Silverman, Silverman, & Eardley, 1984). However, as we have noted, the theory predicts that these structures would be accessible *only* under certain conditions of stress. As a result, several studies have attempted to prime or increase accessibility of dysfunctional beliefs in remitted depressives. We review these studies in Chapter 7, but to illustrate here, several studies have found that remitted depressed individuals, who are presumably vulnerable to depression, differ in dysfunctional thinking from those who are not vulnerable after being primed by negative mood (Miranda & Persons, 1988; Miranda, Persons, & Byers, 1990; Teasdale & Dent, 1987; Miranda, Gross, Persons, & Hahn, in press). Although this work documents a plausible explanation for the failure to find dysfunctional cognitive structures in those who are vulnerable to depression but not currently depressed, prospective studies have not yet been conducted that would establish dysfunctional cognition as a vulnerability factor for depression. We discuss this and related methodological issues in more depth in Chapter 6.

Sociotropic and Autonomous Cognitive Structural Subtypes. More recently, Beck (1987) refined his theory to include two categories of individuals prone to depression by virtue of having more specific concepts represented within cognitive structures. The first is an interpersonal mode known as *sociotropy*; individuals with this concept as a latent cognitive factor value positive interchange with others, and focus on acceptance, support, and guidance from others. The second type is an achievement mode called *autonomy*; these individuals overvalue independence, mobility, and achievement. Stressors congruent with these themes are expected to activate dysfunctional structures and precipitate depression. Recent reviews of the literature on sociotropy and autonomy have been largely positive (Coyne & Whiffen, 1995). However, clear methodological problems exist within this literature. A recent review by Coyne and Whiffen (1995) clearly underscores some of these problems. Particularly problematic is the fact that many participants score high on both subtypes, something counter to the prediction of the theory. Clearly this area is promising, but in need of sounder methodological study.

Anaclitic and Introjective Cognitive Structural Subtypes. Although from a strikingly different paradigm, Blatt (1974) has developed a model with similarities to Beck's depressive typologies. His model is a developmental model of depression rooted in object relations theory. Blatt suggests that depression can be better understood by distinguishing between two types: *anaclitic* and *introjective*.

According to Blatt, anaclitic depression is characterized by feelings of helplessness, weakness, depletion, and being unloved. The anaclitically depressed individual fears abandonment and struggles to maintain direct physical contact with a need-gratifying object. These individuals have intense wishes to be soothed and cared for, helped, fed, and protected. There is a sense of helplessness in being unable to find gratification, and others are valued only for their capacity to provide need gratification. When others are unable to provide for these needs, feelings of being unloved and helpless evolve into depression.

In contrast, introjective depression is developmentally more advanced than anaclitic depression. Introjective depression is characterized by feelings of being unworthy, unlovable, guilty, and having failed to live up to expectations and standards. The person with introjective cognitive structures has a keen sense of morality and self-scrutiny. These individuals have excessive demands for perfection, a proclivity to assume blame and responsibility, and feelings of helplessness to achieve approval, acceptance, and recognition. The introjective person overachieves in order to win the approval which he or she feels is lacking. With any sense of failure or lack of approval from important others (an activating event), the introjective individual is vulnerable to depression.

Blatt (1974) proposes that the genesis of anaclitic and introjective depression cognitive structures resides in impairments in object relations, a theme to which we return in Chapter 9. For Blatt, the nature of the object relations, which emerge out of the affective relationship between the mother and child, serves to organize future experiences of that relationship and future relationships. The failure to establish good relations and adequate levels of internalization of the object results in a vulnerability to depression (Blatt, Wein, Chevron, & Quinlan, 1979).

According to Blatt (1974), anaclitic and introjective depression originate at different developmental levels. He proposes that the origins of anaclitic depression lie in the disturbance of the basic bond with the caregiving person, which occurs at the early substages of separation and individuation. Introjective depression originates in the phallic/urethral phase, which occurs at the later substages of separation and individuation in conjunction with superego formation, sexual identity, and oedipal conflict. Both anaclitic and introjective depression involve the desire for contact with the object. Anaclitic depression is a distorted attempt to maintain satisfying interpersonal experiences, whereas introjective depression is a distorted attempt to establish an effective concept of the self and to gain the approval of others.

Blatt (1974) proposes that different etiological factors predispose to the development of anaclitic cognitive structures as opposed to introjective structures. Anaclitic depression is proposed to be the result of excessive frustration or a failure to have learned how to tolerate and manage frustration effectively and is related to early childhood trauma, particularly loss, and deprivation or overindulgence. An association between depression in adults and reports of depriving childhood experiences has been noted (Blatt, Quinlan, Chevron, McDonald, & Zuroff, 1982; Blatt et al., 1979; S. Jacobson, Fasman, & DiMascio, 1974). An association between early object loss and anaclitic dependency has also been found (Blatt et al., 1982).

Introjective structures, according to Blatt (1974) develop at a later developmental stage than do anaclitic structures. He asserts that they are the consequence of negative conscious and unconscious parental feelings and/or ambivalent or hostile parental behaviors. Such feelings and behaviors promote intense feelings of guilt and worthlessness and a vulnerability to introjective depression on the part of the child.

Blatt's contention regarding the etiology of anaclitic and introjective depression has some support from studies (McCranie & Bass, 1984). Unfortunately, these studies require that currently depressed individuals make judgments about their parents' behavior earlier in their lives, raising the risk that this retrospective methodology is confounded, a possibility that we discuss in Chapter 8. For example, those who are depressed in response to a lost relationship may be described as "anaclitic" and be more likely, because of the recent loss, to describe their parents as not being consistently affectionate.

Blatt developed the Depressive Experiences Questionnaire (DEQ; Blatt, D'Afflitti, & Quinlan, 1976) to differentiate anaclitic from introjective types. Nevertheless, this measure suffers from the same problems inherent in measures of Beck's (1987) sociotropic and autonomous types. That is, although the theory suggests that the two types occur at different developmental times and result in distinctly separate personality types, the scales are highly correlated in most samples. Thus again, measurement issues have hampered the ability of investigators to determine the validity of Blatt's proposals.

Self-Worth Contingencies. Beck's model has also been modified somewhat in a theoretical proposal by Kuiper, Olinger, and MacDonald (1988). In the self-worth contingency model, they suggest that schemas function in much the same way as suggested by Beck, but that several aspects not specified by Beck define more precisely the operation of these schemas. In particular, they suggest that in addition to the content of depressive self-schemas (e.g., negative self-relevant information), the consolidation of this content is an important dimension on which schemas function. Consolidation refers to interconnectedness of the knowledge represented within the schema; consolidated schemas have strongly associated linkages in stored content that results in the efficient processing of information that is consistent with this content.

Another important component of Kuiper and colleagues' (1988) proposals are that the contingencies embodied within the content of depressive schemas serve as the diathesis in diathesis–stress interactions. Specifically, Kuiper et al. argue that the content of depressive self-schemas are quite similar to the types of dysfunctional attitudes suggested by Beck (e.g., "I am a failure if I am not respected by everyone"), which serve as the contingencies that determine whether or not depressive processes will be activated. To the extent that these contingencies are met, then individuals remain nondepressed (e.g., if the person is respected, then he or she will function normally). When not met, however, (e.g., evidence of disrespect is obtained), these cognitions are activated, impinging on self-worth and initiating depression. This proposal is virtually identical to Beck's proposals, but is more theoretically detailed.

Owing to their considerable conceptual similarity, Kuiper and colleagues' (1988) proposals enjoy support comparable to Beck's theory (Kuiper et al., 1988, provide a review of these data). Likewise, the methodological and theoretical issues that apply to research on Beck's model also apply to Kuiper et al.'s theoretical elaboration of this model.

Cognitive Network Theories

Some conceptualizations of depression have focused on theoretical assumptions deriving from experimental cognitive psychology. Although quite similar to conceptualizations relying on cognitive schemas, this approach tends to concentrate on slightly different structural assumptions and to accentuate information processing as the key factor for depression. The basis for this approach can be found in Bower's (1981) model of mood and memory. Bower (1981) argued that associative networks are developed between mood nodules and memory nodules. As a result, mood can precipitate changes in thinking and changes in thinking can precipitate changes in mood.

Ingram (1984) has developed an information-processing model of depression based on a number of constructs developed within the realm of experimental cognitive psychology, including Bower's (1981) associative network model. According to Ingram's (1984) model, the initial experience of depression is conceptualized as resulting from the activation of an affective structure theorized by Bower (1981), specifically a sadness affective structure. Once this structure is activated, cognitions are proposed to recycle through cognitive networks that have previously become associated with sadness and depression. This process not only serves to initiate the depressive episode, but once fully activated, serves to perpetuate depression until the cognitive–affective activity level eventually decays. Vulnerability as conceptualized in this model focuses on the availability of relatively well-developed and well-elaborated cognitive networks that are associated with sadness affective structures. Once activated by any variety of events, sadness thus allows access to more extensive and elaborate processing of depressive information, serving to generate the spiraling from the normative depressive effects experienced by many people into the more significant and debilitating depression experienced by vulnerable individuals who possess such networks. As these networks become better articulated, the universe of depression-triggering events becomes correspondingly larger. A similar model has been proposed by Teasdale (1988).

Interacting Cognitive Subsystems

Recently, Teasdale and Barnard (Barnard & Teasdale, 1991; Teasdale, 1993; Teasdale & Barnard, 1993) have proposed perhaps the most comprehensive information-processing model of depression called the Interacting Cognitive Subsystems (ICS) framework. This comprehensive framework attempts to account for virtually all aspects of information processing (Siegle & Ingram, 1996). According to this system, different aspects of experience are represented by patterns of different kinds of information, or mental codes. For example, at a superficial level, experience is coded in visual, auditory, and proprioceptive inputs. At a deeper level, patterns of sensory codes are represented by intermediate codes. For example, different visual input from objects seen from different perspectives are represented in the object code. At an even deeper level, there are mental codes related to meaning. For example, a sentence conveys one or more meanings. Patterns of these implicational codes represent a deeper level of holistic meaning, which is linked to emotions. This level does not map directly onto language. This is similar to our understanding of a poem at a level that transcends the actual language.

In the ICS framework, emotional reactions are produced when patterns of low level meanings and patterns of sensorially derived input produce emotion-related schematic models. Therefore, production of a depressed state occurs when depressogenic schematic models are synthesized. Depressed mood is maintained when depressogenic schematic models are continually produced. If the production of such models stops, then the depression will lift. Although initial support has been found for some tenets of this very complex model, more research is clearly needed to delineate the validity of the larger model.

Theories Focusing on Cognitive Operations

Self-Focused Attention

Self-focused attention has been shown in numerous studies to be linked to depressive states (Musson & Alloy, 1988; Ingram, Lumry, Cruet, & Sieber, 1987; Ingram & Smith, 1984; Smith & Greenberg, 1981; Smith, Ingram, & Roth, 1985). Consequently, two theoretical approaches to depression have emphasized the critical role of self-focused attention in depression. Before addressing these approaches, a brief definition of self-focused attention is necessary.

Much of the early theoretical and empirical work on self-focused attention derived from Duval and Wicklund (1972) and Carver (1979). Carver's (1979) definition of self-focused attention is as follows:

> When attention is self-directed, it sometimes takes the form of focus on internal perceptual events, that is, information from those sensory receptors that react to changes in bodily activity. Self-focus may also take the form of an enhanced awareness of one's present or past physical behavior, that is, a heightened cognizance of what one is doing or what one is like. Alternatively, self-attention can be an awareness of the more or less permanently encoded bits of information that comprise, for example, one's attitudes. It can even be an enhanced awareness of temporarily encoded bits of information that have been gleaned from previous focus on the environment; subjectively, this would be experienced as a recollection or impression of that past event. (p. 1255)

Ingram (1990) has summarized this definition to suggest that self-focused attention constitutes "an awareness of self-referent, internally generated information, that stands in contrast to an awareness of externally generated information derived through sensory receptors" (p.156).

Perhaps the first specific theoretical account of self-focused attention as this process pertains to depression was proposed in Lewinsohn and colleagues' (1985) revised account of depression, which had previously relied almost exclusively on behavioral constructs. In their revised model, Lewinsohn et al. (1985) accorded a central role to self-focused attention. In particular, they argued that disruptions in a (vulnerable) person's life serve to alter self-schemas and initiate a heightened sense of self-awareness, which results in a reduction in the person's behavioral and social competencies. These competencies are necessary to behave in a way that will ameliorate the negative life events that precipitated the depressive state.

Lewinsohn and colleagues' (1985) proposals for a central role in the self-focused mediation of interpersonal deficiencies is based on a number of studies suggesting both cognitive and behavioral deficits that may be mediated by a heightened level of self-focused attention. For example, N. S. Jacobson and Anderson (1982) found that depressed people referred more to themselves in conversations, a finding interpreted to suggest that depressed individuals' self-preoccupation prevented them from processing the basic task parameters of effective interpersonal interaction and that there was a resulting disruption in these relationships (see also Ingram & Smith, 1984).

As noted at the start of this section, research has consistently supported an association between increased self-focused attention and depression (see Ingram, 1990). Research is also consistent with the role of self-focused attention in depression proposed by Lewinsohn et al.; specifically, that depressed individuals are found to be self-preoccupied and this preoccupation does appear to interfere with adequate task performance. Such appearances aside, however, whether or not self-focused attention as described by Lewinsohn et al. (1985) actually does mediate these processes has yet to be tested directly, perhaps because attention in general and self-focused attention in particular is quite difficult to assess.

In their self-regulatory perseveration model, Pyszczynski and Greenberg (1987, 1992a, 1992b) also accorded a critical role to self-focused attention. They suggested that when individuals experience a disruption in a life domain that is of central relevance for their conceptions of self-worth, an exacerbation of self-focus occurs that in turn instigates a self-evaluation process. Depressed individuals perseverate in this process, which results in the development of a negative self-focused style affecting self-esteem, task performance, affect, and a host of other symptoms of depression. In the face of subsequent events that are negative, Pyszczynski and Greenberg (1987, 1992a, 1992b) propose that this style leads depressed individuals to increase their self-focus, but for positive events they reduce self-focus. Hence, depressed individuals have limited cognitive access to the beneficial effects of positive events, and substantial access to the deleterious effects of negative events.

Empirical evidence for the role of self-focused attention has been mixed. As we have noted, although self-focused attention has repeatedly been shown to be associated with depressive states, many of the predictions concerning the functions of self-focused attention have not been supported. For example, Pyszczynski and Greenberg (1987, 1992a, 1992b) have proposed that self-focused attention underlies the dysfunctional attributions that are frequently seen in depression. Research, however, has not borne this out (e.g., Gibbons et al., 1985). Additionally, numerous data have suggested that self-focused attention is not unique to depression. Indeed, increased self-focused attention appears so ubiquitous across a variety of disorders that it is perhaps best conceptualized as a nonspecific or generalized psychopathology factor. Although this does not diminish the importance of self-focused attention, it does suggest that other variables are required to understand the relationship of this process to such a wide variety of dysfunctional states (see Ingram, 1990, 1991c; Pyszczynski, Hamilton, Nix, & Greenberg, 1991).

Ruminative Response Styles

Finally, a recent cognitive theory of depression has focused explicitly on maintaining rather than precipitating depressive mood. Nolen-Hoeksema (1987) has proposed that persons who maintain depressive mood states differ in their response to original depressive mood from persons who are able to cope effectively with depressive mood states, an approach she has termed the *responses style theory of depression*. Specifically, she proposes that those who ruminate on depressive symptoms and the causes of those symptoms are more likely to maintain depression than are those who distract themselves. Those who engage in distraction focus their attention elsewhere and are more likely to engage in alternate activities. The ruminative response is hypothesized as a causative factor in maintaining the interval and intensity of depression. The responses styles theory of depression is highly similar to self-focused attention models. A key difference is that Nolen-Hoeksema suggests that depressed individuals ruminate on their depressive symptoms, whereas self-focused attention theories are more generalized in the focus of the internal attention.

Several studies have generally supported the notion that those who are depressed engage in more ruminations than do those who are not depressed (Nolen-Hoeksema, 1991), although most of these studies have not directly assessed ruminative thinking. Additionally, and similar to other studies of dysfunctional thinking, a difficult issue is determining whether negative mood precipitates ruminations or ruminations precipitate continued negative mood.

COMMON THEORETICAL ISSUES
IN COGNITIVE MODELS OF DEPRESSION

We began this chapter with a brief definition and discussion of the core element in any cognitive theory of depression; that is, we have operationally defined as cognitive any model that incorporates a major cognitive element within its conceptual framework. Aside from the commonality of this defining feature of cognitive models, several salient issues tend to occur consistently across cognitive models of depression. We conclude with a discussion of these issues. In particular, we examine the issues of self-related information processing, cognitive distortion, and causality.

The Concept of the Self in Cognitive Models of Depression

Cognitive theories of depression are largely theories of information processing pertaining to the self. This can be seen in the theoretical postulates of these models (e.g., the hypothesized importance of the self-schema, or the results of self-focused attention) as well as in the empirical studies that have sought to evaluate these models. For example, studies of cognition in depression have almost uniformly addressed the processing of self-related information such as the occurrence of self-statements or, in incidental recall paradigms, the encoding of information as it pertains to descriptions of oneself.

The self *is* important and will no doubt remain so in subsequent iterations of cognitive models of depression. Yet, the self is not the only important cognitive construct in depression and other sources of "depressive variance" may play an important role. The lack of inclusion of these other sources may have served to diminish the ultimate explanatory power of cognitive models of depression (Hammen, 1992).

What are other cognitive constructs besides the self? In Chapters 1 and 10 we discuss the concept of working models that, while still including representations of the self, also consider information processing pertaining to others and the interactions between the self and others. Such working model conceptualizations are becoming, and we believe will continue to become, increasingly important in theoretical constructs for depression. There may also be other constructs that fit within the parameters of cognitive models that have yet to be theoretically articulated. A conceptual openness to other constructs will serve cognitive models well.

Cognitive Distortion

The notion of cognitive distortion has been integral to many models of depression. Beck (1967) was the first to suggest that depressed individuals make information-processing errors that are distorted in a negative direction. Although the idea that depressed people distorted information was well accepted for some time, research by Alloy and Abramson (1979, 1982) began to cast doubt on this idea. In a series of experiments, they found that depressed college students actually showed evidence of more accurate information processing than nondepressed control subjects, a finding that they suggested characterized depressed people as "sadder but wiser." They dubbed this phenomenon "depressive realism" and argued that perhaps the ostensible bias in information processing in depressed people is apparent only in comparison to nondepressed people who bias their information processing in a self-enhancing and positive manner.

Subsequent research has shown that the depressive realism phenomenon is not as robust as originally thought, and, at the very least, interactions between accurate information-processing level and depression are determined by a complex set of factors that defy generalized conclusions (e.g., "depressed people process information accurately"). Most fundamentally, however, there is still much confusion as to what constitutes distortion. Although accuracy and distortion can be relatively easily defined in a laboratory setting, there is little consensus for how to define distortion. Kendall (1985), for example, has offered an important distinction between cognitive deficiencies and cognitive distortions. In the arena of childhood disorders, he argues that children who evidence cognitive deficiencies (e.g., a lack of impulse control) may represent a fundamentally different set of problems, and present different treatment challenges, than children who cognitively distort information.

Even this distinction, however, leaves the concept of distortion largely undefined. Although in principle, distortion might appear easy to define (e.g., beliefs or the processing of information that does not correspond to reality), such a straightforward definition can be deceiving. The original discussion of cognitive distortion offered by Beck (1967), for example, implies what might be considered a *distortion by commission*. This definition suggests that depressed individuals somehow "change" positive or neutral information into negative information or conclusions in a manner that is consistent with their predominant depressive schema. Indeed, this may be the case. Nevertheless, an equally likely but very different definition of distortion is a *distortion by omission* conceptualization. In this case, depressed individuals may process negative information very accurately while cognitively ignoring positive information. The reverse may be true for nondepressed people who are particularly attuned to positive stimuli, but neglect to focus on information that is more negatively valenced. The *overall* effect of this processing style would thus be distortion, not because information was changed in some manner, but rather because of an imbalance in the information that was actually processed relative to what was available. In such a case, depressed individuals would indeed look very accurate when it came to assessing their processing of negative information, but such a conceptualization would preclude the conclusion that they were cognitively accurate. Whether this or other conceptualizations of distortion are useful, cognitive theoretical models with distortion as a component must clearly define what constitutes distortion.

Cognitive Causality

Although it may seem self-evident on the surface, the definition of causality is anything but clear. For example, causality may be considered the onset of a depressive state or may alternatively be considered to be the maintenance of a state that lasts for many months, as depression tends to do. This distinction and other issues pertinent to the causal spectrum are discussed more fully in Chapter 5. Such distinctions aside, however, virtually all cognitive models of depression are causal models, that is, the cognitive factors they specify are considered to be the primary causal agents of the disorder. Thus, in this regard, structural models view constructs such as schemas or cognitive networks as playing the key causal role whereas product models view certain kinds of thinking processes to be the critical causal factors.

We have briefly commented on the empirical support for these causal propositions earlier in this chapter and will discuss related empirical issues in many parts of the remainder of this volume (see particularly Chapter 7). An extremely large and unquestionable body of research suggests that the kinds of cognitive variables described by cognitive models do indeed characterize depressed individuals. However, to extrapolate from this research and suggest that the causal aspects of these models have been validated would be in error. Indeed, much of the existing empirical data examining the cognitive features of the depressed state may not be relevant to causality, at least to the extent that causality is viewed as the onset of the disorder. As we have noted in this chapter, and discuss in Chapters 6 and 7, these features are ostensibly not stable when depression remits and it is therefore difficult to continue to detect indications of negative or dysfunctional cognition. This is the case to a large degree because much of the extant research assessing cognition in depression is cross-sectional and thus correlational. There is no doubt that depression researchers have developed an impressive knowledge of the nature of cognition within the depressed state. What is less clear is how or whether this cognition relates to the onset and maintenance of depression.

Issues concerning the causal status of cognition in depression have sparked a considerable and, at the very least, spirited debate. Perhaps the most illuminating example of this debate can be seen in a series of articles in a relatively recent issue of *Psychological Inquiry*. In 1991, a consensus conference on cognitive models of depression was held in Banff, about which a final report was prepared and published in this journal (Segal & Dobson, 1992). A number of researchers were invited to comment not only upon the published report from this conference, but also upon the broader issue of the vitality of cognitive models in depression. To illustrate the tenor of the discussion, and to gain a sense of the wide divergence of opinions on cognitive models of depression, one need only sample the titles of several of the responding articles such as "A Consensus Conference without Our Consensus" or "Cognition in Depression: A Paradigm in Crisis."

Perhaps the most critical perspective on the views of the validity of cognitive models expressed at this conference was offered by Coyne (1992), who began his response this way:

> There is a delightful Monty Python skit in which a community develops a novel solution to its housing crisis. Rather than go to the expense of constructing new housing, the community enlists a hypnotist to leave everyone with a post-hypnotic suggestion that they live in a high-rise apartment building. . . . The cognitive approach to depression is facing a serious crisis of another sort, but the entranced participants at the Consensus Development Conference seemed to be more intent on preserving their illusory theoretical high-rise than on confronting what is wrong with their perspective. (p. 232)

Aside from a shared affinity for Monty Python, we have fundamental disagreements with this perspective, specifically that cognitive models of depression have little or nothing to offer attempts to understand the essential characteristics and features of depression. Clearly, criticisms of the cognitive approach to depression have proved to be extremely valuable in leading to theoretical refinements and new research paradigms. In addition, acknowledging the inability of existing cross-sectional and correlational research (the bulk of currently available research) to inform us about causality has been an important outgrowth of this criticism. Nevertheless, we submit that the persistence of cognitive models of depression has less to do with shared delusions among researchers than with the existence of compelling theory and research suggesting that there are important cognitive factors at work in the onset and maintenance of depression. Cognitive models of depression are imperfect, and like all approaches to understanding psychopathology in the foreseeable future, will remain imperfect. But they also provide an important foundation that, through criticism-derived theoretical and research modification, will serve as the impetus for future development. In fact, such criticism of the putative causal statements of cognitive models of depression has driven to a large degree the resurgence of interest in issues such as diathesis–stress perspectives and vulnerability.

SUMMARY AND CONCLUSIONS

Numerous cognitive models of depression have been proposed. One way to organize these models is to cluster them according to constructs suggested by the meta-construct framework. Accordingly, structural and propositional models have been suggested by a number of theorists. The oldest and most well-known of these is Beck's (1963, 1967, 1987) schema model, which was revised somewhat by Kuiper et al. (1988). Models by Ingram (1984) and Teasdale (1988) focused more on the cognitive network approach to depression whereas Teasdale and Barnard (1993) have presented a newer approach that examines the interactions of various cognitive subsystems. Finally, Blatt's (1974) model of introjective and anaclitic depression can also be considered a structural model.

Operational models tend to emphasize the cognitive processes that operate in depression and have been proposed by Lewinsohn et al. (1985), Pyszczynski and Greenberg (1987), and Nolen-Hoeksema (1987). Cognitive product models, which focus more on the cognitions that depressed people experience have been suggested by A. Ellis (1994, 1996) and Abramson et al. (1978, 1989).

Despite the different emphases in these models, there are a variety of issues that occur across virtually all models. All extant cognitive models, for example, are essentially models of the self in dysfunction. Although the principle of the self will remain an important construct, we argue that, in order to maintain their viability, cognitive models will need to evolve to include additional cognitive elements. Distortion or inaccurate information processing is also a construct that is central to cognitive models of depression, with some models proposing that depressed people suffer from these distortions and other models suggesting just the opposite. At least some aspects of these different perspectives may be resolved by articulating explicit definitions of distortion, something that most models have failed to do. Finally, the issue of causality is also an important consideration for cognitive models; although causality is a central tenet of all models, the abundance of currently available cross-sectional research has been unable to test causality claims.

An in-depth examination of cognitive models is clearly beyond the scope of this chapter and this book. Nevertheless, we believe that understanding the central tenets of extant cognitive models is a necessary prerequisite for understanding the issues that are pertinent to cognitive vulnerability to depression. With this theoretical foundation laid, we now turn to consideration of some of the fundamental issues in the conceptualization and study of vulnerability.

CHAPTER 4

Vulnerability Approaches to Psychopathology

To the lay public, the concept of vulnerability is well-known; people are vulnerable to the extent that they are susceptible to being hurt or wounded. Intuitive extension of this conceptualization to psychological domains implies an increased susceptibility to emotional pain and to the occurrence of psychopathology of some type. Yet, as intuitively appealing as this concept has been, few precise definitions of vulnerability are available in the scientific literature. Such definitional impoverishment is the case even though the notion of psychopathological vulnerability has generated a significant body of theory and research, and terms such as "risk" and "vulnerability" are frequently used by researchers investigating a variety of disorders. In a like fashion, discussion of the fundamental conceptual and empirical issues in the study of vulnerability has also been limited in the literature.

In this chapter, we will seek to address the fundamental conceptual and empirical issues as they pertain to vulnerability. The focus of this chapter, however, is not on cognitive vulnerability or vulnerability to depression per se, but on a more general examination of the construct as it can be applied to psychological research. We will start by addressing the origins of the vulnerability construct and then turn to what appear to be some core characteristics of psychopathological vulnerability. These will provide a conceptual foundation for a working definition that will guide our subsequent discussion of cognitive vulnerability to depression.

ORIGINS OF THE VULNERABILITY APPROACH

Any attempt to understand the history and origins of the concept of vulnerability to psychopathology must account not only for the conceptual origins of the vulnerability construct (i.e., early theoretical approaches), but also for its empirical origins (i.e., early empirical findings). We explore in some detail both of these in the next two sections.

Conceptual Origins

The vulnerability construct in psychology originates largely in theory and research on schizophrenia. In his classic paper, Meehl (1962) was among the first to allude to a psychogenic vulnerability to the schizophrenic disorders. Meehl proposed that the onset of a schizophrenic episode is determined by a neural deficit (labeled "schizotaxia") and the individual's particular learning history. Meehl referred to the combination of schizotaxia and learning history as "schizotypia" and suggested that schizotypia represents a vulnerability to schizophrenia. At the same time, however, schizotypia in and of itself is not considered to be a sufficient precipitant of a schizophrenic episode. Indeed, Meehl (1962) suggested that only a subset of schizotypic individuals would eventually decompensate into clinical schizophrenia. This subset is determined by the presence of a schizophrenogenic mother who exposes the child to a developmental climate of ambivalent, unpredictable, and aversive mother–child interactions: "It seems likely that the most important causal influence pushing the schizotype toward schizophrenic decompensation is the schizophrenogenic mother" (p. 830). Meehl's viewpoint thus suggests that the onset of clinical schizophrenia is a function of both genetic (schizotaxia) and psychogenic vulnerability factors (e.g., the individual's learning history and disturbed mother–child interactions).

Since Meehl's (1962) paper, several investigators have alluded to various schizophrenia vulnerability possibilities (e.g., Gottesman & Shields, 1972; Millon, 1969). Among the first to explicitly discuss vulnerability were Zubin and Spring (1977). They argued that research progress on the causes of schizophrenia was at best equivocal, and, as a consequence, investigators were generally dissatisfied with the adequacy of the major conceptual approaches to the etiology of the disorder (e.g., environmental, genetic, developmental, neurophysiological). To begin to resolve this problem, they posited that vulnerability could be viewed as the common denominator that underlies all of the various conceptual approaches to schizophrenia; hence, although each of the major etiological models emphasized different approaches to schizophrenia, all share the possibility that some vulnerability factor might predispose the person to the development of a schizophrenic episode, even though these potential vulnerabilities may also be very different.

Considering these various etiological perspectives as well as the suggestions of other researchers who had anticipated the vulnerability approach (e.g., Gottesman & Shields, 1972; Meehl, 1962; Millon, 1969; Rosenthal, 1970), Zubin and Spring (1977) proposed that vulnerability can consist of both genetic and acquired factors, or as they phrased it, the "inborn and the acquired":

> Inborn vulnerability [is] that which is laid down in the genes and reflected in the internal environment and neurophysiology of the organism. The acquired component of vulnerability is due to the influence of traumas, specific diseases, perinatal complications, family experiences, adolescent peer interactions, and other life events that either enhance or inhibit the development of subsequent disorder. (p. 109)

According to Zubin and Spring (1977), vulnerability is not the only risk factor for the onset of a schizophrenic episode. They also hypothesized that a person's competence level (e.g., "the skills and abilities needed to achieve success") and his or her coping efforts (e.g., "the energy exerted in situations") are involved in the initiation of a schizophrenic episode (p. 114). Together, competence and coping efforts comprise a person's coping ability; "the initiative and skill that an organism brings to bear in formulating strategies to master life situations" (p. 123). Although important, Zubin and Spring (1977) argue that these factors operate independently of vulnerability factors. For instance, they note that, although some (but not all) data have shown that competence is low during a schizophrenic episode, research is unclear as to whether competence deficiencies are a function of premorbid competence deficits or are instead a function of life stress and disorder-induced strains that decrease competence level. Zubin and Spring (1977) do, however, suggest the possibility of an indirect link between coping abilities and vulnerability to schizophrenia. That is, they posit that people whose coping has been compromised in some fashion are more likely to experience heightened stress levels and thus heightened risk for disorder. In a sense then, coping acts as a gate through which high or low stress levels may be moderated.

Even though Zubin and Spring's (1977) vulnerability approach is perhaps the most well known, other schizophrenia researchers have also discussed the concept of vulnerability. More recently, for instance, Nicholson and Neufeld (1992) have proposed a "dynamic vulnerability formulation" of schizophrenia. In line with Zubin and Spring (1977), they suggest that genetic factors underlie the individual's vulnerability to schizophrenia. These genetic factors influence both the person's cognitive appraisal strategies, which are responsible for assessing situations accurately, and his or her coping abilities, which determine how adequately the person can respond to situations appraised as stressful. These factors interact to produce the person's ultimate level of vulnerability. Level of vulnerability is proposed by Nicholson and Neufeld (1992) to affect the level of schizophrenic decompensation; the greater the vulnerability, the greater the schizophrenic symptomatology.

Schizophrenia investigators are not the only ones who have recognized the potential usefulness of the vulnerability construct. Developmental psychopathologists, for instance, have focused considerable attention on the factors that may either predispose or insulate children from psychological problems such as psychological disorders, behavioral difficulties, academic performance deficits, and interpersonal problems (e.g., Felner, 1984; Reid & Morrison, 1983; Rutter, 1988). Similarly, alcoholism (Chassin, Furran, Hussong, & Colder, 1996), bipolar disorder (Depue et al., 1981), and psychopathy (Kandel et al., 1988; Widom, 1977) represent psychopathological states that have been the focus of vulnerability analyses.

Empirical Origins

Vulnerability perspectives have also spawned a considerable empirical literature examining the factors thought to render individuals prone to psychological dysfunction. A general examination of applicable research strategies can help explicate the basic concept of vulnerability. A number of approaches for empirically identifying and studying vulnerable individuals exist, which will be discussed in more depth later in this book. For now we will simply provide an overview of some frequently employed vulnerability strategies to illustrate how research guided by vulnerability constructs has been conducted.

One of the most common strategies for identifying potentially vulnerable individuals is to examine the offspring of parents with a psychological disorder (see Chapters 6 and 8 for a discussion of methodological issues concerning this approach and Chapters 7 and 9 for a review of relevant research using the high-risk paradigm). The assumption of many investigators using this strategy is that offspring can be viewed to be at increased risk for disorder by virtue of their parental interactions, by genetic transmission of neural deficits, or by birth or prebirth trauma. Thus, presumably through either genetic or environmental influences, offspring are at risk for developing disorders similar to their parents. This offspring strategy is nicely illustrated by D. Klein,

Depue, and Krauss (1986) in their assessment of social adjustment as a possible risk variable in the children of parents with bipolar disorder, and Walker and Hoppes's (1984) review of the impact of parental schizophrenia on offspring. In the area of depression, Hammen's (1991a) recent extensive work examining a number of factors in the children of depressed mothers is a comprehensive illustration of this strategy. Blatt and Homann (1992), Cohn and Campbell (1992), Downey and Coyne (1990), and Gelfand and Teti (1990) have provided comprehensive reviews of research employing the strategy of assessing the effects of maternal depression on offspring.

Many of the precursors to the offspring approach can be traced to studies originally reported by Mednick and Schulsinger (1968); Kety, Rosenthal, Wender, and Schulsinger (1968); and Rosenthal et al. (1968), which assessed a number of variables in the offspring of a parent (or parents) with a diagnosis of schizophrenia. These investigators were able to locate a large number of offspring of Danish schizophrenic mothers using extensive registers in Denmark known as the National Psychiatric Register and the Folkeregister. The National Psychiatric Register maintains a record of all psychiatric hospitalizations in Denmark while the Folkeregister is an up-to-date register of the addresses of virtually every resident of Denmark. Using these databases, Mednick and Schulsinger (1968) located a sample of 207 children of schizophrenic mothers and a control group of 104 children who were matched on a range of demographic variables. These offspring were tested on a number of variables and were followed over a period of time. Unfortunately, few investigators have the luxury of access to such comprehensive databases.

Although studying the children of disordered parents approach is a frequently employed methodological strategy, some researchers have sought other ways to identify and investigate individuals vulnerable to psychopathology. For instance, another strategy is to identify vulnerable individuals on the basis of some theoretical or empirical criterion. Using such a strategy, Depue, Krauss, Spoont, and Arbisi (1989), for example, have attempted to identify individuals vulnerable to clinical bipolar disorder based on their responses on self-report questionnaires designed to assess factors hypothesized to reflect risk for the disorder. Once identified in this fashion, investigators using this strategy can attempt to elicit evidence for the existence of increased risk for psychopathology.

CORE FEATURES OF VULNERABILITY

As is evident from the preceding discussion, the vulnerability approach to psychopathology is at least several decades old, albeit recently its conceptual appeal and empirical influence have increased noticeably. Yet, as we have noted, as widespread as this approach is becoming, few precise definitions of vulnerability have been offered. It is possible, however, to garner from previous theory and research the core characteristics of the construct. These characteristics appear to constitute the common themes that emerge in virtually all discussions of vulnerability and can thus help establish a consensus for what vulnerability is, and what it is not.

State–Trait Distinctions: Vulnerability as a Stable Trait

Most discussions of vulnerability regard this variable as an enduring trait. Zubin and Spring (1977) have been among the most specific about the trait nature of vulnerability: "We regard [vulnerability] as a relatively permanent, enduring trait" (p. 109); "The one feature that all schizophrenics have . . . is the everpresence of their vulnerability" (p. 122). Although other investigators have not been quite as specific, the enduring trait nature of vulnerability is implicit in many of their discussions of vulnerability. Such assumptions of permanence are likely rooted in the genetic level of analysis employed by researchers who pioneered this concept. For example, most schizophrenia researchers point to the genetic endowment of individuals who are at risk for this disorder. Meehl's (1962) concept of schizotaxia represents an inherited neural deficit, whereas other researchers such as Zubin and Spring, Nicholson and Neufeld (1992), and McGue and Gottesman (1989) are quite explicit that genetic endowment determines one's level of vulnerability (at least to schizophrenia). Little change is theoretically possible; genetic endowment and thus vulnerability are seen as a permanent characteristics.

Such conceptualizations posit that no decrease in absolute vulnerability levels is possible. This is not to suggest, however, that functional vulnerability levels cannot be attenuated by several factors, such as those that affect neurochemistry. This may very well be the case for medications like lithium, which alter the likelihood of developing the symptoms of a bipolar episode by presumably controlling the neurochemistry of the underlying vulnerability. Similar diminishment of functional vulnerability may be seen in the actions of psychopharmacological treatments for depression with medications such as the various generations of tricyclic agents. Even though functional vulnerability may be altered and individuals may be less likely to develop the disorder, however, the vulnerability persists; in the case of lithium, for example, the probability of developing an episode is increased if the medication is discontinued.

Thus, even though the vulnerability may be controlled, the vulnerability trait itself remains.

The trait nature of nature of vulnerability is perhaps most clearly seen in contrast to the state or episodic nature of psychological disorders. Zubin and Spring (1977), for instance, clearly distinguish between an enduring vulnerability trait and episodes of schizophrenia, which "are waxing and waning states" (p. 109). Hollon, Evans, and DeRubeis (1990), and Hollon and Cobb (1993) also distinguish between (1) stable vulnerability traits that predispose individuals to the disorder but do not initiate the disorder per se, and (2) state variables that represent the occurrence of the symptoms that reflect the onset of the disorder. Thus, whereas enduring traits are predisposing factors, virtually all investigators characterize the disorder as a state. Disordered states can therefore emerge and fade as episodes cycle between occurrence and remission, but the traits that give rise to vulnerability for the disordered state are typically thought to remain.

Although vulnerability is assumed by many theorists to be permanent and enduring, depending on a given theoretical context, this need not always be the case. This is especially true when the level of vulnerability analysis is psychological rather than genetic in nature. As we have noted, assumptions of genetic vulnerability offer little possibility for modification of vulnerability characteristics. Most psychological approaches, however, rely on assumptions of dysfunctional learning as the genesis of vulnerability. Given these assumptions, not only functional but actual vulnerability levels may fluctuate as a function of new learning experiences. For instance, Hollon et al. (1990) have reported data suggesting that depressed patients treated with cognitive therapy, or combined cognitive therapy and pharmacotherapy, are less likely than patients treated with pharmacotherapy to experience recurrence of the disorder over a 2-year period. Hollon et al. (1990) and Hollon and Cobb (1993) argue that the effects of pharmacological treatments may be largely symptom suppressive, whereas psychological interventions such as cognitive therapy are designed to alter depressive cognitive structures and, to the extent that genuine vulnerability is rooted in such structures, may lessen susceptibility to depression. Fewer recurrences of the disorder over time may reflect decreased vulnerability. It is certainly possible that factors other than vulnerability reduction may be at the heart of cognitive therapy's prophylactic effects, but this example does illustrate how, theoretically at least, actual vulnerability levels might be altered.

Of course, from the viewpoint of a psychological level of analysis, vulnerability may *decrease* with certain corrective experiences or, alternatively, may *increase* over time. This latter possibility would be the case if continued exposure to aversive experiences and stressful life events served the function of enhancing the factors that contribute to vulnerability. From a cognitive perspective this would be manifest in experiences that increased the complexity and accessibility of dysfunctional cognitive self-structures.

Stability versus Permanence

The possibility that psychological vulnerability levels can be altered (up or down) suggests a subtle but potentially important distinction between stability and permanence. Stability and permanence are likely to be viewed as synonymous. However, even though the concept of stability clearly suggests a resistance to change, it does not presume that change is never possible. Under the right circumstances, positive changes in an otherwise stable variable may very well occur. Indeed, the entire notion of psychotherapy is based on just this premise. Without intervention or other significant life experiences, however, little change in stable variables should be seen. On the other hand, variables that are considered to be enduring, particularly as viewed within a genetic context, imply a permanence or immutability that is not only resistant to change under ordinary circumstances, but is assumed to offer virtually no possibility of change. At the psychological level of analysis then, it seems reasonable to conceptualize vulnerability as stable, but not immutable.

Vulnerability Is Endogenous

Another conjecture that is possible to glean from extant vulnerability work is that vulnerability represents an endogenous variable. This is perhaps most clearly seen in genetic conceptualizations of vulnerability, but is equally relevant for psychological conceptualizations. That is, whether stemming from inborn characteristics or acquired through learning processes, the vulnerability resides within the person. This can be contrasted to other levels of analysis that might, for example, focus on environmental or external sources of stress that initiate a disorder, or perhaps a focus on interactional styles that may lead to a loss of reinforcement etc. (e.g., Coyne, 1976; Lewinsohn et al., 1985). Although these variables are clearly important, vulnerability processes are typically viewed as emanating from within the person.

Stress

Stress can be defined in a variety of ways. To examine these definitions comprehensively would necessitate an entire volume, and indeed, entire volumes have been devoted to this topic (see Brown & Harris, 1989b;

Cohen, 1988; Lazarus & Folkman, 1984). In general, however, stress can be understood as falling into several broad categories. A number of investigators (Lazarus & Folkman, 1984; Luthar & Zigler, 1991; Monroe & Peterman, 1988; Monroe & Simons, 1991) note that a major category of stress is conceptualized as the occurrence of significant life events that, in the case of psychopathology, are interpreted by the person as undesirable. Another kind of stress can be seen as the accumulation of minor events or hassles (B. P. Dohrenwend & Shrout, 1985; Lazarus, 1990). Luthar and Zigler (1991) also note the importance of socioeconomic status as an index of stress; that is, variables such as low maternal educational status or membership in an ethnic minority group may reflect stressful living circumstances.

Although it is clear from these descriptions that the definitions of stress are many, we can view stress in the present context as the life events (major or minor) that disrupt the mechanisms maintaining the stability of individuals' physiology, emotion, and cognition. In the classic description of stress, Selye (1936) notes that such events represent a strain on the person's adaptive capability that initiates an interruption of the person's routine or habitual functioning. As such, stress interferes with the system's physiological and psychological homeostasis and is thus seen as a critical variable in a multitude of models of psychopathology (Monroe & Simons, 1991), regardless of whether these models focus explicitly on vulnerability factors.

Even though stress is sometimes conceptualized as disruptive internal events, stress is typically seen as reflecting factors operating outside of or externally to the individual—the life events that challenge the person's coping resources. An external orientation does not imply, however, that individuals have no role in creating stress. Although many events may simply befall people, several researchers have persuasively argued that others may constitute the results of a person's own actions (Depue & Monroe, 1986; Hammen, 1991b, 1992; Monroe & Simons, 1991; Rutter, 1986a). For instance, the person with social skills deficits (e.g., inappropriately critical of others) may engender tumultuous relationships with acquaintances, coworkers, and romantic partners that result in the generation of significant levels of stress for the person. Vulnerable individuals may therefore play a role in creating their own stresses, which may then precipitate psychological disorder.

In addition to the complexities ensuing from the recognition that stress can be generated by individuals themselves, investigators have pointed out that it is notoriously difficult to disentangle external stress from cognitive appraisal processes, particularly for individuals who are thought to be vulnerable to or in a psychologically disordered state (Lazarus & Folkman, 1984; Monroe & Simons, 1991). The person experiencing a significant anxiety state, for instance, may perceive relatively safe events as posing considerable physical or psychological danger. From the vulnerability perspective, Nicholson and Neufeld (1992) have argued that vulnerability affects the perceptions of stress, even genetically based vulnerability; they note that "genetic makeup affects cognitive appraisal mechanisms, partly determining how accurately the individual is able to assess a [stressful] situation" (p. 122).

The influence of appraisal processes on what is perceived to be stressful has portended significant methodological difficulties for the objective measurement of stress (Monroe, 1989; Monroe & Simons, 1991). Other problems also exist. For example, distinguishing between stressful events that precede, and are perhaps linked to, the onset of symptomatology from those that follow and are the result of a disorder can be extremely difficult. It may be, for instance, that preexisting disorders precipitate the experience of negative life events rather than, or in addition to, stress precipitating the disorder. Moreover, some investigators have argued that even to attempt to separate stress from a person's life at all is artificial; life events and lifestyle are intrinsically related (Kasl, 1983). Examining the timing of stressful events as they relate to disorder is also problematic. Are, for example, stressful life events that precede a disorder by 2 years (1 month, 6 months, 5 years) related to the onset of the disorder?

In all, the problems with the conceptualization and measurement of stressful events are extensive. Nevertheless, we argue that at a purely conceptual level it makes sense to separate stress from vulnerability and psychological disorder. Such a conceptual separation recognizes the possibility that stress can exist independently of appraisal processes and can be consensually defined and objectively measured; everyone would agree, for instance, that a car accident resulting in permanent confinement to a wheelchair will be stressful for everyone regardless of their appraisal processes. Moreover, separation of the stress and vulnerability constructs facilitates communication about the variables potentially operating in psychopathology; that is, it possible to talk about stress without frequent qualifications due to appraisal processes.

The Diathesis–Stress Relationship

By conceptually separating stress and vulnerability, examining the diathesis–stress relationship becomes possible. The diathesis concept has a long history in medical terminology. In briefly tracing this history, Monroe and Simons (1991) note that the concept dates back to ancient Greeks, and as early as the late 1800s was ensconced in the psychiatric vernacular of the day. Diathesis refers to a predisposition to illness and has evolved from its original focus on constitutional, biological factors to presently also encompassing psychological variables such as cognitive and interpersonal susceptibilities. In line with this concept, most psychological models of depression and vulnerability are explicitly diathesis–stress models. That is, although there is general agreement that vulnerability constitutes an endogenous processes, most models also recognize that events perceived as stressful act to trigger vulnerability processes that are linked to the onset of the disordered state. Psychopathology is thus the interactive effect of the diatheses and events perceived as stressful. Framed within the context of a diathesis–stress conceptualization, stress is integral to virtually all extant conceptualizations of vulnerability.

Vulnerability Is Latent

Virtually all vulnerability investigators have, at least implicitly, categorized vulnerability as a latent process that is not easily observable. From a research perspective, this can perhaps be seen most clearly in the empirical search for observable markers of vulnerability; numerous investigators have sought to find reliable empirical indicators of the presence of the vulnerability. There are a variety of research strategies for identifying markers (which will be discussed later in the book), but in each case they operate under the assumption that vulnerability processes are (1) present in individuals who have few or no outward signs of the disorder, (2) causally linked to the appearance of symptoms, and (3) not easily observable. This is particularly the case in investigations that rely on some kind of stressful or challenging event that makes detection of the vulnerability factor possible (see Shelton et al., 1991, for a discussion of the challenge paradigm as it pertains to the conceptualization of vulnerability and dysregulation). The search for vulnerability markers is thus the search for predictors of the disorder in the absence of symptoms of the disorder, an empirical strategy reflecting a conceptual judgment that vulnerability is present and stable, but latent.

Summary of Core Features of Vulnerability

In sum, review of the extant literature on vulnerability suggests a number of essential features that characterize the construct of vulnerability. Perhaps the most fundamental of the core features of vulnerability is that it is considered a trait as opposed to the kind of a state that more accurately characterizes the actual appearance of the disorder. Although vulnerability is conceptualized as a trait, and psychological vulnerability may be stable and relatively resistant to change, it is not necessarily permanent or unalterable. Corrective experiences can occur that may attenuate the vulnerability, or, alternatively, continued exposure to aversive experiences may increase vulnerability factors. Additionally, vulnerability is viewed as an endogenous process that is typically conceptualized as latent. Finally, while conceptually distinct from vulnerability, stress is a critical "feature" of vulnerability in that, according to many models, vulnerability cannot be realized without stress. This latter feature of vulnerability represents the essence of the diathesis–stress approach that is common among many current models of psychological disorder.

GENERAL ISSUES IN THE STUDY OF VULNERABILITY

The relatively brief history of the vulnerability concept within clinical psychological science has provided a number of important clues as to how to define vulnerability. Having examined some of these core features that appear to characterize this definition, we now turn to a general discussion of issues that will be relevant to how investigators study this construct. Specifically, we will examine psychological conceptualizations of vulnerability analyses, the relationship between the concepts of risk and vulnerability, and the relationship between vulnerability and resilience.

Psychological Approaches to the Analysis of Vulnerability

A variety of different kinds of constructs contribute to theorizing about the basic nature of vulnerability. Much of the original work we have reviewed as the foundation of the vulnerability perspective has focused on vulnerability at the genetic level (e.g., schizotypia). "Acquired" factors have been a more secondary focus in these models, but even these factors tend to be viewed from a biological level. For instance, Zubin and Spring (1977) describe some of these acquired factors as "the influence of traumas, specific diseases, [and] perinatal complications" (p. 109), which presumably cause alterations of biochemistry that render people vulnerable to psychopathology. Acquired factors, of course, can also refer to learned processes (e.g., a learning climate of ambivalence brought about by a schizophrenogenic mother), which are acknowledged even in some predominantly genetic models to play an important, if secondary, contributory role in vulnerability.

Accounts of vulnerability that are primarily psychological in nature emphasize that acquired variables are, in the broadest sense of the term, learned. These variables are quite diverse, ranging from a focus on maternal ambivalence and disrupted early interpersonal relationships to variables such as the person's competence and coping in difficult circumstances. In this latter case, for example, vulnerability may in fact be a direct function of coping processes; those who experience stressful life events but who cannot manage them effectively may in fact be vulnerable because of (presumably learned) coping deficits.

All of these types of processes (e.g., maternal ambivalence, interpersonal disruptions, coping deficits) are either thought to affect how and what people learn or are considered to be the result of some learning process. Factors such as these represent fundamental variables in many psychological analyses of mental dysfunction. We will amplify this theme later in the book but for now it is sufficient to note that studies of vulnerability at the psychological level are broad enough to cover a very wide array of variables.

We point out the relevance of these variables to contrast them from models that specifically rule out psychological factors as meaningful vulnerability variables, or relegate them to secondary status (e.g., Zubin & Spring, 1977). However, it is also important to note in this vein that the conceptualization of vulnerability is heavily influenced by the particular disorder under consideration. Investigations of vulnerability to psychotic disorders such as schizophrenia clearly lend themselves to genetic and neurophysiological levels of analysis that correspondingly downplay the significance of psychological variables. Because much of the original vulnerability work derives from models of psychotic disorders, many existing vulnerability approaches quite naturally lean toward an exclusive focus on biochemistry.

That the focus of this book is clearly on psychological vulnerability is not meant to imply that other levels of vulnerability are not possible or are unimportant. On the contrary, as we suggested in Chapter 1, we argue that a variety of levels of vulnerability analysis, ranging from neurophysiological to sociological, have something to offer to our understanding of disorders, regardless of whether these variables are largely physiological or largely psychological in nature. While recognizing the potential contributions of these varied processes, we will highlight the psychological nature of vulnerability in general, and the cognitive level in particular.

The Relationship between Risk and Vulnerability

The terms "risk" and "vulnerability" are often used interchangeably, and, indeed, there is little doubt that these constructs share substantial conceptual variance. Nevertheless, vulnerability and risk are not synonymous. Recall from our earlier discussion that Zubin and Spring (1977) characterized coping and competence levels as risk factors, but *not* vulnerability factors. We believe that the notion of risk describes factors that are associated with an increased likelihood of experiencing a disorder; the concept of risk is frequently used to predict the occurrence of dysfunction. However, relative to the absence of risk factors, the presence of risk only suggests an increased probability of the occurrence of a disorder but does *not* point to what causes the disorder. Thus, in many respects, risk refers to a descriptive or statistical analysis rather than to a causal analysis.

To the extent that any variable is empirically shown to be related to an increased probability of onset, the variable can be considered to be a risk factor. We can point to a number of variables that describe people as being "at risk" for a psychopathological state such as depression. For instance, Kaelber, Moul, and Farmer (1995) have summarized a multitude of potential risk factors for the occurrence of depression. They distinguish between risk indicators that are (1) highly plausible, (2) plausible, and (3) possible. In the highly plausible category are factors such as being female, experiencing depression in the past, being divorced or separated, living in low socioeconomic circumstances, and having smoked. In the plausible category, factors include being never married, having a family history of depression, losing a mother before age 11, and having small children at home. In the possible category, among others, are living in a city, doing chronic housework, being infertile, or being a Protestant. The number and breadth of demonstrated risk factors is impressive.

Although risk factors suggest an enhanced probability of disorder, and it is therefore important to examine these factors, as a rule of thumb they are relatively uninformative about an individual's vulnerability; that is, they do not tell us much about the actual *mechanisms* that bring about a state of psychopathology. Although a city-living, divorced, Protestant who smokes while doing housework describes a person at heightened risk, there is nothing inherent in these characteristics that causes depression. They inform us that the person is at risk, but tell us virtually nothing about the psychological processes that bring about depression. Similarly, knowledge of such risk indicators is generally unhelpful with regard to intervention strategies (e.g., changing religions [and even gender] is possible, as is ceasing to do housework, but these would be unlikely directly to influence vulnerability to depression).

Alternatively, the propensity to dysregulate a certain neurotransmitter may also be a risk factor, but in this case if the occurrence of psychopathology is rooted in this disruption, then this variable constitutes a vulnerability mechanism or factor. Likewise, if depression is linked to the activation of schemas that influence how information is processed, this comprises a vulnerability factor. The important distinction is that empirical verification that an individual is at risk for a disorder does not necessarily tell us about the vulnerability mechanisms that cause the disorder.

Of course, given this definition of risk, any vulnerability factor must also logically constitute a risk factor, a relationship that is illustrated in Figure 4.1. Vulnerability variables are therefore most properly seen as a subset of risk variables. As such, risk conceptually comprises a much broader network of factors than does vulnerability. The distinction is subtle but important.

It should be noted that a conceptual separation of risk and vulnerability factors does not imply that these variables are empirically unrelated. In pointing out a similar distinction, Rutter (1987) and Luthar and Zigler (1991) have argued that these variables interact with each other to produce the onset of a disorder. Thus, the person who is "at risk" because he or she lives in a particularly stressful environment will see this risk realized in a disorder if he or she also possesses vulnerability mechanisms. Thus, the circumstances of living in poverty may trigger the dysregulation mechanisms that are at the heart of the onset of the

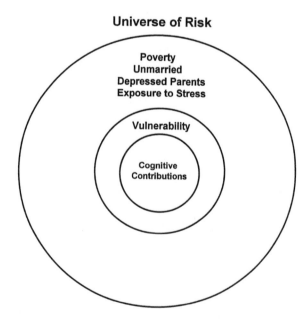

FIGURE 4.1. The universe of risk constructs, including the subset of vulnerability factors.

disorder. This is the essence of the diathesis–stress interaction we discussed earlier. From this perspective, stressful life events can be more clearly seen as a risk but not as a vulnerability factor. This is perhaps even more clearly seen within the context of defining vulnerability as an endogenous variable. Risk can include elements that are external to the person, but vulnerability cannot.

We have argued that risk represents a descriptive factor rather than a causal one, and that as an endogenous factor, only vulnerability can play a causal role. Yet, data have shown that risk variables both can predict the onset of psychopathology and are correlated with vulnerability. Such findings may make it tempting to suggest that risk might have causal significance. Rutter (1988), however, cautions against drawing causal inferences solely from risk variables that appear linked to a disorder. He notes, for instance, that risk and vulnerability are correlated by virtue of their interaction in the onset of psychopathology. To illustrate this point, Rutter (1988) notes findings from his research indicating that test results on a national examination were superior for schools where the children's work was exhibited on the walls (Rutter, Maughan, Mortimore, & Ouston, 1979). Empirically this constitutes a predictor of better test performance, but few would argue that putting children's work on the wall helped their test grades, that is, was the causal factor in getting better grades. Rather, such behavior was simply indicative, and predictive, of an enhanced school atmosphere that had some causal link to better performance. Similarly, the fact that a given risk variable predicts psychopathology (e.g., being unmarried) does not suggest that it caused the psychopathology; it may be predictive for a number of reasons. For example, being unmarried may reflect the state of affairs for an individual whose self-esteem is so deficient that he or she is unable to initiate or maintain romantic relationships. If this deficient self-esteem is a causal (i.e., vulnerability) factor, then lack of marriage may be predictive of psychopathology, but it is a correlate rather than a cause. The cause of the association in this example would be a third variable: the vulnerability. In sum, risk can be an important predictive variable that should be concert with vulnerability, but these constructs are not synonymous.

The Relationship between Vulnerability and Resilience

The flip side to vulnerability has been labeled by various investigators as invulnerability, competence, protective factors, or resilience. Each of these terms suggest invulnerability to psychopathology in the face of stress. Although these terms may reasonably be used interchangeably in some cases, some subtle distinctions also exist. Because, for the most part, we do not believe that most of these distinctions are tremendously important, we prefer the term "resilience" over other terms because it implies a diminished, but not zero possibility of psychopathology. Invulnerability, on the other hand, suggests an all-or-none quality; people are either vulnerable or they are invulnerable. That is, to the extent that individuals are characterized as invulnerable, this implies that they will never experience a disorder. Echoing Luthar and Zigler (1991), another distinction that we believe is important is between competence and resilience. Competence can be used to refer to behavioral competence such as one's ability to complete successfully a variety of tasks ranging from occupational to social functioning. Although it is certainly true that a criterion for psychopathology can be impaired occupational or social functioning, individuals can experience significant distress and still appear, and indeed be, outwardly competent. Thus, a distinction between behavioral competence and psychological competence can be drawn. The two are certainly correlated, but psychological competence can be seen as closely resembling resilience whereas behavioral competence can have to do with a variety of phenomena.

Unfortunately, few empirical data have explored the relationship between vulnerability and resilience. Our working assumption is that resilience and vulnerability represent different ends of a vulnerability continuum. Such a continuum is seen as interacting with stress to produce the possibility that a disordered state will occur. Thus, at the most extreme vulnerability end of the range, little life stress is necessary to result in a disorder. At the resilient end of the range a great deal of stress will be needed before psychopathology develops. To illustrate this idea, we might imagine the case of Viktor Frankl as someone at the far end of the continuum. He was able to maintain a state of mental health even while enduring the horrors of a Nazi concentration camp. On the other end of the continuum would be the person who becomes depressed with even the most minor of life changes (e.g., in one case we know of, depression was reported to have been precipitated by the person's favorite television show going off the air).

The vulnerability–resilience relationship is represented in Figure 4.2. As this figure illustrates, when resilience decreases, the probability that stress will result in a disorder increases. Conversely, when resilience increases, the risk for disorder goes down but does not disappear entirely. Thus, with enough stress, even the most resilient of people will be at significant risk for developing symptomatology, although this sympto-matology will probably be milder than that of the vulnerable person who experiences low to moderate stress, and almost certainly milder than the vulnerable person under significant stress. Zubin and Spring (1977)

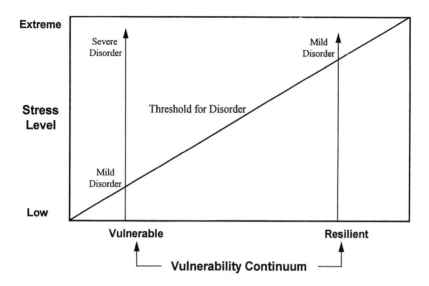

FIGURE 4.2. The relationship between stress and vulnerability in the onset of depression.

suggest that under significant stress even resilient individuals may experience "mini-episodes" of psychotic psychopathology, which are briefer and less intense than those experienced by vulnerable persons. Formal classification systems also recognize that otherwise resilient people can experience symptomatology with enough stress. Under the diagnosis of brief psychotic disorder, for instance, DSM-IV describes a disorder that can be brought about by traumatic events and remits once the stress abates with the person returning to premorbid functioning. Resilience thus suggests the opposite of vulnerability and implies a resistance to disorder, but not an immunity.

SUMMARY AND CONCLUSIONS: TOWARD A GENERAL CONCEPTUALIZATION OF VULNERABILITY

In this chapter we have examined the historical origins of the vulnerability construct within psychology. The notion of vulnerability is relatively recent in the psychological literature and first originated with Meehl's (1962) discussion of the influences of both biological and psychological factors on the development of schizophrenia. Although other investigators also subsequently discussed the idea of vulnerability to schizophrenia, Zubin and Spring's (1977) paper represented another important milestone in the conceptualization of the vulnerability construct as it pertained to schizophrenia. Both the construct's conceptual and empirical origins can be traced to studies of individuals at risk for schizophrenia. The landmark studies in this area were reported by several investigators who were able to locate the offspring of schizophrenic parents using psychiatric registers available in Denmark. These paved the way methodologically for the study of vulnerability to a variety of disorders.

We also examined what appear to be the core features that seem to characterize most if not all, assumptions about vulnerability, and then assessed some of the general issues that must be addressed in the study of psychological vulnerability. Given our comments at the beginning of this chapter about the definitional poverty of this construct, and the material we subsequently discussed, what can we regard as a sensible working definition of vulnerability?

As we noted previously, the extant literature on vulnerability suggest several features that define this concept. Within the psychological domain of inquiry, vulnerability is seen as a persistent and stable trait. As we also noted, however, stability does not imply permanence. Theoretically at least, under the appropriate circumstances, psychological vulnerability levels may be altered. The trait nature of this construct conceptually requires that vulnerability be viewed as residing internally, or within the person. However, risk factors, of which vulnerability is but one instance, can be seen as encompassing external factors.

Our review of the vulnerability literature also suggests that vulnerability is viewed as causally related to, but distinct from, the symptoms of the disorder. In most psychological models of disorder, symptoms are brought about by the interaction between the occurrence of events that are perceived as stressful and the presence of a vulnerability factor, and in this sense vulnerability serves as the final common pathway by which risk factors such as high stress lead to a disorder. Thus, the utility of vulnerability as an explanatory concept must be rooted within a broader diathesis–stress context.

The diathesis–stress context illustrates that vulnerability is latent, which we suggest implies that evidence of vulnerability is observable only under certain conditions. Some writers have suggested that the idea of latent variables all but negates the empirical study of vulnerability (Coyne, 1992). In reality, however, this simply requires investigators to specify the conditions under which vulnerability can be detected (Hollon, 1992; Segal & Ingram, 1994). We will examine some of these conditions in this book when we discuss methodological approaches to the study of both distal and proximal vulnerability variables.

In sum, then, vulnerability can be defined as an internal and stable feature of the person that predisposes him or her to the development of psychopathology under specified conditions such as the occurrence of stressful life events. Individuals who are resistant to the deleterious effects of such events can be considered to possess stable features that render them resilient in the face of these events, although resilience does not imply immunity. In its broadest sense, this is a definition of the vulnerability construct as it appears to apply to psychopathology in general. Each type of psychopathology carries with it its own conceptual and methodological issues, and depression is certainly no exception. Having proposed a broad definition of psychological vulnerability as well as having discussed a number of general issues in the study of vulnerability, we will turn in subsequent chapters to a discussion of vulnerability issues as they specifically apply to cognition and depression.

CHAPTER 5

Conceptual Issues in the Study of Cognitive Vulnerability

Having examined a variety of conceptual and definitional issues that bear on the general notion of vulnerability to psychological dysfunction, we turn in this chapter to a discussion of fundamental assumptions that pertain specifically to cognitive vulnerability and depression. These assumptions allow for the establishment of a guiding conceptual framework for understanding depression from a cognitive vulnerability standpoint. To establish this framework, we examine conceptual issues as they apply to the principal construct examined in this book, that is, depression. We begin by discussing how current definitions and classifications of depression influence both the conceptualization and the study of this disorder. Next we examine some basic assumptions underlying definitions of depression and then address the type of depression that serves as the focus of this book. Once we have examined the conceptual foundation of this depression construct, we discuss assumptions concerning the causal process, particularly these assumptions as they apply to the distinction between the onset and maintenance of depression. Implications of our assumptions for comorbidity, categorical versus dimensional approaches to depression, and generalizability are also discussed, followed by an examination of issues concerning necessary, sufficient, and contributory causes. Relapse and recurrence are explored next, and, finally, the issue of causal specificity and the distinction between distal and proximal vulnerability are introduced.

THE SOCIAL CONSTRUCTION OF PSYCHOPATHOLOGY: THE NATURE OF THE DEPRESSION CONSTRUCT

Taxonomy is an essential element of any scientific endeavor. In Chapter 1 we briefly discussed the idea of a taxonomy as applied to cognitive analysis. In this section we expand somewhat on the construct of taxonomy in general. We then apply taxonomic considerations to two fundamental concerns of this chapter. First, we briefly examine the taxonomy of psychological disorders, and, second, we specifically examine the nature, definition, and classification of depression.

As we noted, taxonomy is an essential aspect of science, and indeed no scientific discipline could proceed without either explicit or implicit taxonomic classification. Ways of viewing phenomena that allow for the differentiation, classification, and categorization of objects underlie any ability to understand the relationships that characterize the functioning of systems and organisms. Natural science offers the most obvious and well-developed examples of taxonomy; for instance, animals can be classified according to their class, order, family, genus, and species. When winnowed to the category of species, substantial further classification is typically still necessary, although not in the case of human beings (e.g., there are approximately 500,000 different species of beetles that have been differentiated and classified, about 10,000 different species of birds, but only one surviving species of hominids). Even beyond the category of species further classification is possible, as a given species, now differentiated from other species, can be differentiated into subspecies and races.

Although differentiation of Homo sapiens is precluded by the fact that there is only one species in existence, intraspecies behaviors, including psychological variables, are amenable to taxonomic classification. Indeed, taxonomic systems are inherent in virtually all efforts to understand psychological functioning, although these are quite crude in comparison to natural science systems. For instance, diagnostic efforts as represented by systems such as DSM-IV reflect the taxonomic attempt to differentiate and then classify dysfunctional behavior. It should be noted, however, that taxonomic systems are not fixed but instead evolve as concepts and paradigms shift and, correspondingly, become more complex with a deeper appreciation of natural phenomena. Indeed, psychiatric taxonomy illustrates just such an evolutionary process; since its introduction in 1952, the DSM has undergone four extensive revisions. There is little doubt that the it will continue to be revised in the future.

What Is Dysfunction?

Before we can classify different types of dysfunctions or psychological disorders it is necessary to have some working framework for operationally defining dysfunction. Various frameworks have been offered and fiercely debated for quite some time (L. A. Clark & Watson, 1994; Gorenstein, 1992; Kendell, 1975; Lilienfeld & Marino, 1995; Szasz, 1960; Wakefield, 1992a, 1992b; Widiger & Trull, 1985). One intriguing framework is offered by Wakefield (1992a, 1992b), who argues that a psychological disorder can be defined as "harmful dysfunction." This idea incorporates two components. The first—the idea of harmful— reflects a social value component. "Harm" is defined as the result of a condition that creates distress or problems for the person as determined by the values and norms embodied by the person's cultural community. Hence, a culture that considers suicide an appropriate action in some situations (e.g., as a protest) would be less likely to view the precipitants of suicide as being harmful in this context. By contrast, Western culture by-and-large considers a person at suicide risk to be suffering from a harmful condition. As this chapter was written, the national media was reporting news of a mass suicide (the "Heaven's Gate" cult) in northern San Diego. The extensive news coverage that is occurring leaves little doubt that this event is considered evidence of extreme dysfunction according to the values of the predominant culture.

The second aspect of the notion of harmful dysfunction relies on a biological criterion that suggests that a condition reflects a psychological disorder if it is caused by the failure of some evolutionarily fashioned mechanism to perform its function, that is, a mechanism formed by the selection pressures that drive evolutionary changes in our species. Dysfunction is therefore conceptualized as the inability of some internal mechanism to do what it evolved to do. According to this view, a mental disorder results when this inability leads to adverse consequences for the person. For example, activation of the evolutionarily efficient "fight-or-flight" mechanism can lead to chronic anxiety when fight or flight is not possible and when the reaction is pronounced.

The idea that dysfunction is defined by the failure of some evolutionarily fashioned functional mechanism (e.g., Wakefield, 1992a, 1992b) is interesting in many respects, but to date there is no consensus on what constitutes the nature of such a mechanism if it exists, nor how or whether the ability of the mechanism to perform its innate function is compromised in depression. For instance, to the extent that such function is biological, genetic, or physiological in nature, there are few, if any, clearly established biological, genetic, or physiological markers that have been identified for what we generally define as a mental disorder.[1] Moreover, with regard to the idea of the breakdown in naturally selected mechanisms, Lilienfeld and Marino (1995) have convincingly argued that few mental functions are evolutionary adaptations, but are instead merely by-products of adaptations, and that some disorders may in fact reflect adaptive rather than maladaptive reactions to stressful or threatening events.

We do not plan in this book to attempt to resolve the debate on what constitutes a mental disorder or what differentiates disorder from nondisorder, but rather to focus on a working definition to guide our efforts to understand vulnerability to depression. In this vein we agree with Lilienfeld and Marino (1995) and Wakefield (1992a, 1992b) that socially determined values must be an integral part of any designation of psychological disorder within a given community. We are also in agreement with virtually all mental disorder theorists that psychological distress is necessary for virtually any operational definition of a psychological disorder. We also find appeal in the notion of harmful dysfunction but we define dysfunction differently and in a much more expansive context; specifically, the idea of dysfunction inherent in our operational definition of psychological dysfunction does not assume the dysfunction of some internal state, but rather reflects a state of dysfunction in the person's life (e.g., impaired social functioning). "Social" is defined quite broadly and includes interpersonal as well as occupational functioning. Examples include the person who is having trouble functioning at work, the student whose optimal functioning at school is disrupted, or the person whose interpersonal relationships or marital functioning may be affected. Thus, dysfunction is a social or behavioral factor rather than an "internal," mechanistic one.

Depression

In theory, dysfunctional behavior can be differentiated from behavior within normal limits. Once dysfunctional behavior is differentiated, all psychiatric taxonomic systems further partition psychological dysfunction into different classes of dysfunctional behavior. DSM-IV lists a

---

[1]This is not to say that there are no established biological mechanisms for any mental disorder. For example, general paresis is recognized as a mechanism of mental disorder that results from syphilis. Such established biological mechanisms, however, are a rarity for psychopathological conditions.

number of specific disorders such as a variety of anxiety disorders, psychotic disorders, substance use disorders, eating disorders, dissociative disorders, somatoform disorders, and of course, depressive or mood disorders.

Psychopathological constructs such as disorders of depression can be thought of in a variety of different ways. Kazdin (1983), for example, notes different levels of reference for psychopathological conditions. Specifically, Kazdin (1983) differentiates between syndromes, disorders, and diseases; syndromes represent constellations of symptoms, disorders are syndromes that are not accounted for by other, more primary syndromes (e.g., a depressive syndrome that is not accounted for by an organic condition), and diseases are disorders where the underlying etiology is relatively well known.

With specific respect to depression, Nurcombe (1992) argues that the term "depression" has been used to indicate a mood state, a symptom or sign, a dynamic constellation of conscious or unconscious ideas, a syndrome consisting of a constellation of symptoms, a disorder that allows for the identification of a group of individuals, or a disease that is associated with biochemical or structural abnormalities. Similarly, Kendall, Hollon, Beck, Hammen, and Ingram (1987) note somewhat different levels of reference to which the depression label can refer; the term "depression"

> has several levels of reference: symptom, syndrome, nosological disorder (Beck, 1967; Lehmann, 1959). Depression itself can be a symptom—for example, being sad. As a syndrome, depression is a constellation of signs and symptoms that cluster together (e.g., sadness, negative self-concept, sleep and appetite disturbances). The syndrome of depression is itself a psychological dysfunction but can also be present, in secondary ways, in other diagnosed disorders. Finally, for depression to be a nosological category, careful diagnostic procedures are required during which other potential diagnostic categories are excluded. (p. 290)

Implied in this description is that the most appropriate way to understand depression, both from a clinical and a research point of view, is to view it as one category among different categories of psychological disorders.

The Categorical Approach to Depression: Implications for Conceptualization and Research

Whereas taxonomic systems typically divide variables into categories, descriptions of psychological disorders can be primarily either dimensional or categorical. Dimensional approaches are inherently quantitative in that they tend to describe disorders as a matter of differences in degree. For example, clinical depression is simply a more severe version of mild depression. Conversely, categorical approaches tend to be defined by qualitative distinctions. Hence, clinical and mild depression would represent fundamentally different psychological states according to this view. Perspectives that rely on qualitative distinctions assume that different disorders represent different conditions with relatively discrete boundaries between these conditions.

A categorical approach to the conceptualization of psychological disorders such as depression has a number of clear advantages. For example, because labels for various mental illnesses can be easily understood, a categorical perspective facilitates communication among mental health professionals and laypeople alike. Indeed, the ability to categorize underlies all language and communication. The categorical perspective also simplifies the conceptualization of psychopathology, at least relative to dimensional approaches, and as such, expedites clinical decision-making processes (Kendell, 1975; Trull, Widiger, & Guthrie, 1990). Indeed, it is much more convenient to speak about an individual as "having" a depressive disorder than it is to try to describe the individual's state according to quantitative variations in depressive symptoms.

The current North American diagnostic standard, DSM-IV, employs a categorical approach to the description of psychological disorder; disorders are depicted as discrete nosological entities that presumably occur independently of other nosological entities.[2] Depression is thus but one of many categories of disorders that is recognizable and consequently diagnosable. DSM-IV also makes clear that disorders such as depression are defined as mental disorders, or mental illnesses, rather than as behavioral or psychological problems.

Like its predecessors DSM-III and DSM-III-R, DSM-IV is careful to point out that mental disorders are not necessarily conceptualized as true categorical variables: "DSM-IV is a categorical classification that divides mental disorders into types based on criteria sets with defining features . . . there is no assumption that each category of mental disorder is a completely discrete entity with absolute boundaries dividing it from other mental disorders or from no mental disorder. There is also no assumption that all individuals described as having the same mental disorder are alike in all important ways" (p. xxii). Although this qualification in the preface of DSM-IV is both important and laudable,

---

[2]ICD-10 uses the same categorical system.

as we just noted the DSM nevertheless establishes a categorical framework for understanding psychological distress.

Such a categorical approach has worked comparatively well in physical medicine where there is little doubt that physical disease entities exist; are frequently (but not always) discrete from one another; and, relative to mental disorders, are easy to identify. Thus, for example, a virus is a microbe that enters the body and precipitates what we define as a disease. In a corresponding fashion, the clinical presence of symptoms can provide useful clues for ultimately identifying etiological processes such as a virus. For instance, virologists are able to identify and categorize new infectious diseases with impressive efficiency and accuracy (e.g., it took only several years to identify and describe the AIDS virus; Garrett, 1995). An infectious disease, of course, is a particular category of disease (that is further divided into subcategories based on the virus), which is in turn differentiated from other categories of disease (with attendant subcategories) such as cancer or coronary disease. Hence, the categorical approach that has worked so well in at least some branches of medicine is explicitly a disease- or illness-based approach and, in a similar vein, implies for many investigators that psychological disorders are manifestations of physical illnesses. Spitzer and Endicott (1978) represent this viewpoint succinctly: "A mental disorder is a medical disorder whose manifestations are primarily signs or symptoms of a psychological (behavioral) nature" (p. 18). Depression is thus viewed by many as a category of medical disorder or illness.

Adherence to DSM criteria and its corresponding categorical approach in the diagnosis of depression is considered a hallmark of model psychopathology research. Indeed, it is difficult to publish research on depression without showing that, on the basis of a structured clinical interview, subjects met DSM inclusion and exclusion criteria for the disorder. When studies are published using research participants selected without adherence to criteria prescribed by the current categorical approach to depression, it is common to see apologetic statements for the use of alternate operational definitions of the construct (Haaga & Solomon, 1993). In fact, in many cases without adherence to a categorical approach with corresponding diagnostic criteria, the use of the term "depression" itself is plainly discouraged. In reference to the use of the Beck Depression Inventory (BDI) for assessing depression, for instance, Kendall et al. (1987) argue that "the term depression should probably be reserved for individuals with BDI scores over 20 and preferably with concurrent diagnoses established by structured clinical interviews. Subjects selected solely on the basis of BDI scores should probably be referred to as 'dysphoric' " (p. 298).

As Haaga and Solomon (1993) have carefully documented, recommendations such as these have substantially affected the ways in to which individuals experiencing symptoms of depression are referred. The clear implication is that individuals with depressive symptoms who do not meet diagnostic criteria (either because an assessment was made and they did not meet criteria, or because no assessment was done) may not "really" be depressed; they may instead be people who are simply having a bad mood day. As such, they are considered by many to be unworthy of study. Coyne (1994), for example, suggests that studies with such samples are not only trivial, but that psychologists conducting such studies risk losing scientific credibility.

If frequent apologies or mention of limits to generalizability have become part and parcel of research on "subclinical" or "mild" depression, it is interesting to note that the use of carefully defined and diagnosed depressed subjects for research purposes creates an interesting generalization inconsistency. To select a sufficiently large group of diagnosably depressed subjects for research purposes, investigators must frequently screen a large number of potential research participants. Many of these individuals will not meet sufficient criteria to receive a diagnosis of depression (e.g., major depressive disorder) and many others will meet exclusionary criteria and will not qualify. Some of these exclusionary criteria are built into taxonomic systems (as noted, e.g., sufficient symptoms of schizophrenia rule out depression), whereas others are quite reasonably imposed by investigators (e.g., the coexisting presence of a significant level of anxiety or substance abuse). Such careful screening, however, severely limits generalizability in that generalization is only appropriate to individuals who share the characteristics of this very select subject sample. Results thus cannot automatically be assumed to generalize to the vast number of individuals who may experience significant psychological distress that includes a substantial degree of depressive symptomatology. This is true even for individuals who experience a clinical level of psychopathology (e.g., who have difficulty functioning adequately), but who do not quite meet depression criteria. Interestingly, statements concerning the limits of generalizability, so common in research on subclinical depression, are virtually nonexistent in studies of diagnosed depression.

Persons (1986) has also pointed out the limitations of relying solely on a syndrome approach to define and then study psychopathology. She notes in this regard that theories are often explicitly tied to psychological phenomena. If we limit our study to diagnostic categories, then these important psychological phenomena may be ignored. To take but one example, understanding the phenomenon of suicidality is important. Depressed, anxious, and physically ill people may be suicidal. However, if we study only suicide in depression, or study only depression as a diagnostic category, then important aspects of this phenomenon will be missed. Additionally, the diagnostic syndrome approach implicitly assumes that individuals with the same diagnosis are alike in all important psychological ways, an assumption that is clearly incorrect. Thus, not all individuals with a diagnosis of depression are suicidal. Alternatively, a focus on suicidality allows for the study of individuals who do share this symptom and are thus alike in important ways. Such an approach may thus be better able to understand the mechanisms that underlie disordered behavior and can thus facilitate theoretical development in ways that studying a diagnosable syndrome cannot. A similar symptom-based approach has been recommend by Costello (1993a).

Comorbidity. The issue of comorbidity is closely linked to matters of the categorical conceptualization of depression in diagnostic systems such as DSM-IV. Although comorbidity can be defined in somewhat different ways with different meanings (Lilienfeld, Waldman, & Israel, 1994), a commonly accepted definition of comorbidity is that it reflects the co-occurrence of more than one disorder in an individual at a given time (see Brady & Kendall, 1992; D. Klein & Riso, 1993; Maser & Cloninger, 1990; Maser, Weise, & Gwirtsman, 1995). The term itself is relatively new, having apparently first being used by Feinstein in 1970 to describe medical diseases that can affect other diseases (Lilienfeld et al., 1994). Despite its recent introduction, discussion of the concept of comorbidity and its implications for the conceptualization, assessment, and treatment of psychopathology are prominent in the psychopathology literature (Maser & Cloninger, 1990).

D. Klein and Riso (1993) note that comorbidity does not represent a particularly important issue for dimensional (as opposed to categorical) approaches to psychopathology. For example, unless certain states represent polar opposites, there is nothing inherent in dimensional approaches that suggests that different dimensions cannot coexist. Personality attributes represent a good example of this principle; even approaches that narrow personality into five basic factors (see Goldberg, 1993) agree not only that people have different degrees of each trait, but that these traits quite naturally coexist.

However, how does a categorical system treat disorders that commonly occur together, specifically, for our purposes, the fact that other psychological states such as anxiety statistically covary with depression? The categorical paradigm typically assumes that such covariance reflects the co-occurrence of discrete disorders (Lilienfeld et al., 1994). In a categorical taxonomic system, such comorbidity may result from a variety of factors. Among these factors are the following: (1) high prevalence rates for each disorder lead to the co-occurrence of two disorders by chance or sampling bias, (2) imprecise diagnostic criteria include overlapping symptoms for more than one disorder, (3) one disorder encompasses or leads to another disorder, (4) the coexistence of disorders actually represents another discrete disorder or represent different aspects of the same disorder, or (5) the disorders are a function of correlated causal processes (D. Klein & Riso, 1993). Each of these possibilities assumes the categorical existence of distinct kinds of psychopathology. Note, however, that apparent comorbidity can also result from assessment artifacts such as overlap in items on measures of "different" disorders (Frances, Widiger, & Fryer, 1990). Nevertheless, DSM-IV diagnostically treats comorbidity as the simultaneous occurrence of different categorical disorders; the person who meets diagnostic criteria for both depressive and anxious symptoms is diagnosed as having two disorders.

Diagnostic Organization and Criteria. The categorical approach to the conceptualization of mental disorders leads quite naturally to the specification of comparatively precise criteria for defining depression, for determining the presence and hence diagnosis of a depressive disorder and, in some cases, for excluding the diagnosis of a depressive disorder. This latter, exclusionary characteristic is due to an implicit assumption in many categorical models that disorders can be hierarchically organized in terms of severity. For instance, although a variety of specific categorical arrangements of psychopathology have been proposed (First, Spitzer, & Williams, 1990; Frances et al., 1990; D. Klein & Riso, 1993), the common thread among these is that increasingly severe levels of disorders represent the greatest disturbances in personal functioning and are represented higher in the hierarchy. Specific occurrence of less severe disorders that are theorized to be lower in the hierarchy are thus excluded from diagnostic status (Foulds, 1973; Foulds & Bedford, 1975). Recall that a definition of disorder offered by Kazdin (1983) is that it is a syndrome that is not accounted for by a "higher order" syndrome. Therefore, even if the patient meets the criteria for a depressive disorder, this diagnosis is not made if the criteria for another discrete but more severe (and thus higher) disorder such as schizophrenia or schizoaffective disorder are met. However, disorders that occur at roughly the same hierarchical level are considered to coexist and can be codiagnosed.

Categorical and Dimensional Approaches: Discontinuity and Continuity

Categorical model assumptions of psychological disorders have significant implications for the issue of generalizability. That is, although different types of a disorder may share features (e.g., major depressive disorder and dysthymia), a categorical approach suggests that these disorders are qualitatively different and hence that generalizability from one disorder is unwarranted. This assumption is long-standing (see Depue & Monroe, 1978a; Maher, 1970) and is referred to as the discontinuity hypothesis (see Compas, Ey, & Grant, 1993; Flett, Vredenburg, & Krames, 1997; Kazdin, 1984). The discontinuity hypothesis suggests that differences in symptomatology are not simply due to differences on a continuum from mild to severe; more severe depression is a fundamentally different state. The issue of continuity versus discontinuity has been vigorously argued by a number of well-respected scholars (Kendall & Flannery-Schroeder, 1995; Tennen, Hall, & Affleck, 1995a, 1995b; Weary, Edwards, & Jacobson, 1995).

Issues of continuity versus discontinuity also overlap with issues concerning the appropriate level of psychopathological study. For instance, we previously noted that some investigators have argued for the study of symptoms rather than diagnostic categories (Costello, 1993a; Persons, 1986), a concept to which we will return in the subsequent section on the construct of depression. When examining symptoms of a disorder, for example, several investigators have argued that at least some, and perhaps many, symptoms are continuous extensions of normal psychological phenomena, a point that can be applied to disorders as diverse as from depression (Persons, 1986) to schizophrenia (Bannister, 1968; Cromwell, 1975). The issue of continuity thus needs to be addressed at the symptom as well as the syndrome level of disorder.

Ultimately, empirical verification is necessary to determine whether the truth lies in a continuous or discontinuous view of depression, and correspondingly whether data generalize from one "kind" of depression (e.g., subclinical) to another kind. Such verification requires comparative research, although such comparative studies are difficult to conduct and are thus rarely, if ever, attempted. Reviews comparing the findings of studies using differently operational definitions of depressive states (e.g., "subclinically" depressed individuals versus "clinically" depressed people) are possible and have been reported. Vredenburg, Flett, and Krames (1993) and Flett et al. (1997) for example, have concluded that there is a good deal of similarity in the findings of studies using nosologically defined and syndrome-defined depression. Such data, however, have done little to convince advocates of the categorical approach; (e.g., Coyne, 1994; Grunhaus & Greden, 1994). Alternatively, depression may be characterized by continuities on some dimensions and by discontinuities on others (Flett et al., 1997). This possibility also necessitates empirical verification.

As indicated earlier, the alternative to the categorical approach is a dimensional approach, which assumes that differences in depressive symptomatology are a function of different degrees of psychological distress as opposed to distinctly different types of psychological distress. Generalizability conjectures are quite different for a dimensional approach and its corresponding continuity assumptions. Such continuity assumptions suggest that depressive symptomatology does, or at least can, occur on a continuum. Generalization from one end of the continuum to another is thus not necessarily compromised because the disorder is fundamentally the same, the differences being primarily with the severity of the symptoms. Contrary to the discontinuous view, these differences may result from mechanisms that are intact and functioning, but functioning at the extreme end of the continuum (Evans & Hollon, 1988; Hollon & Kriss, 1984). It is worth reemphasizing that no matter what the assumption—continuity or discontinuity, categorical or dimensional—empirical verification of assumptions is necessary. There is no a priori reason to assume that one approach is more adequate or captures reality better than another; that is, there is nothing in its inherent nature that suggests the categorical approach is superior.

Depression as a Construct

Much of the preceding discussion begs the question as to what constitutes depression. Certainly, phenomena resembling what we label as "depression" have been depicted since the beginning of recorded time (S. W. Jackson, 1986). The Greeks are widely acknowledged to be the first to describe depression, although Hippocrates probably did not have in mind "at least five of [nine possible depression] symptoms have[ing] been present during the same two week period and represent[ing] a change from previous functioning" (American Psychiatric Association, 1994, p. 327). This quote, of course, represents the official DSM-IV criteria for the diagnosis of major depressive disorder. We mention the DSM-IV in this context to illustrate that DSM criteria represent only one possible operational definition of the construct. A variety of potential operational definitions have been proposed, which underscores the fact that depression is a socially derived construct whose "nature" will vary depending on the particular operational definition in use. The fact that the DSM has undergone, and will no doubt continue to undergo, revision does not inspire a great deal of confidence in the ultimate validity of this operational definition (Garber & Hollon, 1991).

In addition to the changing nature of the psychopathological constructs it codifies, a variety of criticisms of the DSM have been made. As summarized by Beckham, Leber, and Youll (1995), for instance, the DSM requirement that a certain number (but not a certain constellation) of symptoms be present for a diagnosis suggests that different conditions may receive the same diagnostic label of depression. The rationale for the particular set of symptoms that comprise the DSM requirement for a diagnosis of depression is also unclear. Sad mood should obviously be considered a critical symptom to diagnose depression. However, some symptoms that are frequently associated with depression, such as hopelessness and social withdrawal, are not included in the diagnostic criteria. No clear rationale for the inclusion or exclusion of symptoms is provided by the DSM.

Although it is easy to be critical of a system such as DSM- IV (or any system for that matter), it is important to note that socially derived conceptions and corresponding criteria such as those used by DSM represent perhaps the only way we have to make sense out of what are phenomena it would otherwise be impossible to comprehend. Consider, for example, that the DSM-IV-defined constellation of symptoms that we call depression most likely has multiple etiologies, considerably different courses, and diverse responses to different kinds of treatment (see Akiskal & McKinney, 1975; Craighead, 1980; Depue & Monroe, 1978a; Kendell, 1968). Moreover, this category of disorder can have very different symptom clusters (Costello, 1993a). As we noted, for example, DSM-IV criteria allow for the same diagnosis of depression for two people who may only share one symptom in common (see Kendall & Brady, 1995). There can also be differences within the symptoms themselves (e.g., the symptom of sleep disturbance can be initial, middle, or terminal insomnia, whereas the symptom of appetite change can refer to losses or gains in appetites). Differences within the quality or experience of symptoms also occur. One person, for instance, may experience sadness in one way and another person in another way, just as one person may experience loss of pleasure in one way and another person in yet another way. Similarly, differences in the temporal relationship between symptoms may also occur; in a diagnosed case of depression some symptoms may arise or be prominent during some points within the disorder, whereas other symptoms may occur or be prominent at other points. Although some have interpreted this diversity of symptoms, etiologies, courses, and so forth to indicate that there are really a "group of depressions," we suggest instead that there are a group of numerous and widely diverse features we group under the construct of depression. Clearly, the complexity of a mental health phenomenon such as depression makes any systematic diagnostic system attractive, irrespective of its flaws.

Symptom-Based Approaches

Recognizing the heterogeneity in the symptoms that characterize depression, some investigators have argued for a symptom-based approach to understanding the disorder (Costello, 1993b) or aspects of the disorder

(Persons, 1986). Costello (1993a), for example, suggests that "the advantages of researching symptoms of depression rather than syndromes of depression are (a) current psychiatric diagnostic systems produce data of questionable reliability and validity; and (b) syndromes, as they are currently identified, are such intricate yet loosely defined concepts that the professional who finds significant environmental and biological correlates of the syndromes does not know what causal mechanisms are involved or even where to look for them" (p. 1). In theory, a symptom rather than syndrome analysis bypasses disagreement about the proper nature of the construct.

Although a symptom-based approach may very well have several advantages over a syndrome-based approach, from the perspective of defining a syndrome such as depression, this approach still begs a crucial question: the question of what constitutes a symptom. In exactly the same fashion as syndromes, symptoms themselves represent constructs we derive to help understand phenomena. Even though there may be a good deal of agreement about when certain behaviors represent symptoms, others are much more ambiguous and provide for considerably less reliable agreement. Indeed, the fact that psychiatric diagnosis tends to be unreliable is precisely because so little agreement about the symptoms to be included exists. There is little consensus regarding how to define and where the line is drawn between behaviors, emotions, and cognitions that are normal versus behaviors, emotions, and cognitions that are symptoms of a disorder (Lilienfeld et al., 1994). Because symptoms such as sadness, crying, fatigue, and so forth can be present in nondepressed individuals, deciding when to designate these as symptoms of depression can be extremely difficult.

Added to these problems is the fact that our attempts at assessment are, at best, imperfect. Self-report measures have been widely criticized on a number of grounds (see Kendall et al., 1987) in favor of structured diagnostic assessments. Such assessments, however, must still rely to a large extent on the individual's self-report, but also add the potential bias that is due to the judgment of the examiner. Even though significant strides have been made to reduce this bias and hence improve the reliability of such assessments, assessment methods are far from perfect.

Reliability and Validity Issues

Even once reliability is strengthened, the issue facing psychopathologists is one of construct validity (see Sattler, 1995, for a general discussion of construct validity and Meehl, 1986, for a discussion specifically relevant to psychopathology classification). Current constructs are based on some consensually defined operational criteria such as the DSM-IV criteria, but as we have noted, these represent one set of operational criteria that must deal with a variety of problems (e.g., diverse symptoms, different etiologies, etc.). Construct validity is notoriously difficult to demonstrate. In fact, some investigators have argued that efforts to increase the reliability of diagnostic systems has come at the expense of construct validity (e.g., Lilienfeld, et al., 1994).

The problems associated with conceptualizing, comprehending, and measuring (i.e., establishing construct validity for) a psychological construct such as depression are indeed thorny. Although certainly a great deal has been accomplished to clarify contemporary conceptions of what is called depression, much of the current conceptualization of depression is based on the assumption of medical model, disease-based entities that employ corresponding diagnostic assessment methods relying explicitly on operational criteria developed by a subset of medicine (i.e., psychiatry). Although beyond the scope of the present chapter to explore in depth, it is worth noting Gilbert's (1992) description of the sociological pressures behind the reasons that psychiatry in general and depression in particular have became so strongly identified with a disease approach to psychological distress. Similarly, the categorical approach employed by the official diagnostic manual of the American Psychiatric Association has had a tremendous impact on the conceptualization of psychological disorders. In both treatment as well as research decisions, enormous sociological and economic pressure exists to adhere to the categorical classification system as described by the DSM system. For example, the economic and professional reinforcement of this conceptualization and corresponding diagnostic/operational criteria required by insurance companies, grant study sections, and journal editors have done much to shape the "kind" of depression that can be respectably examined. Indeed, as we have previously noted, any operational definition of depression that does not explicitly rely on such theoretical assumptions is likely to be viewed as trivial (e.g., Coyne, 1994). At a practical level, however, this eliminates from empirical consideration a vast number of people with depressive symptoms and significant distress who are not diagnostically classified as "depressed."

Reification of the Depression Construct

Reliance on a categorical, medical model-based construct with associated diagnostic criteria has in many respects led to the reification of depression. That is, by developing "objective" formal diagnostic criteria for something labeled major depressive disorder, and by employing a nosological/categorical conceptualization, researchers have tended to remove the idea from the realm of a psychological construct and have given it a separate reality in its own right. We believe, however, that at present far too much ambiguity exists to remove the idea of a depressive disorder from the domain of a psychological construct. Depression is not alone in this regard. Certainly the categorical approach and its implicit (or sometimes explicit) disease assumptions tend to reify all clinical syndromes, as well as personality dimensions (see Kroger & Wood, 1993).

In arguing that the depression construct has been reified, we do not mean to suggest that "objective" criteria be discarded, or even that a categorical way of communicating about psychological states be eliminated. The depression construct is certainly important and helpful. Moreover, measuring the construct in as objective and reliable a manner as possible is crucial. Rather, we mean to suggest that caution is needed in how the construct is conceptually and empirically treated. We suggest that it would be wise for depression researchers to devote more consistent and thoughtful consideration and discussion to the meaning of the depression construct. Even some investigators who provide extensive discourse on the measurement and correlates of depression pay remarkably little attention to the meaning and hence construct validity of the depression concept (e.g., Coyne, 1994; Gotlib & Hammen, 1992; M. H. Klein, Kupfer, & Shea, 1993; Pyszczynski & Greenberg, 1992a; however, see Gilbert, 1992, for a notable exception). Given the existence of objective diagnostic criteria, it is certainly easy to do so. It appears, however, that adherence to such criteria has the unfortunate side effect of discouraging consideration of the meaning of the construct; these criteria reflect an operational definition that has become enmeshed with a conceptual understanding. Thus in many respects the use of such criteria, although important, nevertheless allows investigators to forgo confronting the difficult issues entangled within the meaning of the construct we are studying.

A Working Conceptualization of Depression

We view the construct of depression in a broad fashion. The assumptions that guide the operational definition of the depression construct we address in this volume are that depression (1) is a state of significant emotional distress and turmoil, (2) is psychologically mediated, (3) can reasonably be viewed as having dimensional qualities, (4) is unipolar and reactive to life events, and (5) represents a socially as well as psychologically dysfunctional state.

The symptoms evident in this disorder may or may not be sufficient at any given time to meet formal diagnostic criteria, although in many cases they will. That is, we expect a significant degree of overlap with DSM-IV criteria. We acknowledge, as do other investigators (e.g., Abramson & Alloy, 1990; Abramson, Alloy, & Metalsky, 1988; Abramson et al., 1989) that this may only describe a subset of depressive disorders, although we suspect that it is a rather large subset. No specific set or cluster of depressive symptoms is inherent in this definition, nor is a necessary duration specified for these symptoms to be present; an underlying assumption of this definition is that to be considered a depressive disorder the symptoms must be enduring enough to reflect meaningful social and psychological distress and must be related to impairment in the individual's interpersonal, social, or occupational functioning. A lack of a specified minimum duration of this symptomatology is not meant to imply that this is a transient mood state; we intend to focus on a state that is clinically sufficient to produce significant distress and disruption in the person's life, regardless of the time frame. Each of our assumptions will be briefly commented upon below.

No etiology is assumed for this working definition save for the central focus on psychological mechanisms. Thus, for instance, although DSM-IV specifically rules out bereavement under most circumstances, no such assumptions are made here. Indeed, bereavement is in a class of "social exits" (see Brown & Harris, 1978) that has been shown to be linked to an extensive degree of depressive symptomatology. Beckham et al. (1995) observe the interesting irony that results from the DSM-IV exclusion of bereavement from diagnostic consideration. They note that the woman who experiences significant depressive symptoms because her has husband left her will be considered to have a diagnosable depressive disorder, yet the same woman with the same symptoms resulting from the death of her husband will not considered to have a disorder, even though the underlying processes may be identical.

Psychological Mediation

Our working assumption is that depression is mediated primarily through psychological processes. Indeed, a cognitive approach to this mediational supposition is the focus of much of the remainder of this book. This operational definition is intended to differentiate this construct from depressive disorders that may be mediated primarily through biological processes.

The division between biological and psychological processes is, of course, arbitrary in that all behavioral function is biologically mediated. Hence we do not mean to suggest that biological, genetic, and physiological aspects are unimportant in understanding any kind of disordered or normal behavior. Our intent instead is to emphasize that the critical factors in our operational definition of the depression construct can be best understood from a psychological level of analysis rather than as a reflection of primarily biological dysfunction. The distinction between biological and psychological processes becomes more meaningful in this context if we assume that it is not the depressed individual's biochemical processes that are malfunctioning to precipitate the disorder. Such an assumption reaffirms the importance of psychological constructs in understanding depression in particular and psychopathology in general.

Consistent with our acknowledgment that we are most likely focusing on a subset of affective disorders, it is correspondingly likely that other constellations of depressive symptoms exist that primarily reflect biological dysregulation; a likely candidate is bipolar disorder (e.g., Depue, Kleiman, Davis, Hutchinson, & Krauss, 1985; Depue & Monroe, 1978b). Psychological mediation assumes that biochemical processes are operating as they are intended to operate, albeit perhaps at an extreme range. An analogy to automobile functioning may be illustrative in this regard. Although a driver may be issued a ticket for driving too slow on the freeway (quite likely any speed under 85 in California, but assume in this case 20 mph), the automobile is functioning as it was designed to function. In this situation, however, it is functioning at a lower end of its range, and is judged against the criterion of average freeway speed; driving so slowly would constitute evidence of a disorder. If, on the other hand, the car is going slowly because the fuel pump is malfunctioning, or the condenser has deteriorated, then the internal processes of the car are not functioning according to their design. Similarly, some states of depression may result from internal processes not functioning as they have evolved to function; as we have noted, some theorists have suggested that such internal dysfunction is a critical aspect of any form of psychopathology (Wakefield, 1992a, 1992b). Our contention, however, is that depression as a specific instance of psychopathology is in numerous (and perhaps the vast majority of) cases the result of functionally intact, but maladaptive processes. As Gilbert (1992) argues, depression does not represent the malfunctioning or disease of a biological system but rather a reflection of the potential of biological systems in conjunction with early learning patterns. Hence, whereas a child who is placed at risk for depression most likely has intact learning processes, subsequent depression originates from *what* has been learned. Therefore, while perceptual processes may function as they have evolved to function, at least some cognitive models assume that depression results from perceptual processes that are functionally sound but keyed to negative self-evaluative information (Evans & Hollon, 1988; Ingram & Hollon, 1986).

The Dimensional Qualities of Depression

Our assumptions of dimensionality in depression reflect the hypothesis that depression represents an extension of normal evolutionarily selected processes that, when triggered, precipitate sadness and its associated features, which then spiral into a deeper depression (see Gilbert, 1992). Hence, depression is seen as functioning at the extreme end of a possible range of variation. Some data do, in fact, show consistency between mild depressive states and more severe states (Vredenburg et al., 1993), although as we previously noted dimensionality must still be considered a hypothesis rather than an established fact. The dimensional view supposes that differing levels of severity of depression reflect quantitative rather than completely qualitative differences.

Unipolar and Reactive to Live Events

Much as species can be subclassified into subspecies in natural science, taxonomic frameworks for understanding psychopathology lead quite naturally to the subclassifications of psychopathological constructs. Depression has been the object of numerous subclassifactory distinctions. One distinction that has endured over time, and is widely accepted, is the distinction between unipolar and bipolar depression (Andreasen, 1982; Beckham et al., 1995; Depue & Monroe, 1978b). There is reasonably wide consensus that bipolar disorder reflects a more active role of biochemical mediation. Our theoretical proposals are thus intended to apply to unipolar depression.

Closely linked to many conceptualizations of unipolar depression is the importance of negative life events. Depression that is not triggered by these life events is unlikely to be psychologically mediated. Moreover, because our proposals, and those of most cognitive theorists, explicitly reflect diathesis–stress perspectives, the notion of life events is critical for understanding not only the onset of depression but also the etiological processes that predispose some individuals toward depression.

Social and Psychological Dysfunction

We suggest that any definition of a depression must include social dysfunction to qualify as a disorder. We view the concept of "social" quite broadly in this context and include interpersonal as well as occupational functioning. Examples include the person who is having trouble functioning at work (e.g., the writer who cannot concentrate on writing), the student whose optimal functioning at school is disrupted (e.g., who cannot study effectively), or the person whose interpersonal relationships (e.g., marital relationship) may be affected. Furthermore, this social disruption must be linked to the individual's dysfunctional psychological condition. Thus, although an individual who has poor social skills or who is significantly below average in intelligence may experience social dysfunction, these would not be considered to result from the individual's emotional distress and would not qualify as correlates of depression.

Although examples of social dysfunction can be offered, what constitutes significant social dysfunction is difficult to define precisely. At present few criteria or operational definitions exist for making such determinations, although significant impairment in social or occupational functioning is indigenous to virtually all psychopathology classification systems. As such, judgments as to the degree of social disruption must presently rely on subjective estimates. For example, although DSM-IV provides examples of social disruption, no criteria approaching the preciseness of the various diagnostic criteria are provided, nor are any operational definitions offered.

THE CAUSAL CYCLE: VULNERABILITY, ONSET, MAINTENANCE, AND RECOVERY

Having discussed our working assumptions of the very broad construct of depression, we turn now to a discussion of the fundamental conceptual elements that must be examined in any vulnerability approach to depression.

Conceptions of Causal Variables

The concepts of onset and maintenance are fundamental to any understanding of depression. In terms of causal significance, however, many researchers differentiate between onset and maintenance and tacitly identify the onset or appearance of depressive symptomatology as synonymous with the factors that cause depression. Correspondingly, because they are not viewed as causal, relatively little importance is ascribed to the factors that help maintain the state (see Barnett & Gotlib, 1988; Coyne & Gotlib, 1983). Such factors are frequently dismissed as epiphenomena or consequences of the depressive state with no corresponding causal relevance.

Causality, however, is not synonymous with onset and we thus believe this to be too narrow a conception of the construct of causality. By virtually all estimates, depression is a persistent disorder with symptoms lasting months (sometimes even with effective treatment) and, in some cases, years (e.g., dysthymia). As we noted in Chapter 2, there is a fairly long-standing degree of consensus among investigators that untreated depression lasts between 6 months to a year or, depending on the severity of the episode, for possibly up to 2 years (Dorzab et al., 1971; Goodwin & Jamison, 1990; Keller et al., 1982). Indeed, symptoms that endure over some period of time are most likely linked to the disruption and personal turmoil that accompany depression. In addition, because sad mood is ubiquitous in the human condition, factors that maintain and intensify this mood may indeed be a "cause" of depression. Thus, the factors involved in the perpetuation of depression can be considered to have very real casual significance; not for the onset of the disorder, but for the maintenance of the disorder. We can legitimately ask whether this aspect of causality is any less important than causal onset perspectives. Indeed, from a causality standpoint the entire distinction between onset and maintenance may be more artificial than it is genuinely helpful.

The concept of causality is not limited only to onset and maintenance; we can also emphasize the importance of other causal elements such as the factors that place individuals at risk as well as those factors that facilitate or inhibit decreases in depressive symptomatology (i.e., recovery). Additionally, those factors that are linked to residual depressive symptoms after recovery can also be seen in a causal light. To understand fully the causes of depression, each of these components must be assessed. The focus here is obviously on vulnerability, but as we will subsequently argue, we believe that this construct pervades all other aspects of depression from onset to maintenance to recovery to postrecovery. Hence, rather than limiting notions of causality to onset, a broader view suggests that it is important to examine different aspects of causality as they pertain to different points within the disorder.

Relapse and Recurrence

Extensive data show that improvement in depressive symptomatology is not permanent for many individuals (Hammen, 1991a). Investigators have suggested, for instance, that a sizable number of individuals with an episode of depression will again be depressed in the future, suggesting that many cases of depression can be considered to be chronic (Depue & Monroe, 1986; Keller, 1985). The reappearance of depressive symptoms can be conceptualized as either a relapse or a recurrence.

The distinction between relapse and recurrence is well known and accepted, although whether relapse and recurrence are truly independent of each other is still somewhat unclear (Hollon et al., 1990). Differentiating these two constructs can thus be fairly problematic. Conceptually, relapse constitutes the return of symptoms, suggesting that recovery from the depressive episode is not complete. Recurrence, on the other hand, is considered to be the reappearance of symptoms that reflect a new depressive episode (Frank et al., 1991; Hollon & Cobb, 1993; Hollon et al., 1990). Hollon and Cobb (1993) note that distinguishing these constructs has important implications for understanding therapeutic change processes. Relapse after treatment suggests that treatment mechanisms may be symptom suppressive rather than curative. Curative mechanisms, however, should eliminate the risk of relapse but would be unrelated to the probability of recurrence. Only mechanisms that are curative and prophylactic should reduce the risk of recurrences.

Questions concerning the causal processes underlying the return of symptoms or the recurrence of new symptoms are open, although from a conceptual standpoint they may be related to the differentiation between the causal variables of onset and maintenance. That is, relapse processes should be linked to factors that maintain the disorder, whereas recurrence should be linked to onset factors. As such, our discussion of vulnerability will be relevant not only to onset and maintenance of initial episodes of depression, but also to relapse and recurrence.

Necessary, Sufficient, and Contributory Causes

A critical factor in assessing causal models of depression is the distinction between necessary, sufficient, and contributory causal variables. As Abramson et al. (1988) point out, necessary causal factors are those that must occur for symptoms to develop, but are not sufficient in and of themselves for occurrence. That is, they must be present, but this does not ensure that the disorder will occur; other variables may also need to be present. Additionally, if certain variables are necessary, then symptoms cannot occur in the absence of these causal factors. Sufficient causes are those whose presence assures that symptoms will occur. The converse of this idea is that if symptoms have not occurred, then the causal factor also cannot be present. Contributory causal factors are those whose presence enhances the probability of symptomatology, but do not serve in and of themselves as necessary or sufficient variables.

Various combinations of necessary and sufficient causes are possible. For instance, causal processes can be both necessary and sufficient, necessary but not sufficient, or sufficient but not necessary. The notion of necessary and sufficient causes can also be closely intertwined with different conceptual models of etiology. Presumably, for instance, biological factors are necessary, but not necessarily sufficient for endogenous disorders that are assumed to be mediated biologically. Likewise, cognitive factors are necessary for psychologically mediated models that focus on cognitive variables. This notion, of course, will be explored in depth in much of the remainder of this book.

Concomitant and Consequential Variables

In addition to the concepts of necessary, sufficient, and contributory variables, investigators have also elaborated the ideas of concomitant and consequential variables (e.g., Barnett & Gotlib, 1988; Garber & Hollon, 1991). Concomitant factors are not antecedents of depression, but instead arise concurrently with the disorder. Likewise, although not being antecedent to the disorder, consequential variables are the result of the processes that give rise to depression, or perhaps of the depressive symptoms themselves. Concomitant variables may or may not be linked to the processes involved in the disorder, whereas consequential variables are clearly associated with depression but are viewed as a result of the disorder.

Concomitant and consequential processes are regarded by some investigators as having little causal relevance (Barnett & Gotlib, 1988); this represents a view of causality that is identical to onset, which as we have noted, is too narrow a view of the causality concept. To the extent that variables follow rather than precede the onset of depression, then such variables may be causally linked to the processes that "cause" the depression to be maintained. Teasdale (1988) has made a very similar point in arguing that

> vulnerability to severe and persistent depression is powerfully related to differences in patterns of thinking that are activated in the depressed state. It is assumed that the type of events that ultimately provoke depression of clinical severity in a minority of people would initially produce at least mild or transient depression in most people. . . . Differences in the [cognitive] patterns activated in more severe states will determine whether those states show remission or become chronic and persistent . . . thus, the crucial pattern that determines whether the initial depression will intensify and persist is the pattern of thinking that exists, once depressed. (p. 251)

The potential causal relevance for consequential variables is not limited to cognitive models of depression. Interpersonal models of depression (e.g., Coyne, 1976; Coyne, Burchill, & Styles, 1990), for instance, may fall into this category; once the person becomes depressed, social support seeking is intensified with, eventually, the paradoxical effect of pushing away social support. To the extent that a lack of social support is linked to depression, these processes can be seen as causal; not for the onset but for the maintenance of the disorder.

Specificity of Causal Variables

The issue of specificity of variables interacts with the notion of necessary and sufficient causal pathways. As we have noted, systems of psychiatric classification are typically hierarchically organized. At similar levels of organization within a hierarchy, comorbidity rates are high; that is, covariation is common between disorders. Such is the case between depression and anxiety; depressive and anxious syndromes tend to covary. If a given variable occurs in both depression and anxiety, does it forfeit any claim to causal status? If negative thinking is linked to both depression and anxiety, should the validity of cognitive models that specify negative thinking as an important variable be rejected? Can such a cognitive variable claim to be necessary, sufficient, or even contributory?

In a cogent discussion of the specificity issue, Garber and Hollon (1991) have argued that nonspecificity exclusively rules out the causal status of a particular model only if the model suggests a single (sufficient) causal variable. In contrast, models that specify multiple interacting causal variables are not disconfirmed by the observed nonspecificity of a variable included by the model. Thus, a feature of a causal model can in fact be nonspecific but still not fatal to the model. For example, few investigators would rule out negative life events as a causal factor in a disorder such as depression simply because negative life events also are linked to other disorders. Such disconfirmation would be the case only if a model proposed that negative life events are a sufficient cause of the depression. However, negative life events are incorporated into different causal models of different disorders because they are viewed as necessary and contributory, but not in and of themselves sufficient. Similarly, negative cognitions are commonly found in both depression and anxiety (D. A. Clark, 1986; Dobson, 1985; M. S. Greenberg & Beck, 1989; Ingram et al., 1987). If a single variable cognitive model proposed that negative thinking (also found in anxiety) was the sufficient cause of depression then this finding would invalidate the model because no anxiety could ever exist independently of depression or vice versa.

Other approaches to the issue of nonspecificity have been proposed. Ingram and Wisnicki (1991) and Ingram (1990) have argued that variables can have causal status for different disorders if these are causally linked to the variables that overlap in these disorders. Depression and anxiety, for example, share a variety of symptoms (e.g., difficulty concentrating, sleep disturbance, and fatigue are some of the DSM-specified symptoms that occur in both major depressive disorder and generalized anxiety disorder). If variables are found to be linked to both depression or anxiety, one logical possibility is that these co-occurring variables may be causally linked to the co-occurring symptoms in the two disorders (see Figure 5.1).

Both of these approaches indicate that nonspecificity is not fatal to a given model when certain requirements are met. Our conceptual assumption is that the cognitive models of depression and vulnerability we will address are not single variable models but instead ones that specify multiple and interacting causal variables; that is, variables that are necessary and contributory.

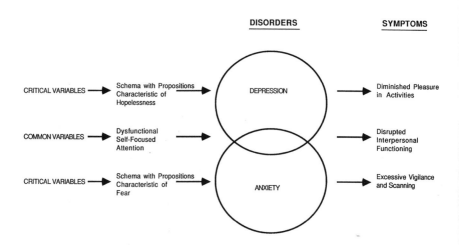

FIGURE 5.1. Representation of causes and symptoms that are unique to different forms of psychopathology as well as common across disordered states. In this example, critical variables that have been hypothesized to be unique to depression or anxiety, or characteristic of depression and anxiety, are viewed as resulting in symptoms that tend to be uniquely characteristic of depression or anxiety. In the case of common variables, these processes are hypothesized to result in the symptoms that occur across both depression and anxiety.

Distal and Proximal Causal Factors

Causal factors can be either distal or proximal in nature. Proximal factors are those that not only precede depression, but also occur temporally close to the disorder. For instance, if a given cognitive model suggests that dysfunctional cognitive interpretations of an event cause depression in response to this event, this would constitute a proximal factor. Distal factors, on the other hand, also occur before the event but are less temporally close in time to the appearance of depression.

Although the distinction between proximal and distal factors is explicitly recognized by some models, different models also view these variables somewhat differently. Figure 5.2 represents a depiction of distal and proximal factors in Beck's (1967, 1987) theory as proposed by Abramson et al. (1988). According to this view, the presence of a negative self-schema is the more distal variable whereas the cognitive distortions and negative cognitive triad that arise from this schema are more proximal causes. This is certainly an accurate representation of the distinction between distal and proximal constructs but these constructs can also be conceptualized on a much more extensive continuum that extends to the developmental antecedents of cognitive vulnerability. For instance, while retaining the negative self-schema construct as a distal feature relative to the negative cognitive triad, the relationship illustrated in Figure 5.3 assumes a much longer continuum between distal and proximal features. Hence, developmental antecedents would represent perhaps the most distal causal or vulnerability factors, that is, the factors that occur considerably before the appearance of a depressive disorder.

For understandable reasons, contemporary cognitive vulnerability research has tended to focus on proximal factors; longitudinal research that is necessary to map the developmental pathways to adult depression

Short-Term Distal - Proximal Continuum

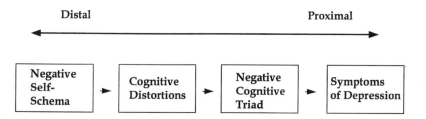

FIGURE 5.2. Example of a short-term distal–proximal continuum.

Long-Term Distal - Proximal Continuum

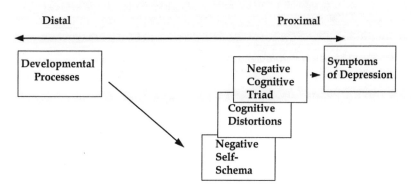

FIGURE 5.3. Example of a long-term distal–proximal continuum that incorporates developmentally determined vulnerability factors.

is not only expensive, but is by definition very time consuming. Nevertheless we will not be able to understand cognitive vulnerability processes fully until we begin to appreciate the need to make these proximal and distal vulnerability distinctions and, more specifically, begin to examine these distal factors.

Onset and Maintenance

The distinction between distal and proximal factors is not limited to the onset of the disorder, although it is this aspect of causality that receives the most attention. Distal and proximal factors can also be distinguished in the role they play in perpetuating depression. For instance, we can search for the variables that, once the disorder is initiated, causes its perpetuation. Several models have explicitly suggested that ruminative cognitive processes serve to maintain depression (Ingram, 1984; Nolen-Hoeksema, 1991; Pyszczynski & Greenberg, 1987; Teasdale, 1983, 1988). These would clearly fall at the proximal end of the continuum. On the other hand, the factors that predispose people to ruminate in response to negative mood states may very well fall more on the distal end. Suggesting that distal and proximal factors can be conceptually distinguished between onset and maintenance, however, is not meant to imply that these factors are unrelated. We suspect that there is probably much overlap between the distal and proximal factors that are linked to onset and those that are linked to maintenance.

SUMMARY AND CONCLUSIONS

In this chapter we have focused on a variety of conceptual issues that pertain to our understanding of vulnerability and the depression construct. We have suggested that the conceptualization of what differentiates normal functioning from dysfunction in general has followed from classification efforts in all scientific endeavors. The more specific application of the idea of classification has, for depression, evolved into the requirement to meet a standard set of criteria specified by DSM-IV. These criteria rely on a categorical approach to the conceptualization of depression that, among other things, suggests that comorbidity is the co-occurrence of two or more different disorders. Such a categorical approach also implicitly assumes a discontinuous rather than continuous view of psychopathology, although this problem has yet to be solved with empirical data.

Although explicit criteria for what constitutes depression have value, rigid adherence to these criteria portend the danger of reifying the depression construct. We propose a working definition of depression as a pattern of depressive symptoms that are dimensional in nature, psychologically mediated, unipolar, reactive to life events, and characterized by significant social and psychological distress. We also noted also that our conceptualization of causality is a broad one that encompasses not only the onset of depression, but its maintenance as well. Following other investigators, we discussed the importance of distinguishing between relapse and recurrence, and necessary, sufficient, and contributory causes. Finally, we noted the critical importance of distinguishing between distal and proximal causal factors. This distinction forms the basis for much of our discussion of cognitive vulnerability factors in depression. With this foundation in place, we now turn to a discussion of methodological issues that are important to consider in research on potential proximal cognitive vulnerability factors.

CHAPTER 6

Methodological Strategies and Issues in the Study of Proximal Vulnerability

$\mathbf{E}$mpirical verification of conceptual proposals regarding either proximal or distal vulnerability must rely on research methods that adequately capture the essential elements of the processes that are thought to underlie vulnerability. To examine the methodological foundations of data on vulnerability, and to provide a context for our subsequent review of proximal cognitive vulnerability data (Chapter 7), in this chapter we discuss several established research strategies for empirically examining issues pertaining to proximal vulnerability. As we noted in more detail in chapter 5, proximal vulnerability is defined as the factors that are linked to the immediate onset (or possibly recurrence or relapse) of depression.

There are numerous research designs that could be brought to bear on the study of various vulnerability-related phenomena. In this chapter we concentrate on several of the major designs that have been applied the study of vulnerability. In particular, the research strategies we examine consist of (1) cross-sectional designs, (2) longitudinal designs, (3) remission designs, and (4) priming designs. Although each of these are discussed as a separate strategy, it is important to note that, depending on the questions of particular research interest, a great deal of overlap among these designs can be found in various studies. In this chapter we devote most of our attention to priming designs, in view of their emerging prominence in vulnerability research.

Because our goal is to examine issues that are of specific relevance to vulnerability research, we will not focus on issues that pertain to general methodological considerations in the conduct of psychological research unless they are particularly relevant to vulnerability considerations. Basic methodological strategies and issues are certainly critical (e.g., confounding, experimenter bias, demand characteristics, etc.), but these are clearly beyond the scope of the present volume. Our assumption is that the principles of sound research design are essential to any area of psychological inquiry and thus serve as the foundation that supports the vulnerability designs we will discuss. Thus, we concentrate on several basic proximal vulnerability designs, discussing both their advantages and limitations. Readers who are interested in research design issues as they apply to clinical research in general or to depression research in particular are referred other sources (Haaga & Solomon, 1993; Ingram, 1989; Kazdin, 1984, 1992; Kendall et al., 1987; Kendall & Butcher, 1982; Sher & Trull, 1996; Smith & Rhodewalt, 1991).

CROSS-SECTIONAL DESIGNS

The current predominant research paradigm for studying cognitive processes in depression is the cross-sectional paradigm. Although there are variations, the general methodological strategy underlying cross-sectional studies follows the established research tradition of studying individual difference variables by dividing subjects according to these variables and then examining subsequent differences on some theoretically specified dimension of interest. In the case of depression research, this typically means selecting a group of depressed individuals and then comparing them on some variable to a control group of nondepressed subjects. In some studies, these comparisons are made as a function of the introduction of a theory-relevant event. In one of many examples of this strategy, for instance, Ingram, Smith, and Brehm (1983) examined differences in information processing between subclinically depressed and nondepressed individuals after they were exposed to either task success or task failure. In other studies, which are more purely concerned with descriptive psychopathology, evaluations are made of existing differences between depressed and nondepressed individuals. The fundamental assumption of this strategy is that, to the extent that these groups differ on a given variable, the variable may play an important role in vulnerability to the depressive disorder.

Somewhat more sophisticated cross-sectional designs attempt to determine the specificity of the various processes studied in depression. In the case of cognitive research, these designs typically assess cognitive specificity (for examples and discussion of this strategy, see D. A. Clark, 1986; D. A. Clark, Beck, & Brown, 1989; Derry & Kuiper, 1981; Ingram et al., 1987; Kendall & Ingram, 1987), that is, the degree to which a cognitive response is specific to depression as opposed to characteristic of psychopathology in general. In these designs, psychiatric or distressed control groups who are not depressed are also assessed, frequently in addition to normal control groups, to try to isolate whether the variable is specifically linked to depression.

The logic behind specificity designs suggests that the variable under consideration should be specific to depression to be meaningful. For instance, given that there are recognized differences between depression and other disorders (see, e.g., L. Clark & Watson, 1991; Watson & Kendall, 1989), an inability to find any cognitive specificity calls into question the ultimate contribution of cognitive conceptualizations of depression. That is, if genuine differences between the etiology and symptoms of depression and other dysfunctional states exist, but the cognitive dysfunctions associated with these states are the same or highly similar, then it is unclear whether dysfunctional cognition can be meaningfully linked to vulnerability to depression. Alternatively, finding specific cognitive factors differentially linked to particular psychopathological states provides support for vulnerability to depression, although, as Garber and Hollon (1991) appropriately argue, causal inferences cannot be made on the basis of specificity alone.

As we noted, even a lack of specificity does not completely rule out cognitive causal contributions. Although specificity is widely considered to be an important criterion for assigning causal status to a measure of cognition, Garber and Hollon (1991) note some exceptions. For instance, a nonspecific variable may play a vulnerability role if it is one of several interacting causal variables or, correspondingly, if it is not presumed to be a sufficient cause of the disorder. Thus, even though a variable in and of itself may not be causal, if it interacts with other variables to produce depression, or if the disorder cannot occur without the presence of the variable (that is, it is necessary but not sufficient), then a "nonspecific variable" may in fact be depressogenic. Ingram (1990) also notes that nonspecific variables can have causal status if they are linked to the processes that overlap among distinct disorders. Hence, even if disorders are reasonably distinct, to the extent that they share some overlapping features, nonspecific variables may play a causal role in these overlapping features. Even with these causal options, however, preservation of the causal integrity of cognitive models of depression vulnerability requires at least some demonstrable cognitive differences between depression and other dysfunctional states.

Although specificity research may represent a more sophisticated cross-sectional design, it is important to note that, even if the variable does not seem to occur in a distressed or psychiatric control group, this does not allow investigators to designate the variable as specific to depression. Such a specificity designation means that the variable occurs only in depression. The problem is the heterogeneous nature of most nondepressed distressed or psychiatric control groups. Because these groups are, in theory at least, composed of individuals with a diversity of psychological problems, investigators can only rule out that a variable is characteristic of psychopathology in general. On the other hand, because a variable may very well be linked to other disordered states that are in fact represented in the psychiatric control group, but compose too little of the group to show up in overall analyses (i.e., psychiatric control group vs. depressed group comparisons), this design is generally unable to detect specificity. Rather, it is most able to rule out that the variable is characteristic of generalized psychopathology. To truly determine that a variable is specific to a disorder, control groups composed of specific psychopathologies (e.g., comparing depression to anxiety) are needed (Garber & Hollon, 1991).

Advantages and Limitations

Cross-sectional designs have generated an enormous, almost overwhelming, amount of data on the cognitive factors that characterize depression and that are presumed to constitute cognitive risk factors (Haaga, Dyck, & Ernst, 1991; Ingram & Holle, 1992; Ingram & Reed, 1986). Hence, as a tool for descriptive psychopathology efforts, cross-sectional designs are invaluable. At the very least, such descriptive efforts can provide numerous and potentially important clues for researchers seeking to understand the causal features of depression.

Just as the database generated from cross-sectional studies is enormous, so too are the limitations of this approach, at least from the perspective of seeking to understand the factors that are linked to the onset of depression. These limitations stem from two basic considerations. The first concerns the type of theoretical model the investigator seeks to assess. By definition within the current context, these are models of cognitive vulnerability to depression. As we noted in Chapter 5, only a subset of individuals labeled as depressed may be so for cognitive reasons. Abramson and Alloy (Abramson et al., 1988; Alloy, Hartlage, & Abramson, 1988; Abramson & Alloy, 1990; Abramson et al., 1989) have persuasively argued that, if this is the case, then cross-sectionally comparing individuals who are selected only on the basis of being depressed is an inappropriate test of such a cognitive model. The problem is that individuals so selected may be depressed for a variety of reasons, some of which may have little to do with cognitive factors. If the proportion of individuals with noncognitive depression is relatively large, then there is likely to be too much error variance in such a sample to conduct any meaningful test of cognitive hypotheses. This concern applies equally to any design that employs depression as the basis for group comparisons. For example, we will discuss remission designs later in this chapter. To the extent that investigators endeavor to assess specific cognitive subtypes of depression, then individuals who are selected merely for having experienced a past depressive episode would not theoretically provide an appropriate test of cognitive vulnerability.

The second limitation of cross-sectional studies derives not so much from the designs themselves as from how the data have been interpreted relative to questions concerning the onset of depression. Confidence in such causal inferences is ostensibly undermined by two closely related considerations. First, cross-sectional designs are explicitly correlational in nature. Such correlational research does not allow for a differentiation between causal variables, consequential variables, or third variable causality (Garber & Hollon, 1991). Thus, although we have begun to develop a fairly clear picture of the cognitive processing patterns of individuals *in* a depressed state, we cannot with any degree of certainty extrapolate these cognitive patterns and apply them to the onset of depression. To infer onset we must demonstrate temporal antecedence; the cognitive feature must precede the onset of the disorder (Garber & Hollon, 1991). Correlational studies that compare currently depressed subjects to nondepressed individuals do not allow for the assessment of temporal antecedence. Such considerations have led some to question whether there is any causal significance whatsoever to cross-sectional studies (e.g., Barnett & Gotlib, 1988; Coyne, 1992, 1994; Gotlib & Lewinsohn, 1992).

The second consideration is that some studies (Dobson & Shaw, 1986, 1987; Fenell & Campbell, 1984; Hamilton & Abramson, 1983; Hammen et al., 1986; Hollon, Kendall, & Lumry, 1986; Persons & Rao, 1985; Segal & Dobson, 1992) have demonstrated that the cognitive features that occur in the depressed state are ostensibly not stable; when the depression remits, it is difficult to continue to detect indications of negative cognition (the logic of remission studies will be described in more detail in the next section). If cognitive factors do not appear to be stable, then how can they play role in the disorder?

Are Any Causal Inferences Possible from Cross-Sectional Designs?

Clearly, whether or not cognitive variables play some role in the onset of depression cannot be determined from these designs. Nevertheless, there is much value for understanding causation in the data generated from such findings. As we noted in Chapter 5, causality is not synonymous with onset, although it tends to be treated that way by some investigators. Given that cross-sectional designs assess individuals when they are in the midst of a depressive episode, one that is presumably being maintained by some factors, such studies may actually be ideal for understanding the factors that are causally linked to the *perpetuation* of depression (recall from our discussion in Chapters 2 and 5 that depression can last, by some estimates, up to 2 years). The cognitive features assessed in the depressed state by cross-sectional designs may therefore have a considerable degree of relevance for vulnerability if we keep in mind the broader perspective that views causality across a broad spectrum. Thus, it is methodologically, empirically, and theoretically inappropriate simply to dismiss any cross-sectional data as representing mere consequences of the depressed state (e.g., Barnett & Gotlib, 1988; Coyne, 1994; Coyne & Gotlib, 1983; Gotlib & Lewinsohn, 1992). Cross-sectional designs can be appropriate to assess vulnerability if the focus of these designs is on vulnerability to the perpetuation of the depressed state.

LONGITUDINAL DESIGNS

Longitudinal designs are well-known methodological designs that comprise a group of strategies that follow a cohort of individuals over time and, at various intervals, assess variables of interest to the investigator. The goal of this approach is to determine which variables predict the subsequent occurrence of other variables such as depressive symptoms. The length of the longitudinal design can vary considerably, ranging from hours to days to months to years (for an example of a longitudinal study spanning almost 20 years, see Zuroff, Koestner, & Powers, 1994). Likewise, assessment intervals can also vary considerably, with a minimum of an assessment at the beginning of the study and one again at the end of the study. Variables such as length and timing of assessment are determined by the theoretical context for the research and the corresponding empirical questions of interest. Pragmatic factors can also play a role in determining length and timing of assessments (e.g., resources available for the research).

Longitudinal designs are appropriate for questions of either proximal or distal vulnerability, and, indeed, a key determinant of study length is whether the proposed vulnerability factors represent distal or proximal factors, with the study of distal factors logically requiring a greater duration. However, because longitudinal designs are particularly appropriate for studying distal factors, we will save the majority of our discussion of these designs, including an examination of advantages and limitations, until Chapter 8 where we examine methodological strategies to assess distal vulnerability.

Although in many instances they are most appropriate for questions of distal vulnerability, longitudinal designs can also be relevant for proximal questions. As we have noted, the duration of the study period is likely to be shorter for questions of proximal vulnerability than for distal vulnerability. For instance, a longitudinal study of college students initiated by Abramson and Alloy (1990) assesses presumably vulnerable subjects over a 2-year period (this design is elaborated on in the section of this chapter on theory-guided operational definitions of vulnerability). Although some proximal factors can operate closer to the occurrence of depressive symptomatology (e.g., immediately proceeding depression onset), a 2-year design is a relatively long time frame and thus assesses factors that are proximal *relative* to the more distal factors possibly formed at childhood. Conversely, longitudinal studies of proximal factors can consist of significantly shorter periods of time. For example, Ingram, Johnson, Bernet, Dombeck, and Rowe (1992) assessed subjects identified as vulnerable over a 10-week period to determine whether these subjects were at increased risk for depressive symptomatology over this study period. Such a short time period reflects a very proximal assessment of vulnerability factors. Similarly, in several classroom settings, Metalsky, Abramson, Seligman, Semmel, and Peterson (1982) and Metalsky et al. (1987) assessed the effects of attributional style on depressive mood following examination feedback. The interval between the assessment of the vulnerability factors and the examination feedback took place over just a few weeks, thus constituting a brief but nevertheless longitudinal assessment.

REMISSION DESIGNS

Remission studies represent another type of research design that can provide important information on cognitive vulnerability. Rather than studying individuals currently in a depressed state, these designs examine individuals who were once, but are no longer, depressed (i.e., in remission).[1] The remission requirement for inclusion in some studies can consist of failing to meet DSM criteria for depression, or in other studies can consist of obtaining a score on a measure of depression, such as the BDI, that indicates a lack of depressive symptomatology. Alternatively, and most thoroughly, studies can also combine these criteria. Once remission is operationally defined, remitted individuals can be identified either through longitudinal analyses where subjects are followed from the depressed state to the nondepressed state (e.g., Gotlib & Cane, 1987; Ingram, 1991a) or retrospectively, where individuals are identified who at some point in the past had a depressive disorder (Ingram, Bernet, & McLaughlin, 1994; Miranda & Persons, 1988; Teasdale & Dent, 1987).

Regardless of how remission is defined, the remission strategy requires that research participants currently be nondepressed. For obvious methodological and theoretical reasons it is inappropriate for subjects to be currently experiencing any other type of psychopathological condition. Correspondingly, although it is necessary that subjects have previously experienced depression, it is wise to exclude these subjects if they have also experienced other psychopathological states (e.g., a psychotic disorder). Ruling this out parallels the methodological practice of many cross-sectional studies that excludes the occurrence of many other DSM-defined disorders (e.g., bipolar disorder, substance abuse disorder, psychotic disorder, etc.).

Conceptually, remission strategies can be treated as separate research designs in their own right, or can constitute a component of other study designs. For example, remission studies frequently represent a subset of cross-sectional studies in that they cross-sectionally compare formerly depressed subjects to nondepressed control group subjects (e.g., Ingram et al., 1994; Miranda et al., 1990; Teasdale & Dent, 1987) and in some cases to currently depressed subjects (e.g., Wilkinson & Blackburn, 1981). As with cross-sectional studies as a whole, designs of this type can evaluate existing differences between formerly depressed and nondepressed individuals in a descriptive psychopathology fashion or can introduce some theory-specified event and then examine subsequent reactions.

The empirical intent of most remission studies is to examine the stability of cognitive variables with a focus on assessing potential causative factors. The assumption that guides this theoretical intent is

---

[1]The term "remission" generally derives from categorical models of depression. Given its wide usage in the literature, we will use this term, although our use of the term does not denote any assumptions about the nature of the depression construct (e.g., whether it is categorical or dimensional).

that causative factors should be stable and hence, if stable, empirically detectable (Barnett & Gotlib, 1988; Lewinsohn, Steinmetz, Larson, & Franklin, 1981).

Advantages and Limitations

Owing to their conceptual overlap, cross-sectional and remission studies share very similar advantages. That is, such studies are ideal for providing descriptive, "post"-psychopathology data. In this regard such data can also be helpful for understanding the longer-term functioning of depressed individuals in a way that purely cross-sectional studies cannot.

Unfortunately, remission designs in and of themselves may not be able to achieve their aims of assessing stability of cognitive factors and, correspondingly, being informative about cognitive vulnerability factors. These data may provide information about the stability of some factors, but only if there is theoretical or empirical reason to believe that the factors assessed are not only stable but are also accessible after remission. In Chapter 1 we discussed the distinction between accessibility and availability: Availability indicates, in the current theoretical context, the presence or possession of certain cognitive factors. On the other hand, accessibility indicates that the factors are not only present, but are accessed and functioning as evolutionarily designed (e.g., to structure information processing). Thus, in the case of cognitive structures such as self-schemas it would be a mistake to conclude that such constructs represent monolithic, static structures that are always accessed; a variety of clinical and social-cognitive perspectives argue that individuals have a diversity of self-representations available but that are not all operative or accessed at the same time. It is therefore important for remission studies attempting to discover potential causative factors to search for factors that are available, stable, and accessible, but not necessarily accessed at all times.

The limitations of remission designs then reside, much as with purely cross-sectional designs, not in the design itself, but rather in how data generated from the design are interpreted. As we noted for the limitations of cross-sectional designs, most remission designs do not take into account the potential existence of cognitive subtypes of depression. From a purely methodological perspective, however, perhaps the most serious issue with how remission design results have been interpreted pertains to the acceptance of null hypotheses. For instance, as we previously noted, in a number of published reports researchers have been unable to detect evidence of dysfunctional cognitive factors once depression has remitted (Dobson & Shaw, 1986,

1987; Fenell & Campbell, 1984; Hamilton & Abramson, 1983; Hammen et al., 1986; Hollon et al., 1986; Persons & Rao, 1985; Segal & Dobson, 1992). This lack of results has been interpreted by some as indicating that cognitive factors are not causal but are instead consequences or concomitants of the depression (e.g., Barnett & Gotlib, 1988b). As with any design, null results can be obtained for a variety of reasons, making it difficult to disentangle whether the hypothesis is not true or whether other factors are obscuring the ability of the design to detect supportive evidence.

In the case of many pure remission studies, the failure to distinguish theoretically and empirically between accessibility and availability strongly suggests that null results may be obtained because these studies have not adequately modeled the genuine complexity of cognitive diathesis–stress models (Hollon, 1992). Thus, as we have noted, rather than viewing depressive schemas as structures that are static and continually operative, even the earliest cognitive depression models (Beck, 1963, 1967) posited that individuals vulnerable to depression possess maladaptive schemas that are dormant until activated in response to stressful life events (Beck, 1987; Ingram, 1984; Teasdale, 1983, 1988). Segal and Shaw (1986) articulate this view by emphasizing that cognitive diathesis–stress approaches view stressful events as activating a "latent but reactive" schema that provides access to an elaborate system of negative content. Once activated, a pattern of negative self-referent information processing that leads to depression is initiated. This is the essence of a diathesis–stress approach to depression and corresponding cognitive vulnerability.

Given such a diathesis–stress conceptualization, to have causal significance it is neither empirically nor theoretically necessary to require that the negative self-representations salient during a depressive episode persist and be equally salient after the episode has remitted. Taken to its next logical step, to contend that (without reference to activating life events) cognitive factors should be always operative, and thus persist after the depressive episode, leads to the conclusion that no remission is possible; if to have causal significance the factors must always be detectable and hence operational, then people should always be depressed. Clearly this is not the case. Overall, then, to assess hypotheses about potential cognitive vulnerability factors by simply assessing individuals after their depression is remitted may not be particularly useful or informative. Rather, dysfunctional cognitions as possible causal agents need to be assessed in the context of the activating features of affectively linked life events. Priming designs, which more closely approximate the complexity of diathesis–stress interactions, are discussed next.

PRIMING DESIGNS

In many, but not all, cases, priming designs can be viewed as a subset of remission designs. Although there are potential variations that we will discuss, many cognitive priming studies expose remitted depressed individuals to an experimental stimulus and then examine subsequent reactions on cognitive variables. A critical assumption underlying this strategy is that remitted individuals, by virtue of their previous depression, possess characteristics that place them at risk for depression. Because the conceptual foundations and empirical goals of priming studies frequently differ from those of straight remission studies, however, we will discuss priming as a separate design.

Conceptual Background, Issues, and Assumptions

Adequate tests of a theory require that the methodological procedures employed model the relationships among variables that are specified by the theory. As we noted in the previous section, remission studies have typically addressed research questions concerning cognitive depression models without considering the diathesis–stress/vulnerability perspective that is integral to these models. The diathesis–stress perspective of current cognitive theories of depression thus necessitates that triggering agents be incorporated into evaluations of the vulnerability components of these models. In order to understand cognitive vulnerability, the logic underlying priming studies is therefore to investigate the activation processes (represented by stress in cognitive models) of hypothesized negative self-referent cognitive structures (the diathesis) (see Chapter 7 and Segal & Ingram, 1994, for reviews). Only fairly recently have cognitive studies of depression, by virtue of relying on priming assumptions, begun to model methodologically the actual complexity of the theoretical proposals they seek to test (Hollon, 1992).

Priming strategies and assumptions are not unique to the assessment of cognitive models of depression. Many hypothesized psychopathology variables are assumed to be discernible only within the context of eliciting stimuli that challenge the homeostasis of the individual. Segal and Ingram (1994) emphasize that the empirical search for many biological markers of depression is methodologically predicated on the need to understand how biological systems respond when challenged. Indeed, Hollon (1992) argues that there is a remarkable similarity between the biological dysregulation models that currently dominate psychiatry research and the assumptions of contemporary cognitive priming studies. For instance, research investigating biological systems that are hypothesized to be linked to affective disorders has established that dysregulation in these systems is apparent only following psychological or pharmacological challenges and not under ordinary circumstances (e.g., Carrol et al., 1981; Depue & Iacono, 1989; Depue et al., 1981, 1985). Interestingly, cognitive diathesis–stress models that underscore the significance of latent but reactive processes predate these increasingly popular biological challenge paradigms by nearly two decades (Hollon, 1992).

Types of Activation

Segal and Ingram (1994) stress the distinction that has been made in experimental cognitive literature between priming through direct versus indirect activation. Direct activation occurs when a cognitive structure is activated by an event whose informational parameters resemble the parameters represented within the structure (see Bower, 1981, and Norman, 1986, for general discussion; and Ingram, 1984, and Teasdale, 1983, 1988, for discussions specific to depression). For instance, to the extent that an individual's loss of a spouse through divorce has cognitive similarities to the death of a parent, which may have given rise to a "loss-related" network or cognitive structure, this network or cognitive structure will become activated (Ingram, 1984).

Indirect activation, on the other hand, develops when an event resembles only one or some of the components of the cognitive network and, through activation spreading via associative linkages with other components, serves to reestablish the network. As an example of this type of priming, suppose that the divorced person in the first example is turned down for a date. There are a variety of reasons for this outcome and for many people the disappointment of being turned down will soon pass. Yet, for the person with a loss-related network, this may activate other elements within the network such as a belief in personal deficiencies and a perceived consequent repudiation of the self by others. Thus, rather than letting the disappointment pass in a timely fashion, this event, through initial activation of some elements, may serve to re-activate the entire network or at least substantial aspects of the network associated with loss and, eventually, depression.

The conceptual difference between direct and indirect activation is, in some sense, a directional distinction. That is, in direct activation a core element is thought to be activated with energy spreading outward to more peripheral elements whereas with indirect activation more peripheral elements, are activated and spread, at least in some cases, toward the core. In theory, experimental activation can be either direct or indirect, depending on the investigator's definition of core elements. If, for example, mood structures are assumed to be central to depression-related cognitive structures (Bower, 1981; Ingram, 1984), then direct activation should occur through procedures that attempt to access this mood as directly as possible (mood priming will be discussed in more detail in a later section in this chapter). Conversely, procedures that attempt to access the structures through activation of elements other than core components represent indirect activation. In a study by Gotlib and Cane (1987), for instance, activation was attempted by asking research participants to listen to and repeat 15 positive and 15 negative content words. To the extent that these investigators were interested in activating a depressive cognitive structure, this procedure depends on the spread of activation through these peripheral channels to enough core features to reinstitute the schema.

Methodological Issues

Types of Priming

Priming studies have most frequently used mood inductions to prime individuals. Although mood priming has been used most frequently, however, no conceptual or methodological reason exists to suggest that other classes of variables cannot be employed to serve the function of re-activating critical cognitive structures. Each type of priming makes certain assumptions that engender issues that need to be carefully assessed. In this section we examine some of these assumptions and issues.

Mood Priming. As we have noted, priming studies have typically employed mood as the prime. This may lead some researchers to question whether cognitive effects are simply mood dependent, and, hence, whether cognition is only a factor that is secondary to affect (see Zajonc, 1980). At a very basic level, mood-priming research can be interpreted as an acknowledgment that cognition is merely the noncausal consequence of affective fluctuations. However, we think such an interpretation is a clear mistake.

Issues concerning mood primacy can be addressed at a variety of conceptual levels. Most generally, and as clearly acknowledged in cognitive theories, affective and cognitive processes are reciprocal and closely intertwined. Cognition is conceptually treated by these approaches as "first among equals" (Haaga et al., 1991). Current conceptual approaches view cognition and affect as intricately embedded within associative webs so that each affects the other (Bower, 1981; Ingram, 1984; Izard, 1993). Therefore, mood priming can conceptually serve as an appropriate activator of depressogenic cognitive processes.

Several models of depressive psychopathology have hypothesized that mood structures are at the core of the activation of maladaptive cognitive structures. For example, several cognitive models place activating mood structures at the center of cognitive networks that are thought to lead to the cognitive deficits and other symptoms that are seen in depression (e.g., Ingram, 1984; Teasdale, 1983, 1988). Specification of these depression models have preceded all reports of mood priming studies in the cognitive-clinical literature. Mood-priming studies thus derive from, and represent logical tests of, existing models. Post hoc conceptual speculations are thus unnecessary to account theoretically for the results of mood-priming studies.

Alternative Types of Priming. A variety of theoretical approaches specify factors other than mood as potential activating agents. For example, a number of researchers have suggested a link between self-focused attention and disorders such as depression (see Ingram, 1990; Pyszczynski & Greenberg, 1987), and, in fact, data have suggested that increased levels of self-focused attention are a risk factor for negative affect (Ingram et al., 1988; Ingram et al., 1992). It would thus be theoretically reasonable to attempt to induce self-focus in vulnerable people and then determine whether depressotypic processing ensues. Indeed, such a strategy has been reported by Hedlund and Rude (1995; see Chapter 7 for a discussion of this research).

Other types of priming variables are also possible. For instance, depression models specifying certain interpersonal events (e.g., expressed emotion, Hooley, 1985; Hooley & Teasdale, 1989; dependency, Zuroff & Mongrain, 1987) as the critical stress components of a diathesis–stress approach would presumably be able to specify the kinds of interpersonal situations that should lead to the activation of depressotypic cognitive structures. Clearly, such situations can be modeled in laboratory settings. In all then, although studies have focused predominantly on mood procedures for priming, a variety of priming possibilities can be derived from various depression models.

Regardless of the type of activating event that is employed, we believe that it is important for investigators to specify their assumptions as to what mental processes priming agents are affecting. Hence, for instance, it is important to articulate the parameters of the experimental activating stimuli as they are proposed to impact vulnerability processes. In cognitive-priming work, for example, studies that use mood inductions typically assume that mood serves as a direct (in contrast to indirect) activating agent when mood structures are postulated to be at the center of depression-related cognitive vulnerability networks. Likewise, studies that employ indirect activating features need to specify the processes as theoretically precisely as possible, including how these processes are affected. Additionally, the parameters of the activating stimuli will vary in terms of their specificity. Some may be quite specific such as the examination of autonomous versus sociotropic life events (Hammen, Ellicott, Gitlin, & Jamison, 1989; C. J. Robins, 1990; C. J. Robins & Block, 1988; C. J. Robins & Luten, 1991), whereas others may be more general, as evidenced by Abramson and Alloy's work specifying a general type of attributional style that places some people at risk (Abramson et al., 1989; Alloy & Abramson, 1990). Other theoretical assumptions may be so general that no particular type of activating events need be specified. It is worth noting that biological challenge models do not necessarily rely on stresses that are specific to a particular theory, but instead tend to focus on "generic" stresses to study the activation of dysregulation, such as exposing subjects to stressful task performance (e.g., math problems; Depue & Kleiman, 1979). Regardless of the level of priming-stimulus specificity, the parameters of this stimulus should be specified and linked to some theoretical account as to why, and hopefully how, the stimulus activates the targeted structure or process.

Assessing the Adequacy of Priming Procedures

Many of the methodological issues that are pertinent to priming studies are extensions of existing psychological experimentation procedures. Some of these procedures have special relevance to priming studies and will be discussed in this context, although general rules of experimental methodology also obviously apply to this research area. In particular, a critical methodological issue for such studies concerns adequate assessment of the effects of priming procedures.

Regardless of the type of priming induction, data must demonstrate either changes in the variables specified to be a function of the prime (e.g., pre–post differences), or at least differences between randomly assigned primed versus nonprimed groups. This is the basic logic underlying manipulation checks; data must demonstrate that the intended (primed) states are actually created.

It is also important to emphasize that these states must be assessed independently of the activation processes that they are presumed to affect. Thus, for example, if a mood prime is used, mood rather than cognitive measures are needed to verify empirically that mood has been affected, either by comparison between pre- and postexperimental assessments, or by comparison to unprimed control groups. In theory, although linked to cognitive processes, measures of mood can be obtained independently. This is the case regardless of the type of induction that is used to activate the relevant cognitive structures. Studies seeking to manipulate self-focused attention, for example, would fall under this same requirement to demonstrate that this self-focused state was in fact induced, something that researchers have frequently failed to do in the past (Ingram, 1991b).

If control groups are used in a between-subjects design, both groups must also evidence the independently derived priming effects, otherwise data are inherently confounded. For example, if a mood-priming procedure is used, recovered and never depressed subjects should show similar levels of sad mood after exposure to the induction. If this is not the case, and only one group experiences sad mood (e.g., formerly depressed subjects), it is impossible to disentangle subsequent cognitive differences: Are such differences attributable to the presence of now detectable maladaptive cognitive structures in vulnerable individuals, or only to the fact that vulnerable but not vulnerable individuals feel bad (or are self-focused, or have experienced expressed emotion, etc.)? This can be a particularly difficult problem in research relying on formerly depressed clinical samples. In some cases such samples report greater levels of negative mood at baseline than do never depressed samples (Miranda et al., in press). Given a mood induction, difference in the level of negative mood at the time of testing may emerge if both groups change at a similar rate. In such cases, statistical procedures will be necessary to control for initial differences.

Ethical Issues

Although ethical issues must be addressed in all areas of research, priming designs carry with them some special ethical considerations. As is evident from our discussion thus far, for example, the diathesis–stress process can be modeled in the laboratory in a variety of ways, and indeed, a number of potentially powerful manipulations are available. Important ethical issues must be considered, however, when stressing, challenging, or inducing sadness in people who are at risk for depression and who, in most cases, have experienced clinically significant depression. Although such issues may not be particularly meaningful from a purely theoretical or methodological standpoint, given our current state of knowledge and technology, they will nevertheless constitute a strong limiting factor in any priming research.

Significant amounts of negative emotion can be generated in experimental situations, which should facilitate the identification of mood-linked cognitive activation if it exists. Clearly, however, this also poses an unacceptable risk to research participants. At present, the best investigators can strive for is an appropriate balance between methodological and ethical concerns. In mood-priming research, this means attempting to create mild and transient sad moods that are nevertheless strong enough to elicit activation of dysfunctional mental processes and then measuring the types of cognitive processing that ensue. Although the focus of this discussion is on mood-related variables, such cautions apply to any kind of laboratory induction intended to model the stress aspect of diathesis–stress proposals.

Advantages and Limitations

The obvious advantage of priming designs is that they are more closely able than other approaches to model the actual complexities of the diathesis–stress assumptions that are integral to contemporary depression models. Priming designs thus enable the study of hypothetically key variables when symptoms are not currently present, allowing a distinction to be made between cognitive processes that are symptomatic of depression and those that may precede, and thus pose a vulnerability to, depression. As we have noted, such interepisode vulnerability variables are theoretically extremely important from a diathesis–stress perspective, but have been notoriously tricky to measure. Moreover, because negative findings that are the result of independent variables that are too weak or insufficiently specified can be dismissed, vulnerability research efforts are strengthened when the hypothesized risk factors are carefully specified and activated prior to assessment. Such activation should thus allow for a more rigorous test of vulnerability hypotheses (Segal & Ingram, 1994). As such, they represent a powerful way to begin to test the proximal aspects of cognitive vulnerability.

Even though we argue that priming designs represent a significant step in an important direction, some clear limitations as to what can be concluded on the basis of priming designs must be noted. The major interpretational difficulty involves the scar hypothesis.

The Scar Hypothesis

The scar hypothesis was first proposed by Lewinsohn, Steinmetz, Larson, and Franklin (1981) and suggests that observed cognitive deficits in depression may represent an effect, or a scar, of the disorder, suggesting that the processes involved in a depressive episode may in some fashion alter people's cognitions. Empirical data thus far have failed to find evidence of depressive scars (e.g., Lewinsohn et al., 1981; Rohde, Lewinsohn, & Seely, 1990; Zeiss & Lewinsohn, 1988), but these data have been generated by straight remission studies, which for the most part, as we have noted, have not modeled the parameters of cognitive diathesis–stress models of depression. Hence, in the absence of a theory-specified evoking event, the failure to find evidence of significant depressive cognition, including cognitive scars, does little to undermine current cognitive assumptions. If scars exist, but are latent, they need to be activated to be detected.

Even though failure to find empirical evidence of scars in remission studies does not negate cognitive vulnerability models, the scar hypothesis itself does present a serious challenge for priming designs, at least with formerly depressed research participants. Coyne (1992), for instance, argues that "with recovered depressed patients, priming may reflect accessing memories of the profound life experience associated with having spent long periods being depressed, rather than the kind of depressogenic thought processes that have been hypothesized. Analogously, recalling serving in Vietnam may affect having responses to a cognitive questionnaire or task, but researchers cannot ipso facto assume that they have isolated the cognitive processes causing someone to serve in Vietnam" (p. 234). Clearly, the precise depressotypic cognitive mechanisms that priming procedures elicit in vulnerable individuals are still unclear. We think it unlikely, however, that activation functions in the fashion Coyne suggests and, moreover, that simply accessing memories accounts for results on the kinds of cognitive measures employed so far (e.g., it is unclear how accessed memories can cause the endorsement of dysfunctional beliefs). Nevertheless, this possibility cannot be ruled out. More generally, we note that, although priming studies have in fact found evidence of depressotypic processing in previously depressed individuals, it cannot be ruled out that this processing merely represents scars that are now detectable, but that have arisen as consequences of having experienced depression rather than serving as vulnerability processes for past and, presumably, future depression.

GENERAL METHODOLOGICAL AND THEORETICAL ISSUES

Although we have discussed a number of methodological issues that pertain to specific proximal vulnerability designs, some methodological concerns are general enough so that they are relevant to all research designs, proximal or distal, remission or priming, and so forth. We turn now to these issues.

Causal Processes

As we noted, the scar hypothesis represents a challenge to the interpretational ability of priming designs as they are currently conceptualized and executed. Closely related to the scar question is the question of cognitive causality. Cognitive models not only posit that vulnerable people possess variables such as latent schemas, but that these schemas are critical causal elements of the disorder. Presently, data have shown that people who are believed to be vulnerable display, in the context of appropriate triggering stimuli, the cognitive characteristics that are predicted by cognitive depression models (see Chapter 7). These data, however, do not demonstrate the next step postulated by these models, that is, that these cognitive characteristics are causally related to the disorder. To do so, data must demonstrate that such characteristics accurately predict the occurrence of subsequent depressive symptomatology. Such results will play a significant role in confirming the actual significance of latent cognitive structures.

Although showing that cognitive variables predict the occurrence of depression is an important step, even this does not establish a cause-and-effect relationship; covariation does not demonstrate cause and effect. Even if it can be shown that cognitive responses do predict subsequent depression, it is frequently difficult to determine if the cognitive variables that are assessed are the actual causal variables. It may be, for example, that correlated with cognitive responses are other primed variables that in reality serve as the causative factors for depression. Thus, even though demonstrating that cognitive responses predict depression is an important step, issues of third variable causality cannot be ruled out. Hence, to have any genuine practical, as well as theoretical, significance, the kinds of cognitive structures that can apparently be activated by priming studies must be shown to be related to some aspect of vulnerability (e.g., to onset or maintenance).

This issue of detecting actual causality applies not only to priming designs, but to all proximal research designs. This issue, however, is not unique to cognitive depression studies, but pertains to virtually all research seeking to establish some factors as having causal significance. Biological challenge studies, for instance, face the same problems; they must show that the dysregulation that occurs in presumably vulnerable individuals as a result of some challenge not only predicts the eventual occurrence of the disorder, but is also genuinely related to the actual disorder.

Disentangling Scar from Vulnerability Factors

As we noted, demonstrating actual vulnerability is likely to be extremely difficult. Showing some causal predictiveness, however, is a useful and important first step in this process. Thus, it will be important to demonstrate that cognitive activation is actually predictive of either the onset or the maintenance of the disorder. Prospective studies that assess activation in vulnerable individuals and can then follow these individuals and establish that obtained markers do predict subsequent depression will go a long way toward demonstrating this predictive ability. Even in the case of individuals who are identified as vulnerable based on past depressive episodes, such demonstrations are appropriate. Conclusions will, of course, be limited to recurrence rather than initial onset, but such effects (if they can be demonstrated) will strengthen the hypothesis that activated depressotypic processing is not an inconsequential result of prior depression and of no real relevance. Moreover, given that recurrence is a serious problem, and perhaps even more serious than initial onset, such data will be extremely valuable.

Operational Definitions of Vulnerability

The study of proximal risk processes in vulnerable individuals obviously requires some type of operational definition of vulnerability. It is difficult to overestimate the importance of credible operational definitions inasmuch as the entire experimental enterprise rests upon the accurate definition, identification, and selection of individuals possessing the vulnerability factors specified by the particular theory under consideration. Several operational definitions are possible. The advantages and disadvantages of these definitions are listed in Table 6.1.

Remission Operational Definitions

As we have noted, many studies operationally define vulnerability by virtue of a previously experienced depressive episode. Several considerations underlie this operational definition. One is a matter of relatively straightforward logic. Individuals who have experienced depression in the past must, by definition, have encountered stimuli (either internal or external) that led to this state. This is not to say that all individuals who experience depression necessarily possess the diathesis features that are characteristic of diathesis–stress models. Most researchers recognize that with enough stress, virtually anyone can experience sufficient symptoms of depression to meet whatever symptom-based diagnostic criteria might be used operationally to define the disorder. As we argued in Chapter 4 (see Figure 4.2), level of vulnerability is likely to be a matter of varying degrees combining with varying degrees of stress to produce depressive symptoms. Undoubtedly, even people without much vulnerability can meet depressive symptom criteria with severe enough stress. Indeed, most sets of diagnostic criteria (e.g., DSM-IV), even for psychotic disorders, recognize this possibility. Nevertheless, it seems clear that at least a subset of formerly depressed people possess vulnerability factors, making them suitable possible participants for vulnerability research.

TABLE 6.1. Summary of Vulnerability Operationalizations Advantages and Disadvantages

Operation-alization	Description	Advantages	Disadvantages
Remission	Assesses individuals who were once, but are not now, depressed. Determined either through retrospective selection of formerly depressed individuals, or longitudinal follow-up	High likelihood that some vulnerability is present	Heterogeneous vulnerability factors: People can be depressed for many reasons
Theory-guided	Selects individuals on the basis of a theoretically defined variable (e.g., specified types of negative cognition; cognitively linked personality such as sociotropy–autonomy)	Provides data relevant to tests of theoretical proposals	Not independent of remission: Presence of a vulnerability variable suggests extremely high likelihood of past depressive states
Empirically guided	Relies on empirical observations of relationship between variables and depression (e.g., parental behaviors) Selects individuals based on these variables	Exploratory analyses are unconstrained by theoretical parameters May provide important information on vulnerability processes May lead to vulnerability theories	Same as for theory-guided operationalizations

The fact that only subsets of formerly depressed individuals are appropriate for psychological vulnerability research suggests that not all types of depression are mediated by the same processes and that these processes, even if similar at some level, are not necessarily related to the same factors. We noted in Chapter 2 that some depressions may be primarily biologically mediated, and hence these individuals need not necessarily possess cognitive vulnerability characteristics. More specific to a psychological level of analysis, as Abramson and Alloy (Abramson et al., 1988, 1989; Abramson & Alloy, 1990) have argued, only some types of depression are likely to have cognitive vulnerability features. Others types of depression may be mediated by other processes. Although the obvious comparison would be biologically mediated depressions, other psychological mediational pathways are possible.

A methodological and empirical issue that follows from these considerations is that vulnerability studies that rely solely on remission operationally to define depression are most likely selecting a heterogeneous group of individuals with regard to causal and vulnerability pathways. Although extant data suggest that there are probably enough individuals who had psychologically (and presumably cognitively) mediated depression in these samples to allow for the detection of group differences (see Chapter 7), heterogeneity can obscure potentially important vulnerability factors. As these sorts of considerations become clearer, investigators and the methodologies they employ must become more precise (Just, Alloy, & Abramson, 1998).

Theoretically Guided Operational Definitions: The Behavioral High-Risk Paradigm

Although remission strategies are commonly used to study proximal vulnerability, other operational definitions are possible, for example, a theory-based definition. Such theoretical definitions are embodied in high-risk behavioral paradigms in which individuals are assessed on the basis of theoretically defined high-risk behaviors. In the present context, these high-risk behaviors consist of cognitive variables that are thought to be linked to vulnerability.

An example of a theoretically defined risk variable is the negative cognition subtype of depression that is hypothesized to be mediated by a dysfunctional inferential style (Abramson et al., 1988, 1989). This hypothesized subtype leads to an operational definition of depression vulnerability that focuses on the identification of individuals who are not currently depressed, and who need not have a history of depression, but who tend to make personal, stable, and global attributions for negative events. Many other examples of theoretically defined risk factors are available. For instance, investigators have examined variables such as *attachment* (Hammen et al., 1995; Ingram, Bailey, & Siegle, 1997; Pearson, Cohn, Cowan, & Cowan, 1994; Roberts, Gotlib, & Kassel, 1996), *dependency and self-criticism* (Blatt et al., 1976; Rude & Burnham, 1993; Smith, O'Keefe, & Jenkins, 1988; Zuroff et al., 1994; Zuroff & Mongrain, 1987), *parental bonding patterns* (Parker, 1979, 1983), and *sociotropy–autonomy* (Hammen et al., 1989; C. J. Robins, 1990; C. J. Robins & Block, 1988; C. J. Robins & Luten, 1991) as theoretically defined vulnerability factors for depression under certain circumstances (e.g., the occurrence of negative life events or negative mood states).

In order to translate a theoretical definition into a testable hypothesis, some measure of the theoretical construct must be used to select research participants. The Temple–Wisconsin Cognitive Vulnerability to Depression Project initiated by Alloy and Abramson (1990) represents a prototypical example of the translation of a theory-driven operational definition of vulnerability to measure this construct. In this project, the Cognitive Style Questionnaire (a revision of the 1979 Attributional Style Questionnaire [ASQ] developed by Seligman, Abramson, Semmel, & von Baeyer) constitutes an operationalization of the negative cognition subtype. Moreover, a revised Dysfunctional Attitudes Scale (DAS; A. Weissman & Beck, 1978) was also employed as an operationalization of the negative schemas proposed by Beck (1967) to place people at risk for depression, and suggested by Abramson et al. (1988) as possibly composing an aspect of the negative cognition depression subtype. Together, these measures were used to select research participants (from a pool of over 5,000) who were not depressed but who tended to display a negative inferential style and a dysfunctional belief system. Similarly, if variables such as level of adult attachment, or the possession of a sociotropic personality style, are hypothesized to place individuals at risk, then some empirical measure of attachment or sociotropy is needed for the assessment of vulnerable individuals to be studied.

Empirically Guided Operational Definitions

Operational definitions do not have to be theory guided. Although the ultimate goal is to develop theoretical models of vulnerability processes, any empirical method that shows promise for detecting vulnerable individuals can be useful, whether or not it is linked to particular theoretical considerations. As we noted in Chapter 4, for example, Depue et al. (1989) used such a strategy to identify individuals at risk for clinical bipolar disorder. They did so by using a self-report measure, the General Behavior Inventory, that has shown promise for identifying vulnerable individuals. When individuals have been identified as at risk in this fashion, investigators can then seek to verify independently that risk is in fact present. In another example of this strategy, Rose, Abramson, Hodulik, Halberstadt, and Leff (1994) used, among other indicators, measures of developmental history to detect individuals vulnerable to depression characterized by negative cognition.

There are a variety of ways that such measures might be developed. One way is to choose factors that have been empirically identified as risk variables (e.g., parental depression, impoverished socioeconomic status, abusive childhood experiences, etc.) and then select subjects for study who fit the risk profile.

Vulnerability Control Groups

In many cases vulnerability control groups embody the acceptance of the null hypothesis. In the case of remission, for example, the assumption is that the nonvulnerable (or nondepressed) control group is composed of individuals who have not experienced depression. This is always a somewhat chancy assumption inasmuch as there are a number of potential reasons that people may be placed in this group. The ideal reason, of course, is that they have not in fact experienced the disorder. Another more problematic reason, however, is that they may have experienced depression, but that the assessment method may not have picked up this experience (perhaps due to the use of a poor measure or an adequate measure poorly administered). Similarly, they may be vulnerable to depression, but have not yet experienced a sufficiently stressful life event to trigger a clinically significant episode of depression. As is always the case with a null hypothesis, concluding that something did not exist can be quite difficult.

Such problems may be exacerbated by assumptions as to what constitutes depression. As we have noted, categorical models assume that if the individual meets a sufficient number of symptoms, then he or she is depressed. Conversely, the person with not quite enough symptoms to indicate depression can be considered to be nondepressed by this definition. Figure 6.1 presents a hypothetical individual who would be considered to meet criteria for vulnerability by virtue of past depression.

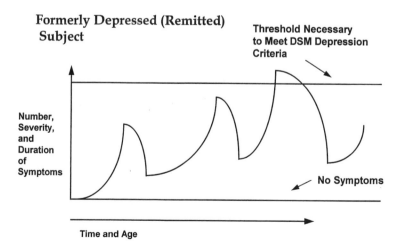

FIGURE 6.1. A hypothetical individual who would meet criteria for a previous depressive episode.

Figure 6.2 presents another hypothesized individual who would not meet these criteria. In theory, this second person could be classified as never depressed and thus placed in a nonvulnerable control group despite the fact that a number of negative affective states and depressive symptoms may have been experienced over a period of time. Such considerations mandate that the selection of control group individuals be based not on whether a person has or has not met criteria, but rather on having a relatively "clean" past psychiatric history. Dimensional approaches to the definition of depression are clearly helpful in this regard.

Independence of Alternative Operational Definitions and Remission

As a general rule, to study vulnerability, individuals must be selected who are presumed to be vulnerable to depression, but who are not currently depressed. Moreover, in cases where measures are sought that not only intend to exclude current depression, but do not intend to rely on remission status, these measures should obviously be independent of remission; that is, they should select people who have not previously experienced depression. However, it may be difficult to find measures that are correlated with depression, but that, by virtue of this correlation, must now be used to detect vulnerable but not currently depressed people. Although difficult, investigators have had success with this methodology. A more difficult methodological issue, however, is the case

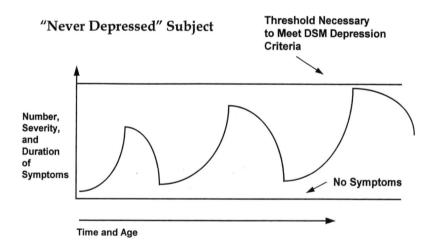

FIGURE 6.2. A hypothetical individual who would not meet criteria for a previous episode of depression despite having a significant number of past depressive states.

in which vulnerability measures are not only intended to tap currently nondepressed people, but are also construed to be independent of remission, that is, of former depression. Unfortunately, measures of genuine vulnerability that do not rely explicitly on remission in their development and conceptualization are nevertheless likely to covary with a history of depression and, therefore, with remission. Empirically, this has in fact been shown to be the case. For instance, employing the original ASQ (Seligman et al., 1979) to select respective high- and low-risk groups of college students who were not depressed, Alloy, Lipman, and Abramson (1992) found that not only were high-risk individuals more likely than low-risk people to have experienced depression in the past, they were also more likely to have experienced more frequent and severe episodes. Logically, of course, this is not surprising; if such measures are genuinely related to risk, then individuals possessing them should have experienced depression. Although this does not represent a problem theoretically (and is, in fact, theoretically desirable), it does represent an empirical problem if the goal is to determine vulnerability in people independently of past episodes of depression.

Several imperfect answers to this problem can be suggested. One that appears appealing, but only on the surface in our view, is to select individuals at a young enough age before they have experienced the onset of depression. College student populations, so criticized by a number of investigators, might be one ideal source for this strategy because many can be tracked at a relatively young age before they have presumably experienced a depressive episode. As we have noted, however, data do not support the lack of previous depression episodes in this group (Alloy et al., 1992). Moreover, this strategy is based on the assumption of a categorical model of depression, with the additional, albeit implicit, assumption that if individuals have not met criteria for depression, then they have not been depressed. As we argue in Chapter 10, we think that a more reasonable assumption is that depression throughout the lifespan represents a cascading series of negative affective states. If the presumed vulnerability factors are truly risk factors for depression, then the individuals in question may have had considerable experience with depressive symptoms, well before they meet criteria for their first "real" episode. The problem of nonindependence of vulnerability operationalization strategies is illustrated in Figure 6.3. Moreover, this problem is exacerbated when individuals are considered who are not currently depressed but who have significant experience with negative mood states and depressive symptoms. Operational definitions of vulnerability that are ostensibly independent of remission may classify these people as not being depressed (and thus not qualifying for remission status), even though they can be considered remitted from the significant depressive symptoms they have experienced in the past (see the example of the "never depressed" person in Figure 6.2).

Another imperfect strategy represents an experimental resignation to the inevitability of previous significant depressive symptomatology in individuals who posses the vulnerability factors. This allows for a combination of remission and other identification strategies. In this type of design, remitted people might be selected and the influence of varying degrees of presumably other vulnerability processes (e.g., attributional processes) might then be statistically examined to discover their influence on the magnitude of subjects' future depressive responses. Perhaps remitted individuals with a history of variables x, y, and z, in comparison to those remitted individuals without a history of these variables, have the most (or least) depressive-like cognitive responses to a priming stimulus, or are more or less likely to experience depression at some time in the future. This allows for some determination of the impact of these factors on vulnerability. The obvious reverse of this strategy would be to select people based on the identified or possible vulnerability characteristics and then examine what impact experience with previous depressive symptoms has on the other depression-linked responses. Neither way is a perfect way to study cognitive vulnerability responses, but given the logical and intricate associations between risk factors and the experience of depression, this may be the best we can hope for at this point, at least for proximal research.

Nonindependence of Vulnerability Operational Definitions

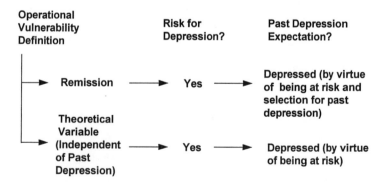

FIGURE 6.3. Even though various operational definitions of vulnerability may be theoretically independent, in many, if not all, cases various definitions are confounded with each other.

SUMMARY AND CONCLUSIONS

Our focus in this chapter was to examine the various research designs that have been used to explore cognitive vulnerability, specifically, cross-sectional, longitudinal, remission, and priming designs. Although all of these designs have been used to study cognitive vulnerability, not all have provided informative results. The design that has perhaps shown the most promise for elucidating cognitive vulnerability is the priming methodology. From a theoretical perspective, priming methodologies have the advantage of more closely paralleling the conceptual parameters of vulnerability as specified by cognitive models of depression. Even though such designs show promise, however, they have thus far not provided answers to such critical questions as to whether or not the cognitive factors that have been detected after priming are, in fact, causally related to depression. Although highlighted by the priming design, this problem plagues not only proximal vulnerability designs, but distal vulnerability designs as well.

One variation of vulnerability research strategies that has received considerable recent attention is the high-risk paradigm. The high-risk strategy selects individuals based on a specified set of vulnerability characteristics and then examines whether the factors inherent in this high-risk constellation are related to the subsequent onset of depression. Although this strategy shows promise in many respects, one of its main premises may be suspect. That is, although such designs have been aimed at examining vulnerability that does not rely on remission, high-risk variables may not be independent of remission due to the very fact that high risk is related to depression. What should be clear from our discussion not only of the high-risk paradigms but of all of these designs is that no strategy is free from problems. Nevertheless, the data generated form proximal vulnerability designs have led to some potentially important information and insights. We now turn to these data.

CHAPTER 7

Cognitive Theory and Data on Proximal Vulnerability

In Chapter 6 we examined the different research strategies that have been employed to study vulnerability to depression from a psychological, specifically a cognitive, standpoint. Whatever their particular strengths or limitations, each method has been employed to test the hypothesis that processing information in a particular way, holding certain beliefs, or relying on specific cognitive styles to interpret one's experience increases a person's risk for depression. In previous chapters we have described some of the ways in which these thinking styles have been defined and operationalized. We now turn our attention to an empirical evaluation of the contribution of cognitive theory and data as they pertain to proximal vulnerability to affective disturbance. A central feature of our discussion focuses on understanding how closely tests of vulnerability have conformed to the models they were intended to evaluate. We will begin by trying to link the different constructs with the theories behind them. We will highlight the two major constructs that characterize cognitive models: schemas and attributions. We will then review the empirical studies that have been conducted in this area, with an eye toward determining how adequately the theories have been tested. In particular, we will review research that has assessed the proposed stability of cognitive processes in individuals who are no longer depressed (i.e., remission studies), and we will examine studies that have used priming procedures and those that have not. Finally, we also examine data from high-risk paradigms that assess proximal cognitive vulnerability features.

ENVIRONMENTAL INTERACTIONS IN COGNITIVE MODELS OF DEPRESSION

As we noted in Chapter 4, cognitive models have always been fundamentally diathesis–stress models, in that they clearly posit that depression is produced by the interaction between an individual's cognitive vulnerability and environmental conditions that serve to trigger this diathesis into operation. Evidence suggests that, under ordinary conditions, persons thought to be vulnerable to the onset of depression are indistinguishable from the general population. Only when confronted with certain stressors do differences between vulnerable and nonvulnerable people emerge (Monroe & Simons, 1991; Segal & Shaw, 1986). As we suggested in Chapter 6, for vulnerable people these life events precipitate a pattern of negative, biased, self-referent information processing that appears to initiate the first cycle in the downward spin of depression. Nonvulnerable individuals react with an appropriate level of distress and depressive affect to the event, but do not spiral into depression. In seeking to explain these differential outcomes in the face of similar life conditions, some models have focused on the dysfunctional cognitive structures and types of thoughts that come to mind in these types of situations. Although these models were reviewed in Chapter 3, we will briefly note them here and comment on data that pertain to these models; we will emphasize data that apply to the vulnerability predictions of these models.

Cognitive Variables: Schemas

Beck's (1963, 1967) initial observations about thinking processes in depressed patients spurred the development of a theoretical model of unipolar affective disorder that features several interrelated cognitive processes, which include a negatively distorted pattern of information processing; an unfavorable view of the self, world, and future; and the occurrence of repetitive and unintended self-referent thoughts that reflect themes of loss. Beck (1967) suggested that these cognitive manifestations of depression originate from maladaptive cognitive structures, such as schemas about the self, that are causally linked to the disorder and triggered or activated by stressful life events. Although definitions vary somewhat, many investigators conceptualize self-schemas as organized representations of an individual's prior experiences. The common principle underlying all accounts of cognitive structures such as schemas is that the basic units comprising these structures are not randomly distributed throughout the memory system, but are instead connected to each other in varying strengths of association. Functionally, the self-schema exerts a significant influence on information processing by selectively screening what information is extracted from both internal and external sources and by affecting both the encoding and retrieval of information (Alba & Hasher, 1983; Kihlstrom & Cantor, 1984).

Cognitive Variables: Causal Attributions

In contrast to the models proposed by Beck, the association between how people explain the occurrence of significant events in their lives and the proximal development of depression is best seen in the hopelessness theory of depression (Abramson et al., 1989), a modification of the original (Seligman, 1975) and reformulated (Abramson et al., 1978) learned helplessness models of depression. In the earlier versions of this model, depression was seen as arising from the lack of control that people had over negative events in their lives and the types of explanations they used to understand this lack of contingency. An important feature of this approach was the specific types of proximal explanations or attributions available about these events; those emphasizing causes that were internal to the individual, stable, and global predisposed people to lowered mood. It is not the presence of the negative event itself, nor even the lack of control over the event, that is seen as critical, but rather the interpretation the person places on the situation.

In their extension of this work, Abramson et al. (1989) propose that hopelessness is a proximal and sufficient cause of depression and that there is a chain of events that builds toward the development of hopelessness in individuals and, subsequently, results in depression. Although no specific link in the chain leads to hopelessness in and of itself, each contributes significantly. The conditions under which hopelessness develops are the presence of a negative life event in an important area of the individual's life coupled with attributions about the event that are stable and global, and have implications for the person's view of him- or herself. The specific cognitive diatheses in this model are a general tendency to explain events in terms of stable and global causes, to view negative events as having extremely negative consequences, and to see negative events as detrimental to self-esteem.

How Good a Fit between the Theory and the Test?

Although investigations of schema-driven or attributional-based cognitive processing during depression have proliferated (Haaga et al., 1991;

Hartlage et al., 1993; Ingram & Holle, 1992; Ingram & Reed, 1986), far less work has been conducted to determine *how* these cognitive structures or products are initially activated. As we argued in Chapter 6, this is a potentially serious methodological omission that limits the extent to which the causal complexity of cognitive theories of vulnerability can be adequately modeled (Hollon, 1992). Knowing that a person's thoughts may follow one pattern over another is no doubt important, but it does not tell us what serves to activate or set off these thoughts, or under which conditions people will react to depressogenic cues by employing one line of thinking over another.

This is especially important for an account of proximal risk factors because what is being described is both the nature of the psychological changes that bias the individual toward the development of a specific disorder and the circumstances that trigger these changes. For example, many studies that have examined cognitive changes in formerly depressed patients (i.e., remission studies) have found that thinking patterns in these patients are largely state dependent and appear to normalize upon recovery (e.g., Barnett & Gotlib, 1988; Segal & Vella, 1990). However, as suggested in our critique of this methodology in Chapter 6, the implications of these findings for theories of cognitive vulnerability remain unclear because few of these studies ensured that the cognitive structures being assessed were activated at the time of assessment.

In providing a better description of the conditions under which maladaptive cognitive processing will be detected, cognitive diathesis–stress models clarify the requirements for empirical refutation and increase the fit between the theory and its test. Individuals at risk for depression should have latent but reactive negative cognitive structures available that will emerge under certain circumstances. One way to strengthen the assessment of proximal cognitive vulnerability, therefore, is to employ strategies capable of activating the constructs one is interested in measuring.

Because many of the earlier studies of vulnerability operationalized depressive cognitive processes in a way that did not represent the causal complexity of cognitive diathesis–stress models, their findings can be interpreted in a number of ways. For example, are negative findings due to a true absence of effect or due to patients not being tested when their negative thinking styles were activated? However, as we noted in our discussion of priming methodologies in Chapter 6, some studies have begun to appear that more closely approximate the notions of triggers and primes as expressed in the diathesis–stress model (for a review see Segal & Ingram, 1994). This is accomplished by empirically attempting to provoke the resurgence of negative thinking in individuals identified as at risk for depression. By using priming procedures, these studies thus seek to examine dysfunctional cognitions as potential proximal agents by assessing cognition in the context of the activating features of affectively linked events, particularly the onset of a sad mood state. Before describing the conceptual parameters of priming as well as findings from proximal priming studies, we note parenthetically that priming can also be employed to test distal features of cognitive vulnerability. We discuss the methodological issues involved in distal priming in Chapter 8 and some findings from this type of priming in Chapter 9.

PRIMING AND CONSTRUCT ACTIVATION IN THEORIES OF COGNITIVE VULNERABILITY TO DEPRESSION

To reiterate briefly our discussion in Chapter 6, priming refers to a collection of procedures intended to activate a hypothesized mental structure, often without the individual's conscious realization that such activation has occurred. Although priming can affect various levels of the cognitive system, this section will focus only on priming techniques that are most likely to affect semantic memory. This memory system enables cognitive representation and is likely the locus in which the hypothesized depression vulnerability constructs (e.g., negative self-representations, self-worth contingencies, etc.) are stored.

As we have argued consistently throughout this volume, a central premise of many cognitive models of depression is that vulnerable individuals possess cognitive risk factors that are largely inactive until the individual encounters adversity in a domain that is tied to his or her sense of self-worth. Because models relying on latent constructs have, at least on the surface, fewer points of contact with empirical data, they run the risk of being perpetually nonfalsifiable, unless the conditions that would permit a more definitive determination of the validity of a cognitive vulnerability formulation can be outlined. For this very reason, ensuring that an individual's vulnerability is activated prior to any assessment of its effects on a specified dependent variable is essential (i.e., the construct is accessed in addition to being available). In the absence of activation, negative findings cannot be used to refute the hypothesis that a particular cognitive variable is a marker of risk for the proximal development of depression because the question of whether the latent predisposition was operative during testing cannot be answered. In the long run, such weakening of a theory's falsifiability works against its utility and promotes a stasis in the field, which is epitomized by equivocal findings and a lack of consensus on its major premises (Popper, 1959).

The use of priming procedures offers one solution to this problem in that the rationale for these procedures is derived from an explicit theoretical model that acknowledges the facilitation that follows from evoking stimulus. Such facilitation is achieved through the interconnection of elements in knowledge structures, so that the entire structure can be brought "online" by activating subfeatures that are part of one's cognitive organization (Bruner, 1957; Erdley & D'Agostino, 1988; Higgins, 1989; L. M. Horowitz & Malle, 1993; Strauman, 1989). In the cognitive science literature, conceptual priming (Meyer & Schvaneveldt, 1971) perhaps comes closest to illustrating the types of phenomena that are relevant to discussions of construct activation in depression. Depressive constructs may come to mind or be processed more easily if they are preceded by constructs that bear an associative relationship to them. In this case, the interrelation among elements would be determined by the individual's past experiences with negative cognition (e.g., self-criticism, Blatt & Bers, 1993; self-blame, Abramson et al., 1989; depressive predictive certainty, Andersen, Spielman, & Bargh, 1992) and dysphoria.

In a nonpathological example of this process, consider that, when greeting a friend who seems to be too preoccupied to engage in conversation and just responds in a cursory fashion, some people may wonder why their friend is so busy and get on with their day. Others, however, may replay the friend's reaction a number of times as they try to figure out what they did or how they could have acted to elicit a warmer response. This may bring to mind thoughts of inadequacy, or the need to engage in social comparisons with others. Eventually, these individuals may find themselves distracted by these thoughts throughout the day. The thoughts may even induce a mild state of dysphoria in which the recall of similar instances of rejection or disregard by significant others is facilitated.

Accounts such as these, in which the activation of interrelated subelements of a cognitive schema is capable of reinstating the entire structure, are consistent with the tenets of a vulnerability model that posits the need for some type of trigger, or releasing variable, to activate an underlying diathesis for emotional disorder. In Beck's cognitive model (1967, 1976), stress in the patient's environment is hypothesized to serve this function, particularly adversity that matches the patient's core concerns or doubts regarding his or her self-worth (Hammen, Marks, Mayol, & deMayo, 1985; Segal, Shaw, Vella, & Katz, 1992). The hopelessness model of depression also stresses that, in the presence of the accompanying attributional style, a general match between a negative event's content and the individual's personal investments may be a particularly powerful condition for the development of hopelessness (Abramson et al., 1989).

As we suggested in Chapter 6, one path by which a person's vulnerability can be activated is through the creation of a mood state that matches the person's state of mind at the time of encoding. Persons and Miranda (1992) have labeled this the "mood state hypothesis" and argue that a stable vulnerability to depression that is cognitive in nature may exist, but that a person's ability to report it is dependent on his or her mood state. Once again, the implication is that people may have ingrained negative views of themselves, but they are not aware of them unless these views are evoked in some fashion (Riskind & Rholes, 1984).

The value of construct activation for cognitive theories of depression therefore lies in its enabling of stronger tests of the vulnerability hypotheses proposed by these accounts. With this in mind, we now turn to an examination of the existing research conducted with depressed and recovered depressed patient samples in which priming procedures were or were not used.

Remission Studies of Depressed and Recovered Depressed Patients

For a measure of depressive cognition to be considered as a marker of risk or vulnerability for the disorder it must satisfy the minimal criteria of *sensitivity* (it should be present in depressed persons), *specificity* (it should be more frequent in depressed samples than in controls), and *stability* (it should always be present in vulnerable individuals, although not necessarily always accessed) (Baldessarini, Finklestein, & Arana, 1983; Garber & Hollon, 1991; Haynes, 1992). Even if these conditions are met, it is still possible that the particular measure may be a "scar" of the clinical state, which either changes more slowly or never changes, but does not actually affect the risk to depression (see Chapter 6). To some authors, familial aggregation is an important additional criterion for any vulnerability marker (Katz & McGuffin, 1993), because studying the proportion of family members showing elevated scores on the measure of interest allows one to step outside the effects of scars or residual symptoms in the proband.

Table 7.1 attests to the variety of research designs that have been used to examine the question of cognitive markers of proximal vulnerability to depression including comparisons between nondepressed and remitted depressed samples, testing depressed samples both in episode and in remission, and using a prospective longitudinal approach to examine whether cognitive variables predispose persons to later depressive episodes. The majority of studies, with two exceptions (Lewinsohn et al., 1981; Nolen-Hoeksema, Girgus, & Seligman, 1992), have examined the problem of risk to recurrence or depressive relapse, rather than risk to initial onset of the disorder. However, as we argued in Chapter 6, it is important to note that, even though "first onset" subjects for these two studies may not have met criteria for a previous depressive

TABLE 7.1. Comparing Depressed and Recovered Depressed Patients on Cognitive Measures: Studies without Construct Activation

Study	Participants	Measure of cognition	Findings
Altman & Wittenborn (1980)	88 Remitted depressed females 88 Normal controls	134-item Self-Descriptive Inventory	62/134 items distinguished between the two groups.
Lewinsohn, Steinmetz, Larson, & Franklin (1981)	63 Depressed S's 115 Remitted depressed S's 154 Normal controls	(1) Attributions for success and failure (2) Expectancies for positive and negative outcomes (3) Irrational beliefs (4) Self-esteem (5) Locus of control	(1) D = RD = NC (2) D > RD = NC (3) D > RD = NC (4) D > RD = NC (5) D = RD = NC
Wilkinson & Blackburn (1981)	10 Depressed S's 15 Recovered depressed S's 10 Recovered psychiatric S's 15 Normal controls	Cognitive Style Test Cognitive Response Test	D > RD = RP = N, on both measures
Fogarty & Hemsley (1983)	14 Depressed S's (tested twice over a 6-week interval) 14 Normal controls	Cued recall of personal memories	Depressed S's recalled more unhappy memories than controls at T1. With return to normal mood at T2, depressed S's recall of unhappy memories dropped and recall of positive memories increased.
Hamilton & Abramson (1983)	20 Depressed S's 20 Psychiatric controls 20 Normal controls (all S's tested pre- and posttreatment)	Dysfunctional Attitudes Scale Attributional Style Questionnaire (composite score)	T1 DAS D > PC > NC T2 DAS D = NC < PC T1 ASQ D < PC = NC T2 ASQ D = PC = NC ASQ and DAS scored in opposite directions
Eaves & Rush (1984)	31 Depressed S's 17 Normal controls (all S's tested pre- and posttreatment)	Dysfunctional Attitudes Scale Attributional Style Questionnaire	T1 DAS D > NC T2 DAS D > NC T1 ASQ (pos.) D = NC T2 ASQ (pos.) D = NC T1 ASQ (neg.) D < NC T2 ASQ (neg.) D < NC
Fenell & Campbell (1984)	100 Currently depressed S's 34 Remitted depressed S's 109 Never depressed S's	Cognitions Questionnaire	D > RD = ND

(continued)

TABLE 7.1. (cont.)

Study	Participants	Measure of cognition	Findings
Silverman, Silverman, & Eardley (1984)	35 Depressed *S*'s (tested in episode [T1] and in remission [T2])	Dysfunctional Attitudes Scale	DAS at T1 > DAS at T2
	63 Depressed *S*'s		BP < D = SA
	10 Bipolar depressed *S*'s		SA = NP/ND/ND = SZ
	19 Schizoaffective *S*'s		
	22 Nonpsychotic/ nondepressive/nonorganic psychiatric control *S*'s		
	12 Schizophrenic *S*'s		
Simons, Garfield, & Murphy (1984)	28 Depressed *S*'s (tested pre- and posttreatment)	Dysfunctional Attitudes Scale	DAS for treatment responders T1 > T2
			DAS for treatment nonresponders T1 = T2
Slife, Miura, Thompson, Shapiro, & Gallagher (1984)	20 Depressed *S*'s (tested pre- and posttreatment)	Differential Recall of Trigrams	At pretreatment, recall of disliked trigrams > recall of liked trigrams. At posttreatment this pattern was reversed.
Reda, Capriniello, Secchiaroli, & Blanco (1985)	60 Depressed *S*'s (tested in episode and in remission)	Dysfunctional Attitudes Scale	DAS at T1 > DAS at T2 = DAS at T3
	30 of these *S*'s (retested 1 year later)		
Blackburn, Jones, & Lewin (1986)	72 Depressed *S*'s	Cognitive Style Test	D > A = NC = RD = RA
	21 Anxiety disorder *S*'s	Dysfunctional Attitudes Scale	
	31 Normal controls		
	29 Recovered depressed *S*'s		
	10 Recovered anxious *S*'s		
Dobson & Shaw (1986)	15 Depressed *S*'s (tested pre- and posttreatment)	Dysfunctional Attitudes Scale	DAS at pretest = DAS at remission
		Cognitive Response Test	CRT at pretest = CRT at remission
			Many depressed *S*'s still showed residual symptoms at time of 2nd testing.

152

Study	Sample	Measure	Results
Hollon, Kendall, & Lumry (1986)	12 Bipolar depressed S's 16 Unipolar depressed S's 12 Substance abuse, depressed S's 17 Substance abuse, nondepressed S's 12 Psychiatric controls 12 Medical controls 32 Normal controls 12 Remitted bipolar S's 13 Remitted depressed S's	Dysfunctional Attitudes Scale	BP = UD = SA/D = PC SA/ND = MC = NC = RB = RD BP = UD > RB = RD
Dobson & Shaw (1987)	24 Depressed S's 14 Remitted depressed S's 14 Psychiatric control S's 14 Normal control S's	Self-Referent Encoding Task (1) No. of depressed content words rated as self-descriptive (2) Rating times for depressed content words (3) Recall of depressed content words	(1) D > RD = PC = NC, on all three measures
Lewinsohn & Rosenbaum (1987)	63 Depressed S's 114 Remitted depressed S's 153 Normal control S's	Recall of parental behavior as assessed by the (1) Rejection, (2) Negative Control, and (3) Firm Discipline subscales of the Children's Report of Parental Behavior Inventory	(1) D > RD = NC (2) D = RD = NC (3) D = RD = NC
Gotlib, Mount, Cordy, & Whiffen (1988)	8 Depressed S's 11 Remitted depressed S's 20 Nondepressed controls	Parental Bonding Instrument: (1) Overprotection, and (2) Parental Caring Subscales	(1) D = RD > NC (2) D > RD = NC
Klein, Harding, Taylor, & Dickstein (1988)	63 Depressed S's 15 Normal control S's (tested at intake and 6-month follow-up)	Depressive Experiences Questionnaire (Dependency and Self-Criticism subscales)	Depen. at intake: D > NC Self-Crit. at intake: D > NC Depen. at 6-mo. follow-up: scores of S's who recovered were significantly lower than their intake scores. Self-crit. at 6-mo. follow-up: scores of S's who recovered were significantly lower than their intake scores.
Seligman, Castellon, Cacciola, Schulman, Luborsky, Ollove, & Downing (1988)	39 Depressed S's receiving cognitive therapy (tested pre-, posttreatment and 1-year follow-up)	Attributional Style Questionnaire (negative composite)	ASQ neg. – pre > post = follow-up

(continued)

TABLE 7.I. (cont.)

Study	Participants	Measure of cognition	Findings
Dohr, Rush, & Bernstein (1989)	*Study 1:* 25 Depressed *S*'s 22 Remitted depressed *S*'s 19 Normal control *S*'s *Study 2:* 12 Depressed *S*'s (tested in episode and in remission)	Dysfunctional Attitudes Scale Attributional Style Questionnaire (failure and success subscales)	*Study 1:* DAS: D > RD = NC ASQ-F: D > RD = NC ASQ-S: D = RD = NC *Study 2:* DAS at T1 > DAS at T2 ASQ-F at T1 > ASQ-F at T2 ASQ-S at T1 = ASQ-S at T2
Bowers (1990)	30 Depressed *S*'s receiving either (1) antidepressant medication, (2) #1 and CT, or (3) #1 and relaxation	Dysfunctional Attitudes Scale	DAS; pre > post for all 3 groups
Hollon, Evans, & De Rubeis (1990)	106 Depressed *S*'s (tested pre-, posttreatment and 2-year follow-up)	Attributional Style Questionnaire Automatic Thoughts Questionnaire Hopelessness Scale	Only ASQ scores at posttreatment predicted relapse/recurrence, once initial level of depression was controlled for.
Imber, Pilkonis, Sotsky, Elkin, Watkins, Collins, Shea, Leber, & Glass (1990)	154 Depressed *S*'s receiving either (1) CBT, (2) interpersonal therapy, (3) antidepressant medications, or (4) placebo	Dysfunctional Attitudes Scale	DAS; pre > post for all 4 groups
Rohde, Lewinsohn, & Seeley (1990)	49 Remitted depressed *S*'s 351 Community controls	28 Psychosocial measures, including behavioral, cognitive, and affective indices	Only 3/28 measures (self-perceived social skills, self-related health, and excessive emotional reliance) distinguished between the two groups.
Whisman, Miller, Norman, & Keitner (1991)	17 Depressed *S*'s receiving antidepressant medication 14 Depressed *S*'s receiving antidepressant medication plus cognitive therapy (*S*'s assessed pre-, posttreatment and 12-month follow-up).	Dysfunctional Attitudes Scale Cognitive Bias Questionnaire	DAS; med. group – pre = post = 6 = 12 DAS; med. and CT group – pre = post > 6 = 12 CBQ; med. group – pre = post = 6 = 12 CBQ; med. and CT group – pre = post = 6 > 12

Study	Sample	Measure	Results
Nolen-Hoeksema, Girgus, & Seligman (1992)	60 Third-grade school children studied over a 5-year period; they were divided into 2 groups: (1) 30 of whom had elevated symptoms of depression and (2) 30 of whom had no depressive symptoms	Children's Attributional Style Questionnaire (composite score)	Before the onset of depressive symptoms 1 = 2 in explanatory style. With the onset of depressive symptoms 1 < 2 in explanatory style. After group 1 showed a decrease in depressive symptoms, 1 < 2 in explanatory style at 6-, 18-, and 24-mo. follow-up.
Thase, Simons, McGeary, Cahalane, Hughes, Harden, & Friedman (1992)	50 Depressed S's receiving cognitive therapy (tested pre-, posttreatment and 1-year follow-up)	Dysfunctional Attitudes Scale	DAS pre > DAS post S's who relapsed within the 1-year follow-up interval had significantly higher posttreatment DAS scores than S's who maintained their improvement.
McCabe & Gotlib (1993)	15 Depressed S's 10 Nondepressed controls (tested twice over a 3-month interval)	Dichotic listening task with a concurrent light probe reaction time task	At T1: Depressed S's took longer to respond to the light probe when negative distractors were presented in the unattended channel vs. positive or neutral distractors
Moretti, Segal, Miller, Shaw, Vella, & McCann (in press)	27 Depressed S's 27 Remitted depressed S's 27 Normal controls	Identification of positive or negative emotion directed toward the self or toward others	*Emotions directed toward self:* RD and NC more accurate in identification of pos. responses. D evenhanded in identification of pos. and neg. responses. *Emotions directed toward others:* D and RD more accurate in identification of pos. responses. NC evenhanded in identification of pos. and neg. responses.

episode, to the extent that they were truly vulnerable to depression, they may have had considerable prior experience with negative affective states. These data may thus have some limitations with regard to factors that truly pertain to the onset of a depressive state.

Very few of the studies reviewed provide information that would allow for estimates of sensitivity, specificity, and stability to be made. At most, comparisons relevant to two of the three criteria are possible (see Hollon et al., 1986, for an exception). The majority of studies seem to have been designed to answer the question of whether scores on a measure of depressive cognition are elevated over the course of the disorder.

With this focus in mind, the findings consistently point to the state dependent nature of most of the measures of depressive cognition employed. In the studies listed, the scores of remitted depressed patients are generally no different from either nondepressed control subjects (Blackburn Jones, & Lewin, 1986; Dobson & Shaw, 1987; Dohr, Rush, & Bernstein, 1989, Study 1; Fenell & Campbell, 1984; Gotlib, Mount, Cordy, & Whiffen, 1988; Hamilton & Abramson, 1983; Hollon et al., 1986; Lewinsohn & Rosenbaum, 1987; Moretti et al., 1996; Rohde et al., 1990; Wilkinson & Blackburn, 1981) or are significantly lower when patients are retested in remission (Bowers, 1990; Dobson & Shaw, 1986; Dohr et al., 1989, Study 2; Fogarty & Hemsley, 1983; Imber et al., 1990; McCabe & Gotlib, 1993; Reda, Carpiniello, Secchiaroli, & Blanco, 1985; Seligman et al., 1988; Silverman et al., 1984; Slife, Miura, Thompson, Shapiro, & Gallagher, 1984; Thase et al., 1992; Whisman, Miller, Norman, & Keitner, 1992).

Evidence in favor of cognitive measures exhibiting trait-like properties is more limited. Eaves and Rush (1984) report that recovered depressed patients' scores on the DAS and the ASQ negative, but not positive, composite differed from normal controls. Dobson and Shaw (1986) found a similar pattern of results for the DAS and the Cognitive Response Test (CRT), but given that many of the depressed patients still showed residual symptoms at the posttreatment assessment it is not clear whether the entire sample was in remission. Gotlib et al. (1988) reported that remitted depressed patients' scores on the Overprotection subscale of the Parental Bonding Instrument (PBI; Parker, Tupling, & Brown, 1979) differed from normal controls, although a cell size of 8 for this comparison requires some caution in interpretation. No differences were found on the Parental Caring subscale of the PBI.

Even if measures of depressive cognition return to normal with recovery, there may exist a subgroup of patients for whom elevated scores indicate ongoing risk for the return of symptoms. In this case, comparisons of group means are less informative than gauging the strength of the predictive relationship between cognitive variables at recovery and the return of symptoms for individual patients, over the follow-up period. If this strategy is pursued, it is vital to isolate the predictive power of the cognitive measure from any association that might be due to residual symptoms the patient may be experiencing. This is important because prediction of relapse may be achieved by the cognitive measure, not through its unique content, but through its intercorrelation with depressed mood. Hollon et al. (1990) and Thase et al. (1992) reported that patients who relapsed during the follow-up periods in their studies had higher ASQ and DAS scores, respectively, than those who maintained the benefits of treatment. Seligman et al. (1988), however, failed to find this pattern with the ASQ. D. Klein, Harding, Taylor, and Dickstein (1988) also found that subjects who recovered had lower scores on the Dependency and Self-Critical subscales of the DEQ than those who were still depressed, at 6-month follow-up.

Finally, the two studies utilizing a prospective longitudinal design reported conflicting findings. Lewinsohn et al. (1981) did not find that adult depressive cognition was a permanent residual feature of an episode, or that it predicted the onset of disorder. Depressed subjects evidencing more negative cognitions, however, were less likely to improve over the course of the study. As we note again in Chapter 9, Nolen-Hoeksema et al. (1992) found that third grade students with elevated depression scores were no different from nondepressed peers in terms of their explanatory style before the onset of symptoms, but differed once they felt depressed. Following a decrease in their depressive symptom endorsement, however, this group continued to exhibit a more global, internal, and stable explanatory style over a 2-year follow-up.

Conclusions from Remission Studies

An inescapable conclusion from the majority of these studies is that depressive cognition is largely state dependent. Little evidence was found for the existence of an enduring proximal predisposition to depression that does not change with treatment. Some data point to the utility of considering posttreatment scores as predictors of future course of depression (e.g., Hollon et al., 1990), but even these findings are controverted by other studies (e.g., Seligman et al., 1988). On the face of it, negative results stemming from this work can present a serious challenge to cognitive theories of depression because they cast doubt on the basic premise of a psychological vulnerability that operates through the information-processing system (Coyne, 1992).

If we look more closely, however, two things stand out. Although the sheer number of studies that have been conducted to date is impressive, a straightforward acceptance of the implications of their negative findings is premature because the majority of studies offered rather weak tests of the proximal vulnerability hypotheses and, as we noted in our discussion of the limitations of remission studies, encountered the interpretational difficulty resulting from acceptance of the null hypothesis (Chapter 6) . This inadequate testing of proximal vulnerability is due to a number of factors including (1) the lack of attention paid to the effects of treatment on cognitive measures, (2) heterogeneity in measures of depressive cognition, (3) inconsistent criteria for the timing of posttreatment assessments and the determination of remission, and (4) perhaps most importantly, the absence of strategies that would make negative modes of thinking more accessible before their assessment.

The fact that depressed patients received treatment in many of these studies suggests that an interaction between the modality of treatment and its effects on cognitive measures of vulnerability may be present. Evidence for differential effects on DAS scores as a function of treatment are reported by Imber et al. (1990; Need for Approval subscale only) and Whisman et al. (1992). Even in comparisons between remitted depressed and nondepressed control subjects, the history of past treatment for the former group is rarely mentioned. Testing for potential treatment by measure interaction effects is important because data bearing on the state dependency of a risk marker, derived from posttreatment comparisons between patients receiving different treatments, could be misleading. In light of distinctions that have been made among different levels of the cognitive system (Ingram, 1990), we find that many of the measures employed in this research assess cognitive products, rather than cognitive processes or structures (e.g., CRT, Cognitions Questionnaire, expectancies for negative outcomes; Hollon & Kriss, 1984). This point is relevant because cognitive theories predict changes in cognitive products with remission, but specify that the enduring predisposition to depression exists at the level of cognitive processes or structures (Segal, 1988). Seen in this light, some of the negative findings may derive from the fact that these studies relied on measures of cognitive products or content, which are considered to be unlikely markers of vulnerability, by the very cognitive theory they are intended to validate.

The absence of a standard approach for the determination of recovery or remission is also problematic. In some cases, patients were still experiencing residual symptoms at the time of the posttreatment assessment (Dobson & Shaw, 1986), whereas in others (D. Klein et al., 1988; Fogarty & Hemsley, 1983) patients were simply retested after a certain time interval had elapsed, regardless of whether or not recovery had been achieved (6 months and 6 weeks, respectively). Other studies used varying criteria for judging remission such as a score of less than 10 on the Hamilton Rating Scale for Depression on two consecutive occasions (Eaves & Rush, 1984) or discharge from hospital (Hamilton & Abramson, 1983). In light of the potential biasing effects that residual low mood can have on cognitive measures, the adoption of standard criteria for determining recovery and remission, such as those proposed by Frank et al. (1991) would be a step in the right direction.

Finally, it is unclear whether the questions addressed by this body of research bear a sufficiently close resemblance to those articulated by the cognitive theories themselves, that is, by ensuring the activation of the putatively stable cognitive features that comprise the proximal predisposition to depression. Negative findings in the absence of attempts to enhance the accessibility of these depressive cognitive patterns can still be interpreted as the outcome of poor design, rather than reflecting the inadequacy of the cognitive theory. Persons and Miranda (1992) have written that

> patients treated with antidepressant medication "appear" to show changes in dysfunctional thinking during treatment. However, the mood-state hypothesis proposes that these patients still retain their dysfunctional attitudes; the attitudes are simply not reported because patients are in a positive mood at the time their attitudes are assessed . . . the dysfunctional attitudes are present, but they are . . . inactive, and unavailable for report . . . the mood induction (or other activation procedure) "turns on the light" that allows the investigator to observe real differences between groups that are hidden from view. (p. 497)

Although recourse to latent variables as an explanatory strategy has drawn criticism to cognitive theories of depression (e.g., Coyne, 1992; Coyne & Gotlib, 1983, 1986), this hypothesized explanation for previous negative findings is both testable and falsifiable. Specifically, the possibility of dormant causal pathways can be empirically evaluated, rather than merely added post hoc. The strongest tests of theses theories will be those studies that include priming as a precondition for the assessment of vulnerability variables. We now evaluate this small, but growing, literature.

Remission Studies with Priming/Construct Activation of Depressed and Recovered Depressed Patients

It should be noted at the outset that, relative to remission studies, few studies have employed priming methods to examine whether cognitive measures are stable during a depressive episode and during remission. This is no doubt due to the recent focus on priming strategies, along with the recently revitalized emphasis in cognitive models on diathesis–stress processes. Despite this, enough studies exist to warrant consideration of their implications for theories of cognitive vulnerability to depression. These studies are summarized in Table 7.2.

As we have argued in Chapter 6, the logic underlying priming studies is to study the activation processes of negative self-referent cognitive structures in order to understand cognitive vulnerability. In theory, activation can be brought about by any number of factors. In practice, priming studies have typically relied on inducing a negative mood in individuals who should have the requisite vulnerability factors (e.g., people who have previously experienced a clinically significant episode of depression). Perhaps the first study to use a priming procedure to examine postdepression cognitive processes was reported by Blackburn and Smyth (1985). They reported no evidence on either the DAS or the Cognitive Style Test of differences between remitted depressed subjects and normal controls following a mood induction. However, the remitted depressed group appeared refractory to the mood induction; without an adequate mood induction in the key group, these results are therefore inconclusive. Quite possibly, individuals who have recently recovered from depression are motivated to avoid negative mood states, thus making the hypothesis difficult to test.

Using a modified version of the Stroop Color Naming Test, Gotlib and Cane (1987) tested a group of depressed subjects during an episode and again at discharge. Subjects were asked to name the ink color of depressed, manic, or neutral content targets. The priming procedure was adapted from the work of Higgins and colleagues (Higgins, King, & Mavin, 1982) and consisted of presenting subjects with a series of positive or negative prime words, which subjects were asked to listen to and repeat. Following this, the Stroop Test was administered with the same valence of material as was used in the priming condition. Results indicated that, while in episode, depressed subjects were slower in color naming depressed content than nondepressed content words, but that this difference was no longer apparent when subjects were retested at discharge. One problem with this study is that the priming manipulation did not work. As is the case with the Blackburn and Smyth (1985) study, these findings are inconclusive with respect to the question of whether priming can alter the accessibility of negative constructs in formerly depressed patients.

An adequate mood induction in vulnerable subjects was reported by Teasdale and Dent (1987). These authors found that recovered depressed subjects did not differ from never depressed subjects in a

TABLE 7.2. Comparing Depressed and Recovered Depressed Patients on Cognitive Measures: Studies with Construct Activation

Study	Participants	Measure of cognition	Type of prime used	Findings
Blackburn & Smythe (1985)	10 Remitted depressed S's 10 Remitted anxiety disorder S's 10 Normal controls subjects (tested in neutral and induced negative mood)	Dysfunctional Attitudes Scale Cognitive Style Test	Velten Depressed or Neutral Mood Induction	For RD group: DAS in neutral mood = DAS in depressed mood CST in neutral mood = CST in depressed mood Findings inconclusive; hypothesis could not be tested due to failure of the independent variable manipulated. RD group appeared refractory to the depressed mood induction.
Gotlib & Cane (1987)	34 Depressed S's (tested pre- and posttreatment) 14 Psychiatric controls	Stroop Color Naming Latencies for adjectives with (1) Depressive, (2) Manic, and (3) Neutral content	Subjects were asked to listen and repeat 15 positive-content and 15 negative-content prime words	D at T1; $1 > 2 = 3$ D at T2; $1 = 2 = 3$ PC at T1; $1 = 2 = 3$ PC at T2; $1 = 2 = 3$ D versus PC at T1: $1 > 2 = 3$ D versus PC at T2: $1 = 2 = 3$
Teasdale & Dent (1987)	32 Remitted depressed females 21 Never depressed female controls	Incidental Recall of Self-Descriptive Adjectives	Musical induction of depressed mood	Normal mood: RD < NC on recall of positive adjectives RD = NC on recall of negative adjectives Depressed mood: RD < NC on recall of positive adjectives RD = NC on recall of negative adjectives RD > NC on recall of negative adjectives endorsed as self-descriptive
Dent & Teasdale (1988)	53 Depressed female S's (tested twice over a 5-month interval)	Number of global negative trait adjectives related as self-descriptive	Measures taken in depressed mood to predict non-depressed status	Differences in the number of negative adjectives endorsed as self-descriptive when S's were depressed predicted who was still depressed 5 months later.

(continued)

TABLE 7.2. (cont.)

Study	Participants	Measure of cognition	Type of prime used	Findings
Miranda & Persons (1988)	43 Female community based S's, 30 of whom had a prior history of depression	Dysfunctional Attitudes Scale	Velten Depressed or Elated Mood Induction	(1) Baseline DAS > elated mood DAS (2) Baseline DAS = depressed mood DAS (3) Regression analysis indicated that only for S's with a past history of depression, DAS scores increased as negative mood increased.
Williams (1988)	Longitudinal design in which the same measure was administered to nondepressed university students who were tested in both neutral and sad mood. S's were then followed for 1 year	Differential recall (positive vs. negative) of self-descriptive adjectives at T1, in two mood states	Musical induction of depressed mood	Differential recall in depressed mood, but not in neutral mood, of ratio of positive to negative adjectives predicted who became depressed 1 year later.
Hartlage (1990)	91 Depression-prone students 89 Nondepression-prone students Depression proneness determined jointly by low BDI and high ASQ score	Modified semantic priming paradigm: S's had to decide whether a briefly presented target cause was due to "internal" or "external" factors.	Brief computer screen presentation of a life event (e.g., fail test)	Depression-prone subjects showed greater facilitation for internal attributions for negative events and external attributions for positive events. Non-depression-prone subjects did not show the expected opposite pattern.
Miranda, Persons, & Byers (1990)	14 S's with a prior history of depression 27 S's who had never been depressed	Dysfunctional Attitudes Scale	Diurnal mood variation	In subjects who were vulnerable (prior history) to depression, DAS scores increased with negative mood. In subjects who were not vulnerable (no prior history) to depression, scores did not change with negative mood.

162

Study	Sample	Measure	Induction	Results
Ingram, Bernet, & McLaughlin (1994)	45 Formerly depressed S's 44 Never depressed S's	Dichotic Listening Task	Musical induction of depressed mood	Normal mood: FD = ND in number of errors for shadowing both positive & negative information Depressed mood: FD > ND in number of errors for shadowing negative information FD > ND in number of errors for shadowing positive information
Hedlund & Rude (1995)	18 Never depressed S's 15 Formerly depressed S's 20 Currently depressed S's	Stroop Color Naming Task Scrambled Sentence Task Incidental recall	Self-focus induction	Stroop: FD = ND = CD Scrambled negative sentences: ND < FD < CD Incidental recall, negative words: FD > ND, FD = CD
Roberts & Kassel (1996)	88 Remitted dysphoric S's	Dysfunctional Attitudes Scale Automatic Thoughts Questionnaire Negative Automatic Thoughts Self-Esteem Measure	Naturally occurring positive and negative affect	Negative affect: Significant correlations between cognitive measures and mood for remitted group only Positive affect: Weak correlations between affect and cognitive measures for both groups
Miranda, Gross, Persons, & Hahn (in press)	33 Formerly depressed women 67 Never depressed women	Dysfunctional Attitudes Scale	Film negative mood induction	Increased negative mood increased DAS in FD Increased negative mood decreased DAS in ND
Dykman (1997)	60 Remitted depressed S's 60 Never depressed S's	Dysfunctional Attitudes Scale	Velten Depressed or Elated Mood Induction	Normal mood: RD = ND Positive mood: RD = ND Negative mood: RD = ND

(continued)

TABLE 7.2. (cont.)

Study	Participants	Measure of cognition	Type of prime used	Findings
Ingram & Ritter (1998)	35 Formerly depressed *S*'s 38 Never depressed *S*'s	Dichotic Listening Task	Musical induction of depressed mood	Normal mood: FD = ND in number of errors for shadowing both positive and negative information Depressed mood: FD > ND in number of errors for shadowing negative information
Segal, Gemar, & Williams (1998)	25 Depressed patients recovered with CBT 29 Depressed patients recovered with antidepressants	Dysfunctional Attitudes Scale	Musical induction of depressed mood	Normal mood: Antidepressants = CBT Depressed mood: Antidepressants > CBT Cognitive reactivity regardless of treatment received predicted relapse up to 30 months later.
Smith, Teasdale, & Cowen (1998)	15 Formerly depressed women 12 Never depressed women	Attributional Style Questionnaire Dysfunctional Attitudes Scale Autobiographical Memory Bias	Tryptophan Depletion Paradigm	Patients whose drop in mood approached levels of clinical relapse were significantly *more positive* in their response measures of depressive cognition. Patients whose drop in mood was extreme showed a trend toward endorsing more negative content on these measures.

normal mood state on measures of adjective recall. When a negative mood was induced, however, recovered depressed subjects recalled more negative adjectives that had been endorsed as self-descriptive than did never depressed subjects. In a related study, Dent and Teasdale (1988) tested 53 depressed female subjects twice over a 5-month interval. Differences in the endorsement of negative adjectives during a depressive episode predicted who would remain depressed and who would recover. To the extent that these endorsement patterns can be considered a marker of a negative cognitive structure, they suggest that such cognitive structures place people at risk for increased persistence of their disorder, a possibility that has been suggested by several researchers (e.g., Kuiper et al., 1988; Teasdale, 1988).

Analogous results have been reported by Miranda and Persons (1988; Miranda et al., 1990; Roberts & Kassel, 1996) who, using the DAS, examined the endorsement of dysfunctional attitudes following a negative mood induction. Such attitudes are presumably a content aspect of the depressive cognitive process. Their results indicate that mood predicts the occurrence of dysfunctional attitudes *only* in people who have a history of depression; as negative mood increases, people with a history of depression are more likely to endorse dysfunctional attitudes. In people without such a history, little evidence of a relationship between mood and dysfunctional attitude endorsement was found. Thus, people who are vulnerable to depression, as operationalized by having a previous episode, do seem to possess distinctly depressotypic attitudes, but these attitudes do not appear accessible unless they are assessed in the context of a triggering event, in this case a mild depressed mood.

Miranda et al. (in press) reported a replication of their earlier work with a sample of 33 formerly depressed and 67 never depressed women. They used a film-based negative mood induction procedure as the prime and examined responses to the DAS before and after subjects watched the film. As in previous studies, increases in negative mood led to the increased endorsement of dysfunctional attitudes in formerly depressed subjects, whereas in never depressed subjects the effect was, surprisingly, in the opposite direction.

R. M. Williams (1988) used a longitudinal design to examine vulnerability to depression in a student sample. Subjects' recall of positive and negative self-referent adjectives was measured under two conditions, neutral mood and induced sad mood. Subjects were then followed for a period of a year to determine who experienced a significant episode of depression. Results indicated that differential recall (positive vs. negative adjectives) in neutral mood did not predict depression status. Differential recall under conditions of induced negative mood did predict subsequent depression. Subjects who recalled more negative than positive self-descriptors in mildly sad mood were more likely to become depressed over the subsequent 1-year follow-up.

A failure to replicate the relationship between construct activation and dysfunctional attitudes in vulnerability was reported by Dykman (1997). In this study, never depressed and formerly depressed individuals participated in a Velten (1968) Mood Induction Procedure used to prime mood. In the negative mood induction condition, Dykman (1997) reported a lack of differences in DAS scores between never depressed and formerly depressed individuals. In general, such findings must be judged in the context of the abundance of available data showing the elicitation of dysfunctional information processing in nondepressed but vulnerable individuals. As such, the failure to replicate may suggest methodological limitations (e.g., the Velten Mood Induction Procedure has several flaws). Yet, because differences in dysfunctional attitudes were assessed across groups but not across mood conditions, it is not completely clear from the data reported whether this study did not in fact replicate some previous findings. That is, when compared to the no mood induction control group (DAS $M = 114.0$; $SD = 25.8$), the formerly depressed individuals in the negative mood condition probably evidenced a significantly greater endorsement of dysfunctional attitudes (DAS $M = 146.9$; $SD = 25.8$). Clearly the data from this study must be considered cautiously.

Diverging from the mood priming methodology, Hartlage (1990, cited in Hartlage et al., 1993) used a semantic priming paradigm to examine the automaticity of attributional inferences in response to life events in groups of never depressed and depression-prone students (i.e., students with high, but nonclinical, levels of depressive symptoms as well as high scores on a measure of negative attributional style—a cognitive measure that theoretically predisposes to depression). Subjects were asked to decide whether a target cause (e.g., "incompetent") was due to internal or external factors, as quickly as possible. The manipulation in this case was the presentation of a prime, describing a relevant life event (e.g., fail test), just prior to the presentation of the target cause. Results indicated a priming effect for the at-risk group only, in that depression-prone students showed greatest automaticity for internal attributions for negative events and external attributions for positive events. Nonde-pressed subjects showed no evidence of automaticity in the formation of internal or external attributions.

Ingram et al. (1994) tested attentional processes in recovered and never-depressed subjects; how attention is allocated is thought to be a schema-driven process that functions to structure information processing (Neisser, 1967, 1976; J. M. G. Williams et al., 1997). By modifying a dichotic listening paradigm, Ingram et al. (1994) sought to test whether

latent cognitive structures could be momentarily activated into operation. Specifically, in one ear subjects heard a story to which they were
instructed to attend while in the other ear distracter words were
presented, some representing positive stimuli and some representing
negative stimuli. Tracking errors served as an index of the diversion of
attentional capacity to task-irrelevant stimuli. No differences between
subjects in the normal mood control condition were found, but when
induced into a sad mood, formerly depressed subjects made more
tracking errors for both negative and positive stimuli than did never
depressed subjects. The number of tracking errors for never depressed
subjects, however, was quite similar in both the normal and sad mood
conditions. These data appear to suggest that the occurrence of a
negative mood does activate a process in vulnerable people that has been
suggested to be schema controlled, that is, the allocation of attention.
This attentional allocation as shown in this study, however, appeared to
be fairly diffuse with regard to emotional cues. Not only did depressive
stimuli receive enhanced attentional resources, but those stimuli that had
positive affective connotations did so as well. At the early, preattentive
processing stage that this task may assess (MacLeod, Mathews, & Tata,
1986; Neisser, 1967, 1976), there was not much discrimination between
positive and negative emotional stimuli; rather, if the input was emotional in nature, it appeared to receive some attentional processing.

Some of the results of the Ingram et al. (1994) study were replicated
in a subsequent study by Ingram and Ritter (1998). Vulnerability was
again operationalized as remission from depression and thus nondepressed individuals who had experienced a previous depressive episode
were compared to nondepressed individuals who had never been depressed. Following a similar mood induction, a dichotic listening task
was again administered. For negative stimuli, the pattern of tracking
errors was identical to Ingram et al.'s (1994) earlier results; that is, in
the control condition vulnerable and nonvulnerable individuals were
indistinguishable, whereas in the negative mood condition vulnerable
subjects made significantly more errors than nonvulnerable subjects.
Unlike in the Ingram et al. (1994) study, however, no differences were
obtained for positive stimuli. Thus, while these data provide further
support for the accessibility of dysfunctional cognitive structures in
vulnerability, they temper to some degree previous findings that these
structures may be more emotionally diffuse. Building on these findings,
Taylor and Ingram (1998) used a high-risk research paradigm to assess
the children of depressed mothers, a group considered to be at increased
risk to develop the disorder. Subjects participated in a memory task that
allowed for a comparison of recall rates for negative and positive
information. Half the subjects were tested following mood priming and

the other half were tested under normal mood conditions. When primed, the children of depressed mothers were more likely to increase their processing of negative information than were equally primed children of nondepressed mothers. These results indicate that cognitive reactivity may be a feature of populations at risk for the development of depression, and not just a characteristic of those who have already experienced the disorder.

Finally, a recent study by Segal, Gemar, and Williams (1998) sought to extend these types of findings by examining whether different treatment modalities produce differential cognitive reactivity to a mood challenge and whether patients who display this reactivity, regardless of the treatment they may have received, are at a greater risk for relapse. Depressed patients who had recovered either through CBT or through pharmacotherapy (PT) completed self-reported ratings of dysfunctional attitudes before and after a negative mood induction procedure. Consistent with other priming data, PT patients showed a significant increase in dysfunctional cognitions following the induction. CBT patients, however, showed no change. A follow-up study reassessed patents several years after initial testing and found that patients' cognitive reactions to the mood challenge were predictive of relapse, even after controlling for the effects of the patients' previous history of depression. These data are among the first to suggest that there may be differential effects of treatment on cognitive reactivity to a mood challenge, and for the link between such reactivity and risk for later depressive relapse.

As we have previously argued, although mood inductions are common ways to prime cognitive processes, other priming procedures are possible. Hedlund and Rude (1995) examined negatively biased information processing in a sample of euthymic, formerly depressed patients following a self-focus manipulation. Formerly depressed, currently depressed, and never depressed subjects were tested on a modified Stroop Color Naming Test, a scrambled sentences task, and an incidental recall task. Results indicated that in the presence of increased self-focus, the groups did not differ on the Stroop test but formerly depressed subjects completed significantly more negative sentences than never depressed subjects and, on the incidental recall task, showed a negative bias in recall and intrusion errors relative to never depressed subjects. Currently depressed subjects completed more negative sentences than formerly depressed subjects and were roughly equal to them on the recall measure. An innovative study by Teasdale et al. (1998) using a Tryptophan Depletion Paradigm (TDP) suggests that remitted depressed patients' responses to negative mood states may differ according to the magnitude of dysphoria being experienced. Formerly depressed subjects for whom the TDP induced a massive shift in mood, to the point of almost equaling levels of clinical relapse, responded by attempting to minimize their negative cognitive responses to their falling mood. In fact, on some measures they were significantly *more positive* than controls. For other subjects who were not experiencing this magnitude of mood shift, their responses trended in the negative direction. What this work speaks to is the possibility that in the face of very strong shifts in mood, remitted depressed persons may resort to conscious, controlled strategies to try and reverse these changes. This study is unique in that it is certainly the first time that the cognitive effects of TDP have been studied. Clearly more work is needed to see whether these effects are reliable.

Conclusions from Priming Studies

Although not completely uniform, results from available priming studies do support the notion that priming prior to cognitive assessment allows for the detection of depressotypic cognitive variables in individuals who are theoretically at risk, but not currently depressed. Moreover, the lack of differences between vulnerable and nonvulnerable subjects in the various control (normal mood) conditions of these studies closely parallels previous research that has failed to find evidence of depressive cognitive processing after the depression resolves (e.g., Lewinsohn et al., 1981); that is, under ordinary conditions depressive cognitive processes cannot be detected after individuals are no longer depressed.

Interestingly, these differences in cognitive variables cut across several different levels of cognitive analysis (Ingram, 1990). For instance, in the presence of negative mood, dysfunctional cognition for those at risk appears evident in cognitive content (DAS scores; Miranda & Persons, 1988; Miranda et al., in press), information encoding and retrieval (adjective recall; Dent & Teasdale, 1988; Hedlund & Rude, 1995; Teasdale & Dent, 1987; R. M. Williams, 1988), and attention (tracking errors in a dichotic listening task; Ingram et al., 1994, 1997). These effects have also been obtained when a semantic, rather than affective, prime was used (Hartlage, 1990; but see Gotlib & Cane, 1987, for an exception). This would suggest that a maladaptive cognitive structure/schema, activated as a consequence of the priming manipulation, may be the organizing construct linked to each of these more specific cognitive effects. Sad mood, in these studies, may serve as an analogue to potent environmental triggers and appears to contribute to activating proximal cognitive structures that, heretofore, have only minimally been involved in online information processing. Furthermore, the data from at least one study (Segal et al., 1998) suggest that such activation may be moderated as a result of psychological treatment. Interestingly, following recovery, patients who continued to respond to a negative mood induction with high levels of dysfunctional thinking were at higher risk for relapse than equally recovered individuals who did not respond with dysfunctional thinking. As Kraemer et al. (1997) have argued, the demonstration of an effect on the course of illness through manipulation of a risk factor, is a strong piece of evidence in favor of its causal role in the disorder.

Perhaps the most direct indication of the importance of priming comes from considering the findings of two studies using similar methods with and without a priming manipulation. McCabe and Gotlib (1993) and Ingram et al. (1994, 1997) examined attentional biases in formerly depressed people (subjects at T2 in McCabe & Gotlib, 1993, and recovered depressed people in Ingram et al., 1994) with the key difference being that the former study did not prime subjects before testing them, whereas the latter studies did. Consistent with the predictions of cognitive models, only the primed groups of remitted depressed individuals showed a performance decrement in the presence of negative content stimuli.

The two studies in which equivocal findings have been reported (Blackburn & Smyth, 1985; Gotlib & Cane, 1987) suggest that the use of construct activation procedures with patients in recovery may not be entirely straightforward. With respect to Blackburn and Smyth, we should not be surprised if patients in at least some cases resist the effects of an induction designed to reinstate aversive states of mind/mood, especially ones from which they are recovering. Yet, it may be that this very unwillingness to experience even small shifts in mood or self-regard under controlled conditions is revealing. Could perceptions of euthymic fragility or lack of control over one's thoughts and feelings unwittingly contribute to the activation of dysfunctional cognitive structures in response to environmental threat or demand? In regard to the Gotlib and Cane study, the positive and negative words chosen as primes bore an uncertain relation to subjects' own connotations of these constructs. Primes were derived from the positive and negative ends on a semantic differential task and, therefore, may have been located more distally in semantic space from subjects' idiosyncratic depressive or manic content. This could be one explanation for the failure of the priming manipulation. Questions such as these, and others, will continue to occupy researchers as they try to gauge the value of including construct activation procedures in depression research.

THE BEHAVIORAL HIGH-RISK PARADIGM

As we have noted, the behavioral high-risk paradigm employs a theoretically defined risk factor and selects people who, by virtue of possessing this risk factor, are assumed to be vulnerable to depression. Although a number of studies have used this paradigm, there are two predominant high-risk approaches that provide data on proximal cognitive vulnerability: the Temple–Wisconsin Vulnerability to Depression Project and the depressogenic personality—life stress congruency approach.

The Temple–Wisconsin Vulnerability to Depression Project

In Chapter 6 we briefly described this program of research, which examines cognitive vulnerability following from work on the hopelessness model of depression. The Temple–Wisconsin project represents one of the more comprehensive studies undertaken in this, or any, vulnerability domain. As we noted, this is an ambitious two-site longitudinal study that seeks to evaluate the etiological postulates of both the hopelessness model and Beck's theory of depression (Alloy & Abramson, 1996). The focus on the prediction of the onset of depression in a sample of first-year college students places this work in a different category than the work just reviewed, which spoke more to the issue of detecting an enduring vulnerability once individuals were no longer depressed (i.e., remission and priming strategies).

The design of this study follows two groups of subjects over time. One group is comprised of individuals who are identified as possessing negative inferential styles or negative self-schemas, and their outcomes are compared with subjects who do not show these cognitive characteristics. An additional aspect of this study is a measurement of life stress that will enable the investigators to study whether the interaction between the cognitive vulnerability and negative life events increases the probability of depression, especially in cases where the type of stress matches the subject's personality style. Compared with previous studies, this study should yield a more complete description of individuals who possess a cognitive vulnerability in terms of their personality features, familial rates of psychopathology, and history of certain developmental variables, such as sexual or physical abuse.

By assessing whether cognitively vulnerable individuals go on to develop depression at a higher rate than their nonvulnerable counterparts, this study will offer one of the strongest tests of the predictive power of cognitive styles. At this point, however, very few data bear on this issue because the study is still in progress. In a preliminary report, Alloy, Abramson, Murray, Whitehouse, and Hogan (in press) have reported on differences in self-referent information processing between subjects who are cognitively vulnerable and those who are not. Subjects classified as being at high or low risk for depression based on their cognitive styles were asked to complete a number of measures of self-referent information processing. The prediction was that the nondepressed, but high-risk subjects would show greater processing of negatively valenced material. This was partially borne out. Relative to the low-risk group, high-risk subjects processed negative self-referent information more fully than positive self-referent information. This effect was found on measures that tapped into more effortful processing, such as ratings or judgments, but was not obtained when the measures reflected more automatic influences (e.g., recall intrusions and recognition errors). Although these data are consistent with the notion that high cognitively vulnerable subjects resemble depressed patients, but are not currently symptomatic, we must await the data from the longitudinal portion of the study before any firm conclusions can be reached about how much this vulnerability actually contributes to the onset of clinical depression.

Congruency between Personality and Life Stress, and Vulnerability to Depression

A different conceptual and operational definition of high risk stems from research seeking to match the occurrence of key life events with specific sensitivities. It has long been recognized that the occurrence of stressful events in a person's life increases chances of suffering from depression (Brown & Harris, 1978). However, this finding, although reliable, has rarely exceeded a small-to-moderate effect size. In an effort to augment its predictive power, the strategy of examining whether specific types of interactions between life stress and personality factors are more likely to result in depression has been advocated by some researchers. Framed within a congruence model, the predictions from this work are that life stress whose content matches the personality characteristics of the individual will be more detrimental than life stress that does not match a person's personal concerns. An example of this would be someone who is very dependent on the approval of others for her self-esteem being more likely to develop depression in response to being rejected by a boyfriend than to receiving a substandard grade in a class.

As more studies have been conducted to test the congruency hypothesis, the evidence in support of this formulation has mounted (e.g., Hammen et al., 1985; C. J. Robins, 1990; Segal et al., 1992). This has led to refinements in both the classification of life stressors and the matching personality styles that would most likely be impacted by these events. In general, two personality types have been identified, one that relies on interpersonal relationships to bolster self worth (sociotropy or dependency) and one that uses the achievement of internal goals or standards to maintain positive self-regard (autonomy or self-criticism; Beck, 1983; Blatt et al., 1982).

Zuroff and Mongrain (1987) outlined the possible relevance of this work for the study of cognitive vulnerability by suggesting that personality can be conceived of as a cognitive style variable and that sociotropy–dependency or autonomy–self-criticism describe cognitive styles that leave people vulnerable to depression. As in the priming work reviewed earlier, the likelihood of observing depressive responses is enhanced following the activation of a cognitive–affective structure or schema that is thought to be related to depression production (Beck et al., 1979; Segal, 1988). Congruent life stress functions as the trigger in this model. Once activated, this cognitive structure and its attendant biases could account for the way in which a competing depressive sense of self exerts an increasingly intrusive influence on information processing and consequent affective regulation.

In reviewing congruency findings from 24 studies, Nietzel and Harris (1990) concluded that the evidence is clearly in favor of matching personality variables and events as placing individuals at greater risk for depression than nonmatching with events of similar severity. They also found that certain types of matches were especially pernicious, so that the combination of elevated sociotropy–dependency interacting with negative social events led to greater depression than an autonomy–self-criticism match or the other two mismatches (e.g., sociotropy–self-criticism). Coyne and Whiffen (1995), in their more recent appraisal of this literature, acknowledge the greater predictive power of personality by life stress matches over mismatches, but are far more skeptical about the relevance of this model to the study of depression vulnerability. We suggest, however, that these findings are clearly supportive of cognitive models of depression that place the proximal cognitive onus on the activation of individuals' meaning and need structures.

SUMMARY AND CONCLUSIONS

In this chapter we have explored some of the ways in which vulnerability to depression can be activated by events happening relatively close in time to episode onset, that is, proximal cognitive vulnerability. One of the central issues in this area has been whether cognitive theories of vulnerability have been adequately tested. More to the point, when tests of cognitive vulnerability models have been conducted in the context of ensuring activation of latent cognitive variables, the findings have generally been consistent with cognitive models, whereas this is not the case for earlier studies in which activation strategies were not featured. Other paradigms for studying cognitive vulnerability, which employ the high-risk paradigm and are informed by the hopelessness model of depression and the personality literature, were also examined. In both cases, support was found for the notion that specific patterns of thinking can lead to depressed mood in persons who are predisposed by virtue of a preexisting explanatory style or an overly conditional view of self-worth. We now turn to an examination of how variables more removed in time contribute to the development of cognitive vulnerability to depression. In particular, in the next chapter we focus on methodological issues and in Chapter 9 we review theory and data as they pertain to the study of distal vulnerability.

CHAPTER 8

Methodological Strategies and Issues in the Study of Distal Vulnerability

In Chapter 6 we examined research strategies for investigating vulnerability from a proximal perspective. In this chapter we turn to methodological issues and research strategies that are relevant to the assessment of the distal components of vulnerability to depression. Recall from our discussion in Chapter 5 that vulnerability can be viewed on a continuum, with the earliest aspects of vulnerability at the distal end of the continuum and the most immediate precipitants of depression on the proximal end. Even though there are potentially many elements of vulnerability at varying points along this continuum, our focus on distal vulnerability tends toward those vulnerability patterns that develop early in life. As such, these early patterns reflect the developmentally determined cognitive antecedents of adult depression. Accordingly, many (although not all) research paradigms relevant to distal vulnerability in this particular context focus on the examination of potential depression vulnerability factors in childhood.

Because the focus of this book is on cognitive vulnerability to depression in adults, before we discuss these strategies, a brief comment is required by the fact many of these strategies are intended to assess variables that are linked to the development of depression prior to adulthood (i.e., the onset of depression during childhood or adolescence). Even though targeted toward children or adolescents in their original design, we believe that many of these designs also offer important opportunities for assessing variables related to vulnerability to depression that occurs later in life. Whether or not there is any continuity in the kinds and quality of childhood depression and adult depression (see Rutter, 1986b), little doubt exists that children who are depressed are at risk for depression as a adults. Thus, much can be gained from examining data on cognition and depression in children, and, correspondingly, those paradigms that are useful for gathering data on these processes, even if the goal is to understand depression in adults.

A variety of distal research designs have been used by investigators, several of which are aimed at assessing functioning in children. To begin our discussion of these designs, we first examine high-risk designs. For the purpose of examining distal vulnerability, high-risk designs can be divided into the more common high-risk offspring design and the quite uncommon high-risk parental design. We next examine the various longitudinal approaches and cross-sequential designs. We conclude with a discussion of retrospective designs, and a subcategory of these designs, experimental retrospective strategies. As in Chapter 6, we again only comment on issues of basic research design as they pertain to methodological strategies that are particular to distal vulnerability research. The advantages and disadvantages of both proximal and distal designs are summarized in Table 8.1.

THE HIGH-RISK PARADIGM: OFFSPRING DESIGNS

Studying the offspring of individuals possessing a disorder is an established research strategy that dates to the very first investigations of vulnerability to psychopathology, specifically vulnerability to schizophrenia. As we noted in Chapter 4, studies by Mednick and Schulsinger (1968) and Kety et al. (1968) investigating the offspring of Danish schizophrenic mothers established this strategy as a way to begin to understand the transmission of the factors that potentially render individuals vulnerable to the disorder. A number of schizophrenia vulnerability studies have employed this strategy; among the most well known high-risk offspring studies are the Stony Brook High-Risk Study (Weintraub, 1987), the Minnesota High-Risk Study (Garmezy & Devine, 1984; Rolf, 1972), and the St. Louis High-Risk Study (Worland, Janes, Anthony, McGinnis, & Cass, 1984).

Offspring of parents with a disorder can be studied for many reasons. A critical assumption underlying this strategy as it applies to the study of vulnerability is that offspring can be viewed as at increased

TABLE 8.1. Summary of Vulnerability Research Designs' Advantages and Disadvantages

Design	Assessment domain	Advantages	Disadvantages
Cross-sectional	Primarily proximal	Provides data on functioning within the depressed state May provide clues to variables operating in depression onset or maintenance	Unable to differentiate between causal variables, consequential variables, or third-variable causality Cannot asses stability of variables
Remission	Proximal or distal	Provides data on post-psychopathological state Able to assess the stability of variables that remain accessed	Unable to assess the stability of latent variables Does not parallel the complexity of diathesis–stress models
Priming	Proximal or distal	Combines the advantages of cross-sectional and remission designs Better able to model the complexity of diathesis–stress hypothesis; can be used to assess latent variables	When used with remission design, unable to distinguish between causal versus "scar" variables
High-risk offspring	Primarily distal	Selection of high-risk children allows for testing of some theoretical variables May assess important developmental variables	Unable to provide data on adult depression processes unless long-term longitudinal assessment is included Typically cross-sectional
Retrospective	Primarily distal	Can provide data on the relationship proximal and distal variables Less time and economic intensity than longitudinal designs	Includes all the limitations of self-report assessment; plus self-reported assessment of past events
Longitudinal	Distal or proximal	Overcomes limitations of many other designs Can assess temporal antecedence Allows for precise timing of assessments Can assess true distal antecedents of adult depression	Extremely complex Time and expense are prohibitive Provides data on correlates of depression, but assessment of causal variables can still be problematic May create reactive assessment
Cross-sequential	Distal or proximal	Combines the advantages of longitudinal and cross-sectional designs and thus allows numerous questions to be tested	Same as for longitudinal designs

risk for developing a disorder similar to that of one or both of their parents. Thus, the offspring of depressed parents should possess the vulnerability factors that make them more likely to develop depression and thus careful study of the functioning of these offspring may lead to clues about vulnerability mechanisms. However, beyond assessing increased risk factors for the development of a specific disorder, offspring designs are also capable of providing a wealth of other data. For instance, even when the interest is in a particular disorder such as depression, this paradigm can also assess whether those offspring who do not emerge with the disorder will experience disruptive events that place them at risk for some other manner of psychological distress, social difficulties (e.g., impaired peer relationships and social support networks), academic dysfunction (e.g., poor school performance), or vocational difficulties.

Methodological Issues

A number of considerations are essential to the conduct of well-executed offspring designs. Some of these represent variations on basic research principles whereas others are relatively unique to this kind of approach to vulnerability. Hammen (1991a, 1995) has outlined a number of these considerations in her superb work on the social context of risk in children of depressed mothers. We summarize these here.

Diagnostic and Demographic Status

The diagnostic and demographic status of both depressed parents and their children represent important considerations in how effectively offspring studies will be able to provide data on the correlates of depression vulnerability in children and, correspondingly, on the correlates of depression when these children have become adults.

Parental Status. It is important for investigators who seek to assess the offspring of depressed parents to provide an explicit description of how depression in parents is defined and to demonstrate reliable procedures that empirically operationalize this definition. As we have noted in discussion in previous chapters, such definitions frequently rely on adherence to DSM criteria. DSM requirements for diagnosis allow for not only inclusion but also exclusion of cases (e.g., bipolar disorder, schizophrenia, etc.), using relatively explicit and reliable criteria.

Depending on the particular question of interest, explicit operational definitions also allow for the inclusion of comparison groups. As we noted earlier, for example, several of the offspring studies assessing schizophrenia vulnerability have used the offspring of depressed parents as controls. Conversely, the offspring of schizophrenic individuals would be an appropriate control group for some studies of depression vulnerability, as would the offspring of individuals with other disorders. For example, Scher and Ingram (1998) employed children of alcoholic parents as a control group to investigate vulnerability in the offspring of depressed individuals. In other cases, comparison groups may consist of individuals without psychopathology but that control for other factors. To control for variables such as hospitalization and family disruption, for instance, Hammen (1991a) employed the offspring of medically ill patients as a control group for the offspring of depressed mothers.

In sum, whatever operational definition of depression is used, it must be explicit enough to allow for comparisons between studies. It must also be explicit enough to minimize overlap in diagnostic status. Given the comorbidity between depression and other problems such as anxiety disorders, explicit operational definitions help to ensure that psychopathology control groups do not evidence sufficient depressive symptomatology to confound comparisons with the depression target group.

The demographic and psychological characteristics of parent samples are also important to assess explicitly. As Hammen (1991a) notes, many studies lump together mothers and fathers without reporting which (or if both) parent(s) meet the depression criteria that have been specified. Whether a father versus a mother is affected may significantly influence vulnerability to offspring developing depression (see Phares & Compas, 1992; Phares, 1996). Similarly, if both parents are depressed, the chances of being vulnerable to depression may be considerably enhanced, akin to an additive, or perhaps even multiplicative, effect. Alternatively, if one parent is depressed while the other suffers from another disorder, the chance of becoming vulnerable to depression or some other psychopathology may be enhanced relative to having one healthy parent. Comorbidity with depression is also a serious issue to be addressed in offspring studies. For instance, a depressed parent who also evidences a personality disorder may differ in the likelihood of producing depressed offspring than a depressed parent without a personality disorder. In this same vein, other psychiatric characteristics are important to examine in offspring studies such as the severity of the disorder, acute versus chronic disorder, past psychiatric history, and so on. Such characteristics may interact significantly with the development of vulnerability to depression in offspring.

In a similar fashion, more typical demographic characteristics such as parents' age, socioeconomic status, education level, and ethnicity may also serve as important correlates of the development of vulnerability. Hammen (1991a) appropriately recommends that either separate homogeneous samples be studied to begin to tease out whether such factors are important, or that large enough heterogeneous samples be studied so that subgroups with differing characteristics can be examined. Given the multitude of variables that may affect the likelihood of offspring becoming vulnerable to depression, for the foreseeable future homogeneous samples will probably be more logistically feasible.

Offspring Status. The same precision and clarity that are needed for adequate assessment of parents in offspring studies are also needed for children. For example, to the extent that diagnostic status is important to these studies, operational definitions and criteria for their diagnostic status must be specified. As with parents, the demographic and psychological characteristics (e.g., age, sex, ethnicity, severity of problems, etc.) are also important to consider in offspring. This is especially important because such characteristics may be correlated with developmental characteristics that interact with other variables. More generally, interaction between the characteristics of parents and the characteristics of their children in these studies may provide important clues as to the development of vulnerability.

Assessment of Mediational Variables for Both Parents and Children

Although demographic and diagnostic status in offspring studies can provide important information, this information is limited in its power to elucidate causal relationships. That is, although quite important for descriptive purposes, such data are generally only able to provide information about the correlates of vulnerability, but not the actual mechanisms of vulnerability. Demonstrating, for example, that the offspring of depressed mothers are more likely to exhibit depression does little, in and of itself, to reveal why this is the case. This is true even if a particular causal theory predicts that offspring will be at increased risk for the disorder for a given set of reasons. For example, genetic theories predict that offspring would be more likely to develop depression because of the transmission of genetic vulnerability factors. However, the mere fact that offspring are more likely to experience depression does not tell us what the genetic mechanism is, or even if a given genetic mechanism rather than some correlated variable (e.g., another undiscovered gene, dysfunctional communication patterns between disordered parent and child, etc.) is causally implicated. Likewise, even though some cognitive theories might predict that offspring will be vulnerable to depression by virtue of learned cognitive patterns, the fact that offspring are more likely to become depressed does not in itself validate these theories.

Additional strategies and variables are therefore necessary to examine mediating factors within the context of offspring designs and to thus ferret out the possible mechanisms of vulnerability to depression. Using again the example of genetic variables, researchers interested in this level of analysis can extend offspring studies to assess different concordance rates for depression in monozygotic versus dizygotic twin offspring (e.g., Torgerson, 1986). Given the different degrees of genetic overlap between these types of twins, inferences can then be made as to the degree of involvement of genetic factors. Supplemental genetic strategies to assess mediational variables are also available. For instance, to separate genetic from environmental causal factors further, investigators can compare offspring who are reared apart to those who are reared together (Bouchard, Lykken, McGue, Segal, & Tellegen, 1990). Such approaches to offspring studies are necessary so as to move beyond merely observing correlates of depression to begin to discover mediating, and hence actual, vulnerability mechanisms.

Because of the importance of truly establishing vulnerability mechanisms, depression offspring studies should carefully consider including the assessment of cognitive mediating variables that might be hypothesized to provide the crucial links between offspring and cognitive vulnerability. To the extent that investigators are interested in schema-driven processes, for instance, the inclusion of variables believed to assess the presence of depressotypic (or -genic) schemas of both parents and children would be a crucial dimension of these studies. Likewise, investigators interested in attributional tendencies would need to include measures of such tendencies. Hence, some measure is necessary of whatever the proposed cognitive mediating variables might be. Cognitive investigators cannot assume that cognitive mechanisms are necessarily involved simply because the offspring of depressed parents are more likely to develop depression than are the offspring of nondepressed parents: Explicit cognitive assessment is necessary.

Advantages and Limitations

Offspring studies have the clear advantage of allowing for the assessment of vulnerability processes from a very early point in individuals' developmental history. To the extent that this history is important, as many investigators strongly suggest that it is (Dodge, 1993), then assessment of these historical factors provides a crucial opportunity to begin to understand vulnerability. More specifically, the careful and thoughtful inclusion of mediating variables allows for the opportunity to gain a glimpse of some potential causally relevant mechanisms. Thus, to be truly informative, assessing the adult–child interactions and behavioral patterns that may create vulnerability processes regardless of parent diagnostic status per se is important. Indeed, the call for assessing mediational variables (e.g., Hammen, 1991a) addresses precisely this issue. The fact that offspring designs allow investigators to assess mediational variables in an at-risk sample is a clear advantage.

Some of the limitations of this approach for assessing distal vulnerability are determined by the age range of the vulnerable people in which investigators are interested. As we noted previously, many designs that are useful for understanding distal vulnerability emanate from research paradigms that are intended to study childhood depression factors. Considerably fewer limitations of this design are inherent for investigators who seek to understand childhood depression; investigators are able to select vulnerable subjects in an age range that corresponds to their level of interest. Because the age of the depression vulnerability that is studied is closer to the ultimate target of interest (depression in children and perhaps adolescents), offspring studies may yield important clues about causal variables at this stage in life.

Certainly such clues are important. However, for investigators interested in the distal vulnerability factors that lead to adult depression, this design may offer considerably more limited utility. Because offspring studies are typically cross-sectional, they are unable to take into account the almost certain reality that vulnerability processes occurring early in life as the result of depressed parents are affected by developmental and social processes that occur as children mature into adults. This is also true even for offspring studies that seek to study the adult offspring of depressed parents. Even though these vulnerable individuals are closer to the target age range for investigators interested in vulnerability to depression in adulthood, there is little way to account in a purely offspring design for the intervening influences that occur as individuals become adults. Thus, numerous modifying processes may take place in vulnerability factors as children progress from childhood to adulthood. To place knowledge obtained from offspring studies in a context that is valuable for understanding adult depression, these factors must be assessed over time. Thus, although offspring studies constitute a good starting point, to understand distal factors that operate in adult depression they must be combined with longitudinal research strategies.

Another potential limitation is that the sample chosen for offspring studies may be aberrant with regard to the factors that typically function in the disorder. For example, whereas the offspring of depressed parents are, in fact, at increased risk for depression and other psychological problems (Hammen, 1991a), certainly many people develop depression whose parents do not have diagnosable psychopathology. Gottesman and Shields (1972) note that the schizophrenia studies that pioneered the high-risk offspring approach also demonstrated that approximately 90% of individuals with schizophrenia do not have a schizophrenic parent. Hence, because offspring studies are by definition limited to studying samples of depressed parents and their children, important factors may be missed by not assessing nondepressed parents and their children who eventually become depressed. Some of these parents may suffer from other kinds of disorders (e.g., personality disorders, alcohol abuse, etc.), but many may not show any evidence of a psychiatric disorder at all.

PARENTAL DESIGNS

If the offspring design suggests that it is potentially informative to study the offspring of depressed parent, the reverse is also certainly true; that it is equally important to study the parents of depressed offspring. Of course, the same methodological considerations that apply to offspring designs apply to parental designs (e.g., careful consideration of not only the descriptive characteristics of depressed children and their parents, but also the assessment of theoretically determined mediational variables for both children and their parents).

The value of the high-risk parental approach can perhaps best be considered within the context of comparisons to offspring designs, although it is important to note that advocating the importance of such designs is not intended to suggest that studies of depressed parents' offspring are unimportant. Indeed, such studies may provide important information as to the kinds of behaviors that place children at risk. Rather, the issue is that these behaviors also need to be studied in samples of nondepressed parents. For example, the interactions between depressed parents and their potentially depressed offspring and the interactions of nondepressed parents and their potentially depressed offspring may differ or be similar on important dimensions that provide clues as to why some children of depressed parents do not become depressed and why some children of nondepressed parents do become depressed. Relatedly, the "kind" of depression (e.g., symptom profile, underlying vulnerabilities, cognitive vs. noncognitive subtype, etc.) that is elicited by depressed parents may differ from the "kind" that may be linked to nondepressed parents. This recognizes the heterogeneity of what we call depression (see Chapter 5) and suggests the possibility that depression may have different causal pathways when linked to depressed versus nondepressed parents. Is it possible, for instance, that there is a larger genetic component in the depression suffered by the offspring of depressed parents? Answers to these questions will not be forthcoming until more heterogeneous parental characteristics and behavioral patterns (ranging from psychopathological to relatively healthy) are studied than is currently the case in studies that are limited to the offspring of depressed parents.

LONGITUDINAL DESIGNS

In Chapter 6 we discussed the fundamental methodological framework of longitudinal designs; studies that follow a cohort of individuals over time and assess relevant variables at various intervals. Such designs can be applied to study either proximal or distal factors. We noted in Chapter 6 that the length of longitudinal designs can vary considerably, but of theoretical and empirical necessity the time frame for longitudinal designs examining distal vulnerability factors will be longer than for studies aimed at assessing proximal factors. Despite these varying time frames, however, the fundamental aspects of these designs are virtually the same. Thus, the basic description of this strategy that we provided in Chapter 6 for proximal research is equally applicable to distal research. In this chapter we note some theoretical considerations that guide longitudinal designs, and then discuss some different types of longitudinal designs that can be applied to the study of distal cognitive vulnerability factors.

Before discussing theoretical considerations and different types of longitudinal designs, it is important to note that the methodological considerations that we discussed in reference to offspring designs apply equally to longitudinal designs. That is, explicit operational definitions and assessment of diagnostic, psychological, and demographic status of samples as well as the assessment of mediational variables are critical to consider if longitudinal designs are to yield useful distal vulnerability information. Depending on the conceptual questions, additional considerations will need to be taken into account such as developmental stages, ages, sex differences, and so on. For an excellent in-depth discussion of the issues to evaluate in conducting longitudinal research, readers are referred to the volume assembled by Rutter (1988).

Theoretical and Empirical Guiding Considerations

In principle, longitudinal research can be atheoretical. Hence, investigators interested in studying distal cognitive vulnerability can administer a large number of symptom and cognitive measures, follow an unselected group of subjects over time, and then determine which variables predict vulnerability to the occurrence of depressive symptomatology. Large-scale epidemiological studies tend to follow this strategy. Although there are also some examples of similar strategies by researchers investigating psychological processes, for most investigators a variety of factors make such a strategy impractical and too expensive to yield a sufficient number of participants who will eventually develop depression, thus, it is difficult to learn anything meaningful about the disorder. Instead, longitudinal research is typically theoretically and/or empirically driven.

Theoretical Considerations

Given the expense and logistical difficulties of atheoretical longitudinal research, theoretical considerations are frequently employed to help guide the choice of samples to be studied and measures to be used. To illustrate, to the extent that an investigator has a theoretical rationale to believe that child abuse leads to cognitive vulnerability and thus adult depression outcomes (Briere, 1992; Browne & Finkelhor, 1986), this rationale would suggest the kind of sample to be followed longitudinally and the choice of cognitive measures that would be used.

In Chapter 6 we discussed the Temple–Wisconsin Cognitive Vulnerability to Depression Project (Alloy & Abramson, 1990). We can also point to aspects of this project as an illustration of theoretically driven, partially distal cognitive vulnerability longitudinal design. Theoretical considerations in this design guide the choice of variables to be studied and thus go hand in hand with the choice of samples. For example, the theoretical framework of this project specifies the need to obtain measures of subjects' attributional tendencies. Given that we described this design in the chapter on proximal research, we should parenthetically note that, relative to distal vulnerability designs that address the developmental antecedents of vulnerability, this research is certainly closer to the proximal end of the vulnerability spectrum. Nevertheless, inasmuch as this project assesses vulnerability variables over a several-year period in individuals who may have had little previous experience with clinical depression, this study can also be regarded as a distal design. The fact that the classification of this design as proximal in some respects and distal in others illustrates the idea that distal and proximal represent only different endpoints on a continuum, with many research designs assessing variables that fall in between these extremes.

Empirical Guiding Considerations

Theoretical considerations are not the only factors that can guide the choice of samples and variables in longitudinal vulnerability designs. Even though not predicated on any existing theoretical basis, empirically observing a relationship between a variable and vulnerability to depressive symptomatology may provide important clues as to which samples and variables to study. For instance, the empirical observation that stress is linked to the onset of depression (see Monroe & Simons, 1991) constitutes sufficient reason in and of itself to study this in subsequent longitudinal research. In such a case, although perhaps desirable, a guiding theoretical framework is unnecessary for the construct of this research (although, once adequately documented, theories specifying the reasons *why* stress is linked to depression will eventually be needed).

Types of Longitudinal Designs

Several standard types of longitudinal designs can be employed to study distal vulnerability factors (for an extensive discussion of these longitudinal designs see Rutter, 1988). These designs consist of (1) prospective designs, (2) catch-up designs, (3) follow-back designs, and (4) register designs.

Prospective Designs

Prospective longitudinal designs identify samples and variables thought to be linked to vulnerability in individuals who are not yet depressed. Prior to the onset of depression, participants are then followed and assessed over some time period specified by the investigator based on theoretical and empirical considerations. The Temple–Wisconsin Cognitive Vulnerability to Depression Project represents an example of a prospective design to assess cognitive vulnerability. Prospective longitudinal designs are ideal for examining the temporal antecedents of variables that Garber and Hollon (1991) have argued to be important for demonstrating at least some types of causality.

Catch-Up Designs

Catch-up designs make use of data previously collected for another purpose to assess a given variable longitudinally. For instance, data potentially relevant to vulnerability that may have been collected when individuals in the sample were young can be examined at a later date to determine if these data predict depressive symptomatology. In Chapter 6 we briefly noted a longitudinal study reported by Zuroff et al. (1994). This study examined data from a study of 5-years-olds first reported by Sears, Maccoby, and Leven in 1957. When the sample was 12, data on self-criticism were collected and later, when the sample was 18 and 31, data were collected on interpersonal relationships, achievement, and general adjustment. Although data on depression have not been collected on this sample, a catch-up design would assess depression (both current and past) and determine whether any of the variables collected earlier, for different purposes, predicted later depression.

We are unaware of current cognitive studies of distal vulnerability to depression that specifically employ this approach. For the purposes of assessing cognitive vulnerability, researchers would need to identify data relevant to cognitive vulnerability collected when individuals were children or adolescents, and then locate (catch up with) these individuals to determine the existence of depressive symptomatology and the cognitive vulnerability patterns that presumably accompany this symptomatology. The study reported by Zuroff et al. (1994) is again an example of how this design could be implemented to assess distal cognitive vulnerability specifically. Given that self-criticism is a cognitive variable that has been proposed as a risk variable for depression (Blatt & Homann, 1992; Blatt et al., 1982; Blatt & Zuroff, 1992), if investigators caught up with this sample later and collected data on depression, then the question of whether this proposed cognitive vulnerability factor was in fact distally related to depression might be answered.

Although clearly preferable, even variables assessed from an earlier time that are not necessarily cognitive in nature may provide some information on cognitive vulnerability. For instance, some of the priming studies that we described in Chapter 7 could be considered a more proximal variant of the catch-up design; many of these studies identified individuals who had previously experienced a depressive episode that, according to extant cognitive models, presumably indicated a vulnerability to depression. By assessing these individuals sometime after the occurrence of the episode, these studies were to some degree "catching up" with the variables of interest. The difficulty with these studies from a catch-up design perspective, aside from the fact that they do not assess earlier cognitive variables, is that in many cases the data on past depression are obtained retrospectively rather than at an earlier time. Retrospective designs are discussed in a subsequent section of this chapter. We noted earlier that there can be considerable overlap among different types of designs. This example illustrates how boundaries between different designs (from distal to proximal and from longitudinal to nonlongitudinal) can blur substantially.

Follow-Back Designs

Follow-back designs represent the logical opposite of catch-up designs. These designs assess individuals on a particular variable and then look for data that may have been collected earlier that may help explain the variable. School records provide an illustration of data that may be used for such purposes. In the context of cognitive vulnerability to depression studies, these designs would identify a group of participants with depression and then look for relevant cognitive data that may have been collected earlier for other purposes but that may be associated with vulnerability.

Register Designs

More a mechanism than a strategy, registries are still relevant for longitudinal designs. Register designs rely on registries of relevant information to assess longitudinal questions. The high-risk studies described in Chapter 4 using Denmark's National Psychiatric Register and the Folkeregister (Kety et al., 1968; Mednick & Schulsinger, 1968; Rosenthal et al., 1968) represent an example of this approach. Thus, if an investigator wishes to assess the offspring of depressed individuals to search for cognitive vulnerability factors, a register (if available) would help locate these offspring. Once located they can be assessed using one of the longitudinal designs previously discussed.

Advantages and Limitations

The advantages of longitudinal designs for studying cognitive vulnerability are considerable. For example, the ability to demonstrate the necessary prerequisite of temporal antecedence (Garber & Hollon, 1991) for determining vulnerability and causality is a fundamental aspect of many longitudinal designs, particularly prospective designs. As such, to the extent that temporal antecedence can be demonstrated and shown to be correlated with study variables, such designs can provide powerful inferences as to the vulnerability, and hence potentially causal, mechanisms of depression. Such designs, again particularly prospective designs, also allow for the relatively precise timing of the assessment of critical events and of variables that coincide with these events and subsequently play a role in the development of vulnerability to depression. Longitudinal designs also allow for the analysis of subgroups (e.g., groups who do and do not develop depression) and the variables such as cognitive vulnerability that potentially differentiate these groups. Finally and most generally, longitudinal studies represent the only designs truly able to tap distal vulnerability that take into account vulnerable individuals' developmental histories.

From a purely theoretical or empirical perspective, the limitations of longitudinal studies are few. One potential empirical problem, however, may result from subjects being tested on more than one occasion (particularly in prospective designs), raising the possibility that repeated testing will alter subsequent test results by creating reactive assessment (see Kazdin, 1992). Unfortunately, from a practical point of view the limitations of longitudinal designs can be substantial. Given the inevitable complexity of issues to be addressed over some period of time, longitudinal vulnerability designs are difficult to conduct adequately. To justify the time and effort required to construct a longitudinal vulnerability study, considerable care is needed to ensure adequate representation of key variables in the study. The difficulty of this task is likely to be exponentially magnified by the length of the study period and the fact that these variables may change over time.

Another practical limitation is that longitudinal designs are, by definition, time consuming and thus apt to be expensive in terms of both resource and labor requirements. This is the case even when data have been previously collected as in catch-up designs; locating individuals from whom data have previously been collected can be an extremely difficult task. Longitudinal designs are also vulnerable to problems in the collection of data, such as high drop out rates for research participants. In turn, such problems raise issues regarding the treatment of data and the interpretation of results. Such designs are thus not for the faint of heart, researchers without adequate funding, or the untenured.

CROSS-SEQUENTIAL DESIGNS

Cross-sequential designs emanate from developmental psychology research and were thus developed with the idea of assessing developmental changes over time (Vasta, Haith, & Miller, 1992). In structure, cross-sequential research designs reflect a combination of cross-sectional and longitudinal designs. As in cross-sectional designs, different groups or cohorts are selected for study. As in longitudinal designs, these different cohorts are followed over some specified period of time. A variety of different comparisons are possible from this design. To illustrate a classic developmental cross-sequential design, for instance, groups of 2-year-olds might be studied along with groups of 4- and 6-year-olds. As illustrated in Figure 8.1, three types of comparisons can be made. First are the typical cross-sectional comparisons; 2-year-olds would be compared to 4-year-olds and 6-year-olds, and 4-year-olds compared to 6-year-olds. Second, longitudinal comparisons can also be done; each cohort can be studied after a specified interval. Thus, the changes that have occurred in the 6-year-old group after 2 years (now 8-year-olds) can be evaluated. Third, and unique to this design, cross-sectional/longitudinal comparisons can also be done. For example, after 2 years the original 4-year-old cohort can now be compared with the original 2-year-old cohort (now 4-year-olds). In theory there is no limit as to the number of cohorts that can be studied, although practical constraints

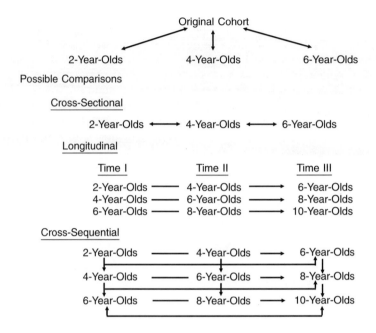

FIGURE 8.1. Comparisons possible using cross-sectional, longitudinal, and cross-sequential designs. Cross-sequential designs combine and extend the comparisons that are possible using either a cross-sectional or a longitudinal design.

will reduce this to a number that the investigators deem not only as theoretically important, but also as practically manageable.

As with some of the longitudinal designs (e.g., catch-up designs), we are unaware of cross-sequential designs that have assessed cognitive vulnerability to adult depression. The daunting and time-consuming task of conducting a cross-sequential study of sufficient length to track distal cognitive variables into adulthood appears quite likely to be responsible for the lack of such data.

Advantages and Limitations

Cross-sequential designs compensate nicely for many of the design limitations of cross-sectional studies. In the case of offspring designs, for example, recall that we noted that many of these studies are cross-sectional and therefore unable to account for how vulnerability processes related to depressed parents are affected by the intervening developmental and social influences that occur over the period of time during which children become adults. In principle, cross-sequential designs allow investigators to track changes over time in the different-age offspring cohorts of depressed parents and to track corresponding changes in cognitive processes.

Most generally, a well-designed cross-sequential study of cognitive vulnerability provides a powerful method for beginning to understand critical aspects of cognition as it pertains to the development of depression. Thus, cross-sequential designs provide a potent technique for tracking cognitive changes over time, determining if some of these changes are associated with later depression, and/or assessing whether cognitive variables that become prominent at certain times in the developmental process are related to vulnerability and, hence, depression.

Cross-sequential designs provide the opportunity to evaluate not only conceptual questions of interest to investigators, but also methodological questions. For instance, cross-sequential designs allow investigators to determine if observed variables are an artifact of the particular group of subjects being studied. Consider two groups of 15-year-old subjects in a 5-year longitudinal study, one assessed when they entered the study at age 15 and one that was initially 10 and was assessed 5 years later. Meaningful differences in the data from the two 15-year-old groups would suggest evidence of a cohort effect, which could not be detected in cross-sectional, longitudinal, or retrospective designs. Because potential cohort effects can be assessed in a cross-sequential design, this design has a unique advantage for answering some questions. Similarly, cross-sequential designs can be used to assess whether subjects are affected by repeated testings, an issue that cannot be readily resolved in longitudinal designs.

As with longitudinal designs, the limitations of cross-sequential designs stem not so much from theoretical or methodological sources, but from practical considerations such as the amount of time necessary to track meaningful processes. Although true for developmental psychopathology studies, this problem is significantly exacerbated for studies seeking to assess adult cognitive vulnerability; that is, as the time frame for cross-sequential studies lengthens, as it inevitably will for studies assessing distal cognitive vulnerability, the practical limitations will be magnified.

RETROSPECTIVE DESIGNS

Retrospective designs seek to understand the influence of distal cognitive vulnerability factors by examining the later recall of information about times in the past when these factors were thought to be operating. In adult depression, this entails asking individuals to recall certain earlier events (from childhood or perhaps adolescence) that the investigator hypothesizes are related to cognitive vulnerability to depression. Presumably the individuals who are asked to recall these events are those that are currently depressed (and who possess some vulnerability) or, if not depressed, are determined by some other means to be vulnerable to depression. To the extent that information about these possible distal vulnerability factors can be adequately and reliably gathered, they provide a potentially critical means for understanding the impact of these variables on adult depression. Hence, for example, the recall of traumatic events (e.g., abuse; Kuyken & Brewin, 1995; Rose & Abramson, 1995) proposed to be linked to cognitive vulnerability may be sought as a way to understand the effects of these events on factors that are related to the subsequent development of depression in adults. Similarly, if certain parenting behaviors are proposed to be linked to depression vulnerability, then recall of these behaviors would be assessed in retrospective studies (Brewin, Firth-Cozens, Furnham, & McManus, 1992; Gerlsma, Emmelkamp, & Arrindell, 1990; Kuyken & Brewin, 1995). In the arena of cognitive vulnerability, of course, the focus of retrospective studies must necessarily be on examining the recall of earlier factors that are thought to be linked to the development of cognitive variables that are related to depression.

Retrospective designs may also help understand the link between distal vulnerability factors and more proximal factors. For instance, retrospective research reported by Brewin et al. (1992) examined the association between recalled dysfunctional parenting (a factor potentially related to distal vulnerability) and excessive self-criticism as an adult (a potential proximal cognitive risk factor). Because distal vulnerability represents the foundation from which proximal vulnerability must be developed, assessing the relationship between distal and proximal vulnerability is key to any genuine understanding of how people become depressed.

Experimental Retrospective Designs

A subset of retrospective designs can be categorized as experimental retrospective designs. Whereas the typical retrospective design aims to examine vulnerability factors by examining the recall of early experiences by (typically) depressed individuals, experimental retrospective designs can impose experimental conditions to examine somewhat different aspects of presumed distal vulnerability. These experimental conditions thus far have pertained to priming paradigms, although other conditions are possible.

Priming: Past Depression and Putative Vulnerability Factors

As we noted in our discussion of priming methodologies in Chapters 6 and 7, priming paradigms seek to examine under theory-specified conditions the resurgence of potentially depressogenic cognitive processes. We also noted in these chapters that as they have typically been conducted (e.g., studying individuals with a past history of depression), priming studies share some characteristics with distal designs. However, the extant parameters of the priming approach allow for an even more explicit focus on distal vulnerability. Several variations are possible.

Primed Recall of Distal Vulnerability Features. Cognitively oriented priming designs typically assess depressotypic thinking following the priming task. Depressotypic thinking is not the only type of dependent variable possible; such designs also permit assessment of the recall of possible distal vulnerability factors. For instance, disrupted bonding experiences with parents have been hypothesized to serve as a vulnerability factor for depression (see Chapters 9 and 10). However, it is possible that such disrupted patterns may be difficult to detect for vulnerable individuals who are not currently depressed, and, therefore, examination of such recollections under priming conditions may represent a way to assess the presence of vulnerability-inducing interactions, if they exist. Put simply, vulnerable individuals who have been primed may be more able to recall these disrupted interactions. Of course, this procedure runs the risk of inducing biased recollections, particularly if the priming condition is one of an induced negative mood (a general risk that will be discussed in the section on advantages and limitations). Nevertheless, in principle such a procedure at least has the potential to generate data that might not otherwise be available.

Theoretically Defined, Retrospectively Assessed Priming Approaches. As we noted in Chapter 6, although studies of vulnerability have frequently operationalized vulnerability by virtue of a past depressive episode, other operational definitions are possible. One example of an alternative operationalization consists of a theoretically defined high-risk group. We noted the examples of attachment, dependency and self-criticism, parental bonding patterns, and sociotropy–autonomy as theoretically defined high-risk factors for depression. From a distal point of view, several of these constructs must be assessed through retrospective reports (e.g., recollections of past bonding experiences). Once assessed, these variables may become important elements in a priming paradigm. Thus, for example, if disrupted attachment (retrospectively assessed) is the variable of interest, priming may be employed to examine whether the kind of cognitive processes that have been hypothesized to be linked to depression, which are not apparent in the nondepressed state, become evident in individuals with disrupted bonding once they have been primed. In essence, this strategy employs the same priming experimental tactics, but assesses a theoretically defined group of individuals rather than a group who are deemed vulnerable because they have been depressed in the past.

Retrospectively Assessed Mediational Variables. Whether empirically derived (e.g., past depression history) or theoretically defined (e.g., disruptions in attachment patterns), risk variables are rarely mutually exclusive. Consequently, the assessment of more than one risk variable allows for not only mediational analyses but also for a more precise cognitive risk analysis. For instance, when a past episode of depression constitutes the operational definition of vulnerability, other vulnerability variables may also be assessed to determine whether they might mediate depressotypic cognitions in response to a priming induction. Hence, investigators interested in past bonding disruptions would retrospectively assess this variable *in addition* to previous depression history and determine whether the bonding variable accounted for any variance in the cognitive responses of previously depressed research participants after they were primed. If such bonding did mediate depressotypic cognitive responses (e.g., those with poor bonding evidenced the most negative cognitions), then this would provide evidence for poor bonding as a distal vulnerability factor.

Theoretical Considerations

As with all of the designs we have discussed in this chapter, the choice of distal experiences to be examined is a function of the theoretical framework from which the investigator is operating. For instance, theorists interested in examining the role of attachment experiences on cognitive vulnerability to adult depression (e.g., Bowlby, 1973, 1980) will seek to assess recollections of the quality of parental care as it pertains to attachment patterns between the subject as a child and his or her parents. Likewise, investigators interested in specific kinds of traumatic experiences such as sexual or physical abuse (e.g., Miller, 1983) would seek to assess recollection of these distal variables and then assess the relationship of recalled experiences to later depression. Of course, in addition to these theoretical considerations, the importance of choosing adequate measures and samples applies just as much to retrospective designs as it does to the other types of designs that we have discussed in this chapter. These will be guided by the cognitive constructs the investigator wishes to examine.

Advantages and Limitations

A clear advantage of retrospective designs is that they provide access to an abundance of data on early experiences that may constitute distal vulnerability factors. Moreover, they do so without the expense and practical difficulties involved in conducting longitudinal research. However, although potentially providing a wealth of such information, these designs are also vulnerable to criticisms that retrospective reports are likely to be unreliable and thus invalid. Brewin, Andrews, and Gotlib (1993) have provided an detailed review of these concerns. They classify concerns over memory reliability into three categories: normal limitations in memory, memory deficits associated with psychopathology, and mood-congruent memory processes. According to Brewin et al. (1993), concerns over normal limitations in memory suggest that memory for such distal events is likely to be unreliable because of the passage of time and is thus not valid. Adding to this possible problem, concerns with memory deficits linked to psychopathology suggest that disordered states in particular interfere with accurate memory processes. This may lead to false conclusions. For example, a depressed adult may look to his or her childhood to explain current troubles and, thus, be motivated to "remember" poor parenting. Finally, research on memory processes in depression finds that depressed people are inclined to remember events whose affective connotations are consistent with their current mood state. This may lead to a biasing of memories for events in a more negative direction than as the events actually occurred, or increased remembering of negative events for depressed versus nondepressed individuals, even if the occurrences were similar.

Based on an extensive review of research, Brewin et al. (1993) argue that data generally do not substantiate these concerns. For example, although changes in memory do take place over time, data suggest that individuals have fairly good recall of salient facts, which in turn contributes to relatively good recall of the general aspects of events. Additionally, research does not suggest actual memory deficits in depressed people so much as that depressed individuals may not exhibit much effort to recall events. Finally, research reveals that fluctuations in the mood or diagnostic status of depressed people do not appear to affect the consistency of their reports of childhood experiences.

Although these data suggest that retrospective reports can be accurate, it is unlikely that these reports will ever be completely free of such problems. Accordingly, Brewin et al. (1993) offer several suggestions to strengthen the validity of these data sources. For instance, they suggest that supplementing retrospective reports with information from other informants can lead to a more valid picture of childhood events. Citing data that parents' accounts of events are almost always more positive than children's, they caution against parents serving as these other informants. Although not problem-free, siblings may provide a better informant group, ideally from same-sexed, similar-aged siblings. Depending on the vulnerability question that is being asked and availability, independent records obtained by outside sources may also provide a reliable account of childhood circumstances; note that this represents the follow-back design that we previously discussed. Brewin et al. (1993) also suggest that carefully structuring the manner in which recall is assessed can improve the validity of these reports. Structured or semistructured interview methods allow investigators to elicit information that may clarify the validity of memories.

To assess cognitive vulnerability, of course, these design considerations must be combined with valid and reliable cognitive measures, which will be easiest to obtain for currently depressed (or vulnerable) individuals. Equally or perhaps even more important, however, are cognitive variables that are retrospectively reported; for example, recall of the types or content of thoughts individuals had at an earlier age. Although the reliability and validity of such measures will be harder to achieve, they may still provide very informative data on distal vulnerability factors.

While offering much potential, retrospective reports as a vulnerability design present problems that are in some respects mirror images of the problems of offspring studies. That is, whereas offspring studies narrow their focus to the depression that may result from having a depressed parentretrospective studies, by virtue of starting with a groups of adults who have been identified as depressed (or vulnerable to depression), narrow their focus to behaviors that are associated with these depressed or vulnerable individuals. Whether these recalled behaviors also result in normal adult functioning cannot be assessed. That is, if groups of never depressed individuals were studied, similar results might be found. This is true even when a normal control group is also used; even though the behavioral patterns may be different between depressed and normal controls, this does not assure researchers that other nondisordered people did not have experiences similar to the depressed subjects.

In a closely related fashion, it is difficult to determine the specificity of these behaviors to depression; that is, whether they are specifically associated with depression or are also related to other psychopathologies. This is the case even if psychopathology control groups are used. As we noted in Chapter 6, the heterogeneous nature of most psychiatric control groups does not allow us to conclude that a variable is specific to depression, even if it does not characterize the psychopathology group. Rather, at most what can be concluded is that the variable does not seem to characterize generalized disturbance. To suggest that the occurrence of certain recalled behaviors is linked primarily to depression, psychiatric control groups ruling out specific alternative disorders (e.g., anxiety) must be used.

GENERAL METHODOLOGICAL ISSUES

Many of the methodological concerns addressed in our discussion of proximal vulnerability research designs apply equally to distal designs. Of prime importance are issues of establishing the actual mechanisms of vulnerability, that is, causality; as with many proximal designs, although distal research strategies may inform us about the cognitive correlates of depression, genuine cognitive causality must still be established. As advocates of longitudinal research have cautioned, these designs, although potentially quite powerful for providing data on risk *indicators,* do not necessarily inform us about risk *mechanisms* (Rutter, 1988). Likewise for offspring studies, questions of causality are extremely difficult to address; even if a strong relationship can be shown between variables related to both maternal and offspring depression, in the absence of other information, this tells us little about how the vulnerability operates. Thus, for instance, even though researchers testing explicit theoretical predictions and using well-established and valid measures of cognitive structures may find similarities between, say, the cognitive schemas of depressed mothers and the cognitive schemas of their offspring, these data do not necessarily allow us to conclude that these offspring's cognitive schemas serve as authentic vulnerability factors.

A final problem is that some of these designs are particularly susceptible to ethical issues. For instance, in a longitudinal study of at-risk individuals, investigators would expect to find that a substantial percentage of subjects develop depression at some point. From a methodological perspective, the onset (or recurrence or relapse) of depression may disrupt longitudinal research plans to study cognitive vulnerability. At the same time, and of primary importance, investigators have an ethical obligation to ensure that the subjects receive treatment. Treatment, of course, (ideally) confounds the natural history of the disorder and, thus, for many hypotheses, may alter substantially the research questions that can be asked. We know of no methodological way around this issue, save for withholding treatment, which is obviously ethically unacceptable.

SUMMARY AND CONCLUSIONS

The various proximal and distal vulnerability designs, along with their advantages and disadvantages are summarized in Table 8.1. As with proximal vulnerability research, a number of specific types of distal vulnerability designs can be articulated. The high-risk, offspring design assesses the children of individuals with depression to determine the factors that place these children at risk. Longitudinal designs include a variety of subtypes of longitudinal assessment such as prospective strategies, catch-up strategies, follow-back approaches, and register approaches. Cross-sequential designs reflect a combination of cross-sectional and longitudinal (specifically prospective) designs and, because these designs can compare individuals both across groups and over time, they represent a powerful method for understanding psychological change. Cross-sequential designs thus incorporate the strengths of both longitudinal and cross-sectional approaches. Retrospective approaches assess distal vulnerability factors by examining the later recall of information about the time that these factors were presumed to be operating. A subgroup of retrospective designs, dubbed experimental retrospective designs, incorporate experimental manipulations of retrospectively assessed variables to determine the effects of these variables on theoretically relevant cognitive factors.

Each of these designs has clear strengths and can provide important data for understanding distal (and, in many cases, proximal) cognitive vulnerability. In many respects, their weaknesses derive not so much from methodological considerations but from logistical and pragmatic concerns; for example, distal research is complicated, time consuming, and expensive. These considerations likely account for the relative paucity of distal research on cognitive vulnerability to depression in the literature. Additionally, such designs also suffer to some degree from the inability to track precisely the actual causal factors that may be linked to the onset of depression. As we noted, showing that certain variables are correlated with the experience of depression does not necessarily show that they are causal. Such limitations aside, distal research designs have nevertheless enabled the study of what may constitute several meaningful long-term cognitive vulnerability factors. We review the key aspects of this research in Chapter 9.

CHAPTER 9

Cognitive Theory and Data on Distal Vulnerability

As childhood and adolescent depression have become increasingly recognized as a serious problem (Compas et al., 1993; Nurcombe, 1992; Petersen et al., 1993; Speier, Sherak, Hirsch, & Cantwell, 1995), research examining depressotypic cognitive processes in children and adolescents has grown substantially (Compas et al., 1993; Garber, Quiggle, & Shanley, 1990; Kendall, Stark, & Adam; 1990; Malcarne & Ingram, 1994; Prieto, Cole, & Tageson, 1992; Thurber, Crow, Thurber, & Woffington, 1990). Not only are theory and research on cognitive vulnerability factors in childhood and adolescent depression tremendously important in their own right, but such perspectives may ultimately provide significant clues about cognitive vulnerability to depression in adults. That is, available conceptual and empirically derived data may aid in understanding the distal cognitive factors of adult depression.

Although important distal vulnerability information may be derived from cognitive conceptual and empirical work with children and adolescents, these are not the only sources of information concerning these vulnerability factors. Several theoretical perspectives and a number of studies specifically intended to be applicable to adults also are potentially quite informative about distal cognitive vulnerability factors. Because there tends to be a somewhat different set of theoretical assumptions as well as distinct methodological strategies for such approaches, adult-based work examines the problem from a different point of view that may add valuable perspectives to our understanding of distal vulnerability variables.

In order to assess child, adolescent, and adult work that provides information about distal vulnerability, in this chapter we will investigate several sources of theory and data. First, because aspects of childhood may provide us with clues to adult cognitive vulnerability to depression, we summarize the relationship between depression in childhood and in adulthood. Next we will briefly comment on childhood events that pertain to cognitive vulnerability. We then examine theories that explicate cognitive vulnerability factors. These theories fall into two broad categories relevant to distal vulnerability: (1) adult-based conceptual statements and (2) developmental theories.After an examination of these theoretical approaches we will review research findings pertinent to distal cognitive vulnerability. Such findings include not only data on adults but data garnered with children and adolescents that may have some value in understanding adult vulnerabilities.

RELATIONSHIP OF CHILDHOOD DEPRESSION TO LATER DEPRESSION

Relapse and recurrence of depression in children has received less attention than similar phenomena in adults. Nevertheless, the data that are available clearly suggest that childhood depression predicts subsequent depression. Kovacs et al. (1984), for example, found a cumulative 72% probability of children having a second episode of major depression within 5 years after the onset of a first episode. Garrison, Addy, Jackson, McKeown, and Walker (1991) found that current depression predicted future depression in a 3-year follow-up of children who were 11–12 years of age. Similarly, McCauley, Mitchell, Burke, and Moss (1988) showed that 61% of children and adolescents experienced a recurrent depressive episode within 3 years. In a sample of hospitalized, depressed children, Asarnow, Goldstein, Thompson, and Guthrie (1993) found that 35–45% of children diagnosed with a depressive disorder were rehospitalized within 2 years after they were discharged. Clearly, children who are depressed are at significant risk for future depression.

Examining the probability that childhood depression will be related to future childhood depression is, of course, only one way to assess subsequent depression risk. In this regard, two major studies have assessed the impact of childhood depression on adult depression. In the first, Zeitlin (1985) used a follow-back design to assess the likelihood that currently depressed adults had a depressive disorder when they were children or adolescents. Zeitlin found that 84% of these patients had, in fact, experienced such a disorder. Harrington, Fudge, Rutter, Pickels, and Hill (1991) conducted an 18-year retrospective study and found that postpubertally depressed youths reported depression rates that were approximately twice as high in adulthood as compared to prepubertally depressed youths. This finding clearly suggests that postpubertal depression may be the strongest predictor of adult depression. Although Rutter (1986b) warns that there may be important differences in the depression experienced by children/adolescents and adults (even when these are the same people), little doubt exists that early depression does predict subsequent depression. Having established at least some empirical evidence for a continuity between the experience of depression from childhood to adulthood, we turn now to a brief discussion of the events that may precipitate childhood depression.

CHILDHOOD EVENTS AS DISTAL VULNERABILITY

Do childhood events create cognitive vulnerability to depression in adults? Much as there is a substantial body of work showing that adult depression is linked to the occurrence of stressful life events (Monroe et al., 1992; Monroe & Simons, 1991), a reasonably substantial body of work also suggests that depression in adulthood is related to the occurrence of negative events in childhood. Bemporad and Romano (1992) have reviewed a number of studies suggesting that individuals depressed as adults report greater numbers of negative events when they were younger than do nondepressed individuals. However, the variety and interacting nature of such events is so complex as to preclude any definitive conclusions about the precise nature of the link between these events and later depression. Childhood maltreatment, for example, is commonly found to be linked to an increased incidence of adult depression (Browne & Finkelhor, 1986; Kendall-Tackett, Williams, & Finkelhor, 1993). Even within this specific category of events, however, there are considerable differences. For example, maltreatment can be physical, sexual, or emotional. To make matters yet more complicated, these variables can and frequently do occur in differing combinations, making attributions to any single form of maltreatment somewhat problematic.

Other categories of stressful events such as childhood bereavement, have also been shown to be linked to vulnerability to adult depression, but here again the relationship is anything but simple. Brown and Harris's (1978) well-known finding that the loss of a mother before age 11 is associated with adult depression has not been confirmed in all subsequent studies (see Brown & Harris, 1989b). Brown and Harris (1989a) have suggested that one key to resolving such inconsistent findings is to examine the contextual factors surrounding such losses.

For instance, they found that individuals who suffered a parental loss, but who had the benefit of coming from better socioeconomic backgrounds were less likely to experience subsequent depression than those from more impoverished socioeconomic backgrounds. Even this finding, however, suggests a bewildering array of possible mediational variables such as attending quality daycare, completing an education, and waiting to become pregnant until an older age. Although the nature of these events might suggest intuitive reasons for not becoming depressed later on, the exact mechanisms by which they are related to resilience (and, correspondingly, which attributes of low socioeconomic living conditions are related to increased vulnerability) are unclear and have not been empirically tested.

The potential *cognitive effects* of such events, which may serve as the mediational basis for future depression vulnerability, are even more murky. That is, although some conceptual explanations have been offered to establish a cognitive bridge between the multitude of negative events in childhood and subsequent adult vulnerability to depression, these tend to be quite speculative. We will explore some of these relationships in Chapter 10. To provide a conceptual basis both for such speculations in Chapter 10, and for our discussion of possible distal factors in this chapter we now turn to a discussion of theoretical models that might guide our theorizing about the nature of these processes.

ADULT-BASED THEORIES RELEVANT TO DISTAL COGNITIVE VULNERABILITY

As is apparent from our discussion in previous chapters, contemporary cognitive theories of depression have typically been directed toward understanding depression in adults and its corresponding proximal vulnerability. However, many models assume that childhood events create a cognitive vulnerability to depression. Therefore, these theories provide a conceptual basis for examining the distal factors that may predispose toward adult depression. Although some of these models only briefly allude to distal vulnerability (e.g., Ingram, 1984), others have provided more detailed descriptions of possible factors, as have two of the major cognitive theories of depression, Beck's (1967) cognitive schema model and the hopelessness theory (Abramson et al., 1989)

The Cognitive Schema Model

The overwhelming theoretical discussion devoted to the model originally proposed by Beck in 1967 has been directed toward the development and course of depression in adults (see Engel & DeRubeis, 1993; Haaga et al., 1991; Sacco & Beck, 1995). Likewise, virtually all research that has attempted to test various aspects of the model has been conducted with adults (Haaga et al., 1991; Ingram & Holle, 1992; Ingram, Scott, & Siegle, in press). Yet, at the core of this model is the idea that vulnerability to depression develops through the acquisition of cognitive schemas concerning stressful or traumatic events in childhood and adolescence. Specifically, Beck suggests that when such events occur relatively early in the individual's development, these individuals become sensitized to just these types of events. The corresponding generation of negative schemas to process information about these events leads to the subsequent activation of these schemas and to corresponding depression, if and when similar events occur in the future (in adulthood, for our purposes):

> In childhood and adolescence, the depression-prone individual becomes sensitized to certain types of life situations. The traumatic situations initially responsible for embedding or reinforcing the negative attitudes that comprise the depressive constellation are the prototypes of the specific stresses that may later activate these constellations. When a person is subjected to situations reminiscent of the original traumatic experiences, he may then become depressed. The process may be likened to conditioning in which a particular response is linked to a specific stimulus; once the chain has been formed, stimuli similar to original stimulus may evoke the conditioned response. (Beck, 1967, p. 278)

Thus, although most commonly viewed as a theory of adult depression, Beck's (1967) model specifically and centrally incorporates the concept of development of distal vulnerability factors.

Hopelessness Depression

Beck's is not the only adult depression model that has been applied or extended to encompass distal cognitive vulnerability factors. Rose and Abramson (1992) have recently elaborated upon the developmental antecedents that may underlie the hopelessness theory of depression. They suggest that children who experience negative events seek to find the causes, consequences, and meaning of these events. Under some circumstances, the factors involved in this process lead to the development of the negative attributional style that is proposed to be critical to some kinds of depression. They further suggest that young children have a tendency to make internal attributions for all events, including negative events. Such internal attributional inclinations, however, are insufficient to lead to the hopelessness attributional style that is thought to be associated with depression. To the extent that unpleasant events are repetitive and occur in the context of significant relationships with others (e.g., parents), these events begin to undermine the child's basic need to maintain both a positive self-image and an optimism about future nonnegative or hopeful events. Moreover, the continuation of such events (such as neglect, or emotional, physical, or sexual abuse) along with the degradation of positive self-image are hypothesized to produce a pattern of attributions for negative events that tend to be, and become over time, stable and global. Once this attributional pattern for situational contexts becomes more trait-like, the foundation is set for hopelessness responses in the face of future stressors, which are in turn linked to the onset of hopelessness depression.

DEVELOPMENTALLY BASED THEORIES RELEVANT TO DISTAL COGNITIVE VULNERABILITY

The cognitive schema and hopelessness models are focused on adult depression. Therefore, their accounts of proximal vulnerability are naturally more thoroughly articulated. Several models have been developed specifically with distal cognitive vulnerability in mind. Many of these models stem from psychoanalytic traditions in general, and object relations perspectives in particular (see M. J. Horowitz, 1988; E. Jacobson, 1964; Kernberg, 1976; Wachtel, 1987; and, of course, virtually any of Freud's work). Perhaps the most important and influential is attachment theory.

Attachment Theory

Attachment theory as developed by Bowlby (1969, 1973, 1980) addresses variables and processes that shape the capacity of individuals to form meaningful and enduring emotional bonds with significant others throughout their lives. The development of this capacity is thought to begin virtually at birth and to continue as the infant grows and matures. Although the shaping of attachment processes does not terminate with the end of infancy and childhood, several investigators have argued that once developed, attachment patterns are relatively stable and persist into adulthood (Ainsworth, 1989; Bartholomew & Horowitz, 1991; Doane & Diamond, 1994; Ricks, 1985). Indeed, Bowlby suggests that attachment is a process that extends from "cradle to grave".

The primary determinants of the individual's attachment patterns are thought to be both the quantity and the quality of contact with caretakers (Ainsworth, Blehar, Waters, & Wall, 1978). Specifically, consistently nurturant, affectionate, and appropriately protective interactions with caretakers (such as parents) promote the development of the child's ability to form cognitive, behavioral, and emotional connectedness to others. The capacity to form these positive bonds facilitates the subsequent development of genuinely trusting, dependable, and secure relationships with others throughout the lifespan. Attachment patterns are therefore postulated to have profound consequences for both the child's current sense of security as well as for later behavior, adjustment, emotions, and interpersonal regulation (Doane & Diamond, 1994).

The capacity to develop attachments to others serves to maintain bonds between people at a variety of stages of development and life circumstances, beginning at birth. Indeed, from a phenomenological perspective, virtually any mother or father can attest to the tremendous sense of emotional bonding that takes place with their child at birth. This bonding helps to ensure that caretakers will undertake the necessary commitment not only to provide for the child's basic needs but to provide nurturance and guidance throughout development. Beyond interactions with caretakers during childhood, attachment capabilities are also essential for the maintenance of proximity between mature members of the same species. This idea and its relevance for the core features and the development of distal vulnerability will be articulated more fully in Chapter 10.

The ability to form attachments would seem to be the necessary prerequisite for successfully developing relationships with others; however, this does not mean that attachment always functions normally. For instance, when normal developmental processes are disrupted in some fashion, a variety of deviations from secure attachment have been proposed to result. Bowlby (1969) has suggested that disruptions in the attachment process can result in a variety of insecure attachments that he has labeled "insecure-ambivalent" attachment, "insecure-avoidance" attachment, or "insecure-disorganized" attachment. In a similar fashion, Bartholomew and Horowitz (1991) conceptualize disrupted attachment as resulting in either ambivalence, fearful-avoidance, or dismissive-avoidance. These categories of insecure attachment overlap significantly (but by no means completely) with those proposed by Hazan and Shaver (1987) and Main, Kaplan, and Cassidy (1985). Despite any differences in the specific proposed form of attachment-related insecurity, there is widespread agreement that significant developmental stresses lead to some form of disruption in the attachment process. The concept of attachment disruption, therefore, reflects the general dimension or factor underlying more specific types of dysfunctional attachment patterns.

In childhood, these insecure or dysfunctional attachment patterns have been posited to serve as risk factors for a diversity of problems (e.g., Bemporad & Romano, 1992; Cummings & Cicchetti, 1990; Wilson & Costanzo, 1996). In line with these proposals, data have shown that insecure attachment in children and adolescents is related to peer rejection, social competence deficits, problematic self-control, conduct disorders, and alcohol abuse (see Cole & Zahn-Waxler, 1992, and Doane & Diamond, 1994, for reviews). These data are quite consistent with theoretical proposals that suggest that disrupted attachment constitutes a risk factor for later psychological problems (e.g., Bowlby, 1988). Of particular interest for our purposes are the links that have been suggested not only between disrupted attachment and depression, but most significantly, between these variables and cognitive factors.

In particular, the risk that appears to originate from dysfunctional attachment patterns may stem at least in part from cognitive variables. Theoretical discussions of attachment have emphasized the importance of internal working models (see Chapter 1). Working models reflect the cognitive representation of relationships that have been generalized through early interactions with key figures in the individual's life. Attachment theorists have proposed that once developed, these internal working models subsequently guide the processing of information and the cognitions individuals experience about relationships with others. Similarly, if attachment is insecure, this will be reflected in the organization and functioning of the individual's working models, leading to an increased risk for disrupted interpersonal functioning and stress as information about interpersonal interactions is distorted (see Bowlby, 1988). Given our central premise that cognitive variables play a critical role in the onset, course, and remission of depression, a mechanism that helps to explain the link between cognition, developmental processes, life stress, and depression has substantial explanatory and integrative implications.

The possible link between disrupted attachment and increased risk for depression can be seen clearly in the conceptual similarity between the working model construct and the schema models that characterize much contemporary theory and research on depression. Both cognitive and interpersonal depression theorists (Gotlib & Hammen, 1992; Safran & Segal, 1990, respectively) have posited that the cognitive schemas of individuals with disrupted attachment patterns may be correspondingly disrupted, at least to the extent that they may facilitate the maladaptive processing of information. As pointed out earlier, a significant amount of research has demonstrated that depressed individuals and individuals who are vulnerable to depression show maladaptive processing of information. To the extent that individuals process information nonadaptively, then this information processing, and the schematic structures that presumably underlie the processing, may constitute at least one mechanism by which attachment disruptions may lead to increased risk for depression.

Object Relations Theories

Object relations theory derives primarily from the psychoanalytic viewpoint and, from a developmental perspective, examines the perceptions of infants and children as they view significant objects in their lives (e.g., parents). Bowlby's work on attachment theory stems from an objects relations perspective. Many of these core ideas of object relations and the basic concepts suggested by Bowlby have been elaborated upon by other theorists. For example, Westen (1991) has built on these ideas, as well as contemporary theory and research on social cognition, to suggest a synthesis of psychoanalytic and contemporary social-cognitive perspectives. This synthesis converges in the clinical significance of unconscious information processing in clinical disorders.

As regards the present context of examining distal cognitive vulnerability to depression, Westen (1991) suggests that individuals at risk for psychopathology develop working models that contain conflicting elements, some or many of which are not consciously available to the individual. Depression, then, is the result of working models that conflictually distort the processing of information about others, as well as the self in interactions with others, in ways that lead to significant interpersonal disturbance. For example, when (objectively nonthreatening) others are viewed as threatening and harmful because their actions are interpreted through the model developed by past negative experiences with ostensibly similar people at developmentally sensitive times, then the person will naturally perceive and fear potential harm. The perception of harm elicits an "appropriate" response, and hence the individual will most likely behave in ways that will significantly undermine these relationships. Consider the deep-rooted conflictual nature of this cognitive process for the individual in this example—he or she has a fundamental need to maintain connectedness with others of the species, and, simultaneously, cognitive processes are operating that push others of the species away. As we discuss in more detail in Chapter 10, such a cognitively mediated disruption of interpersonal functioning and social bonds is very likely to result in depression.

Baldwin (1992) likewise provides an elaboration of the idea of working models that incorporate not only views of the self, but also views of others in interaction with the self. Termed "relational schemas," Baldwin's (1992) theory proposes that people internalize abstractions (e.g., develop working models or schemas) about their relationships with significant others that result in cognitive representations of the regularities in patterns of relating to others. In particular, relational schemas are composed of representations of oneself, representations of important others, and scripts for how interactions with important others are expected to proceed. Relational schemas comprised of relatively positive experiences with important others in the past will subsequently facilitate successful interactions and the development of positive relations with those who become important in the future. Conversely, if the person has encoded and cognitively represented predominantly negative interactions with important others, subsequent relationship information will be processed in ways that lead to the disruption and dissolution of potentially important new relationships. In colloquial terms, the person will bring the (cognitive) "baggage" of old relationships to bear on possible new relationships, usually with ill-fated results. These cognitively mediated relationship disruptions provide fertile ground for breeding vulnerability to depression.

Summary of Theoretical Approaches Relevant to Distal Cognitive Factors

Attachment theory represents perhaps one of the most powerful theoretical approaches for examining the cognitive elements, which, through disrupted developmental relationships, potentially form the basis of distal cognitive vulnerability. Accordingly, attachment theory has seen a rebirth of interest among researchers interested in psychopathology, including adult psychopathology. Although attachment theory is perhaps the most widely known, other approaches stemming largely from the same theoretical ancestor (i.e., object relation theory) have also begun to describe cognitive factors that may play a significant role in vulnerability to depression, especially factors that converge on descriptions of the functioning of cognitive structures. Among the most notable theoretical work in this regard is that of Westen (1991) and Baldwin (1992), who have described cognitive schemas that incorporate content and processing assumptions about the self and others.

There is also a growing body of empirical work examining variables that are relevant to distal cognitive vulnerability, some of which has grown specifically out of these theoretical perspectives, and some of which has not. We turn now to this work. In particular, we will describe results from retrospective and high-risk studies. Much of the research we will examine deals with potential vulnerability factors in children. As we noted earlier, although our focus is on adult vulnerability, we review this research for clues that it may provide regarding the formation of factors that seem likely to play a later role in cognitive risk for depression. Such an assumption, of course, will ultimately need to be empirically tested, most likely employing longitudinal designs.

RESEARCH FINDINGS ON DISTAL
COGNITIVE VULNERABILITY

As we noted in Chapter 8, distal vulnerability research strategies can fall into several categories: longitudinal, cross-sequential, high-risk, and retrospective designs. Both longitudinal and cross-sequential designs are rare in this area of research. Specifically, longitudinal research, while perhaps representing the most powerful set of strategies is also among the most expensive, time consuming, and difficult. It comes as little surprise then that very few longitudinal data on distal cognitive vulnerability in adults have been reported, and there are no data of which we are aware from cross-sequential designs that combine cross-sectional analyses with longitudinally collected data. Correspondingly, the bulk of research on cognition and adult depression vulnerability comes, not surprisingly, from retrospective studies.

Retrospective Adult Studies

Retrospective studies generally consider one of two variables as the possible genesis of distal vulnerability: parental interactions and early abuse experiences. Before discussing these studies, a potentially important caveat is in order. Virtually all of these studies have relied on university students with ages generally around the late teens and early 20s. The problem in examining these studies for information on adult distal vulnerability factors is, of course, that for many individuals around these ages the line between adolescence and adulthood is blurred considerably. We discuss these studies for two reasons. First, at present these studies represent the closest to adult data that are available. Second, and more conceptually important, even though these samples tend to be young they reflect an age range during which individuals are at significantly heightened risk for the first clinically significant episode of depression (Burke, Burke, Regier, & Rae, 1990; Lewinsohn, Duncan, Stanton, & Fischer, 1993). In this regard, studies with such research participants may be particularly appropriate and valuable for assessing distal cognitive vulnerability factors.

Parental Interactions

As we have noted, attachment is considered an important function of parental interactions, and several studies have assessed the link between attachment and depression. For example, Hammen et al. (1995) examined attachment cognitions in high school girls to determine whether these cognitions predicted an increased incidence of depression or other disorders. Over the course of a year they found that attachment cognitions in conjunction with interpersonal stressors significantly contributed to the prediction of depressive symptoms, although the effects were not limited to depression. Pearson et al. (1994) also examined the relationship of attachment to depression, but contrasted different aspects of attachment. Specifically, they differentiated among people who had always had a secure sense of attachment versus those who currently had good levels of attachment, but had overcome early patterns of difficult relationships with parents (e.g., "earned security"). They found that people with continuously secure attachment had lower levels of depressive symptomatology than did those with earned secure attachment, whose depressive symptoms were comparable to those who had never had secure attachment. Likewise, studies by Randolph and Dykman (in press), and Roberts et al. (1996) found that the link between indices of attachment and depressive symptoms in college students was mediated by dysfunctional attitudes, a construct central to cognitive theories of depression. Together, these studies suggest that early attachment patterns do appear to play a key role in long-term functioning, regardless of events that may subsequently intervene.

A number of the studies examining the impact of parental interactions on depression have assessed the recall of these interactions with the Parental Bonding Instrument (PBI; Parker et al., 1979). The PBI is important in this regard because it not only appears to be a valid and reliable measure of recalled parental interactions, but also because the two scales that comprise the PBI are based on a relatively well-articulated theoretical rationale for the development of adult dysfunction as a result of these styles. Specifically, the PBI assesses the recall of parental caring and overprotectiveness by both one's mother and father. Parker (1979, 1983) suggests that low levels of parental care can be evidenced by either neglect or by overt rejection, and that this leads to future vulnerability by disrupting the child's self-esteem. He further suggests a cognitive mediation aspect to this vulnerability in that deficient self-esteem elicits the interpretation of communications in adult interpersonal relationships as rejecting or demeaning. This is the case even when such negative comments are insignificant or even nonexistent. In contrast to low levels of expressed care, overprotectiveness is thought to operate on vulnerability also through too little care, not because of rejection or neglect but because the parent is so anxious or intrusive that a genuine caring relationship cannot be established with the child. Parker proposes that, rather than being mediated through low self-esteem and consequent cognitive disruptions in interpersonal information processing per se, children who have experienced high levels of overprotectiveness simply do not develop the skills necessary to negotiate a successful relationship outside of the family.

Certainly other dimensions of family interactions may be important for the genesis of psychopathology, but there is wide agreement that lack of care and overprotectiveness are core dimensions. Reviews by Blatt and Homann (1992), Burbach and Borduin (1986), and Gerlsma et al. (1990) demonstrate the presence of a substantial body of literature showing that disruptions in early interactions with parents are indeed linked to a greater likelihood of experiencing depression. Studies that examine the cognitive component of this link between disrupted interactions with parents and depression, however, are much less common. Moreover, even those that do examine cognitive factors tend to examine these factors more as proximal vulnerability variables rather than as being associated with the occurrence of depression itself. That is, they tend to examine associations between the recall of parental interactions and the current occurrence of putative proximal risk factors, but not whether these factors are actually linked to depressive symptoms. Nevertheless, these studies may be helpful in understanding both proximal and distal variables.

In several recent studies employing the experimental retrospective approach, Ingram and colleagues have assessed the link between depressotypic cognitive processes and the possible vulnerability variables of attachment and parental bonding. In the first, attachment was conceptualized according to scores on the Revised Adult Attachment Scale (Collins & Read, 1990), a measure that, when combined with interpersonal stressors, has been found by Hammen et al. (1995) to predict depression over the course of a year. Ingram, Bailey, and Siegle (1997) found that nondepressed individuals who showed evidence of dysfunctional attachment on this measure were more prone that "normally" attached individuals to attend to negative stimuli after they had experienced a negative mood induction. Poorly attached individuals who were not primed with a negative mood induction were indistinguishable from normally attached individuals. These data provide further evidence consistent with the idea that attachment serves as a vulnerability factor for depression. Most notably, however, they suggest that one of the mechanisms through which vulnerability may be translated into disorder is via cognitive means, that is, the activation of cognitive processes that appear to be sensitive to negative stimuli. Although the relationship of such cognitive responses to actual depression is still speculative (see chapter 6), these results are compatible with the idea that cognition mediates the relationship between attachment disruptions and depression.

In another study using an experimental retrospective paradigm that employed a priming strategy, Ingram and Ritter (1998) operationalized vulnerability in much the same way that other investigators have done so, specifically by virtue of studying nondepressed individuals who had previously experienced a depressive episode. In line with previous research, and as we noted in Chapter 7, Ingram and Ritter (1998) assessed attention to negative stimuli using a dichotic listening task, with the result in brief, that vulnerable individuals displayed more negative errors when they had been primed by a sad mood then did unprimed vulnerable people or primed nonvulnerable subjects. Unlike previous studies using this paradigm however, Ingram and Ritter (1998) were also interested in the possible impact of individuals' perceptions of the quality of parental care when they were young. Thus, before the negative mood priming procedure was administered, the PBI was given. Results using this measure showed some evidence of mediation of this pattern by PBI scores. Specifically, ratings of maternal care were negatively associated with errors on the negative stimulus aspects of the dichotic listening task, suggesting that lower levels of perceived maternal care were associated with the processing of more negative information when vulnerable individuals were in a negative mood. These data may therefore point in the direction of early interactional patterns leading to cognitive processing that may ultimately be linked to depression. More specifically, these data may suggest that a perceived lack of caring by the mother may set the stage for the development of a depressive self-schema. Such interpretations do not suggest that fathers are unimportant in these possible vulnerability functions, but rather only that these data were unable to detect a role for fathers.

In the final study to use the experimental retrospective paradigm by Ingram and colleagues, Ingram, Bailey, and Siegle (1997) used the same negative mood priming paradigm but conceptualized vulnerability in terms of bonding patterns as indicated by scores on the PBI. In particular, an index was created by selecting individuals reporting that they had mothers and father who tended to be the least caring and the most overprotective ("affectionless control"; see Parker, 1983). To assess potentially dysfunctional information processing, research participants were asked to perform a Stroop task comprised of both negative and positive stimuli. As with the original Stroop procedure, the participants' task was to respond to each word in the task by naming the color in which the word is printed, with the length of reaction times suggestive of the level of interference caused by the semantic content of the word. Thus, for example, if people are processing positive information this will interfere with their responses for naming the color of the positive words, and their reaction times will be slowed. In fact, the only significant effect that was found was an interaction for positive information in which the good and poor bonding individuals in a neutral mood responded relatively similarly, but in the negative mood condition secure bonding individuals showed slower reaction times while poor bonding individuals showed faster reaction times.

There is a variety of potential interpretations of these results. For example, these findings may suggest that positive information processing is the first to deteriorate as dysfunctional schemas start to become activated. Researchers tend to focus a great deal of attention on negative information processing, but it may be that the first sign of a depressogenic schema is an inability to focus on positive information. If depression is thought of in terms of a spiraling process as several investigators have suggested, then perhaps the first part of this spiral is that people are unable to appreciate positive information, an interpretation similar to that offered by Ingram et al. (1983) in their investigation of depression and the processing of positive self-referent information. Such interpretations are certainly speculative, but, if true, suggest that the current predominant focus on negative information processing may be somewhat misplaced. What is less speculative is that these experimental retrospective studies all point to disrupted information processing as a possible variable that may mediate the relationship between depression and early experiences.

Recall from our earlier discussion that self-criticism has also been proposed to serve as a distally developed cognitive vulnerability factor. Several studies have assessed this variable. For example, McCranie and Bass (1984) found that among young women nursing students, an overcontrolling mother was associated with greater dependency needs, whereas for students who had both a mother and a father who were overcontrolling, a greater tendency toward self-criticism was found. Likewise, Brewin et al. (1992) found among young medical students (average age 19.8) that higher levels of self-criticism were related to reports of inadequate parenting. This was particularly true for individuals who consistently reported high levels of self-criticism over time. Similar results have been reported by Blatt et al. (1979). Because both dependency and self-criticism have been discussed as possible (proximal) cognitive vulnerability factors, and have been shown in other studies to be associated with depressive states (Blatt & Zuroff, 1992), these data may be relevant for eventually understanding the cognitive diathesis of depression.

As we noted, with the exception of several recent experimental retrospective studies, relatively little research has assessed the relationship between the perceived quality of parental care, cognitive variables, and depression. A study reported by Whisman and Kwon (1992) did examine these questions for mild levels of depression. Specifically, in a sample composed primarily of female undergraduates, Whisman and Kwon (1992) found that lower recalled levels of parental care were associated with a higher level of depressive symptoms. More importantly from a cognitive vulnerability perspective, they also found that this relationship was mediated by depressotypic attitudes and dysfunctional attributions. The extant evidence thus does suggest that disturbed parent–child interactions may create risk factors that are cognitive in nature.

Early Abuse Experiences

Just as research has shown consistent relations between perceptions of the quality of parental care and later depression, data have also suggested a consistent relationship between reports of abusive experiences, particularly sexual abuse, and depression (for reviews, see Browne & Finkelhor, 1986; Cutler & Nolen-Hoeksema, 1991; Kendall-Tackett et al., 1993). Research on distally determined cognitive variables that may mediate the relationship between abuse and depression parallels research on parental interactions, in that there is a paucity of such data. In one of the few studies that did investigate cognitive variables within the context of abuse and depression, Kuyken and Brewin (1995) assessed memory retrieval in a sample of depressed patients, some of whom who had experienced sexual and/or physical abuse as children. Kuyken and Brewin's (1995) data indicated that depressed women who had been sexually (but not physically) abused showed an inability to recall specific memories in response to both positive and negative cues, suggesting the possibility that avoidance of key memories and disruptions in working memory may play a role in the relationship between abuse and depression. Interestingly, they also found that parental indifference was related to this inability to recall specific events.

From a very different perspective, Rose et al. (1994) also examined the mediational effect of cognitive variables on the relationship between sexual abuse and depression. In assessing the possibility of different subgroups of depressed individuals, they found that one group that had experienced childhood sexual abuse was characterized by negative cognitive styles, as measured by the DAS and a modified ASQ. They speculated that these adverse early experiences lead to the development of negative cognitive processing patterns that are linked to vulnerability to depression. This speculation was further supported in a study by Rose and Abramson (1995) showing that, for depressed individuals who were maltreated as children, the greater the maltreatment, the more dysfunctional were their cognitions. Taken together, the data reported by Kuyken and Brewin (1995), Rose et al. (1994), and Rose and Abramson (1995) suggest that a history of early adverse experiences such as sexual abuse may produce distal cognitive patterns that lead toward the later development of depression.

Although our focus is on vulnerability, it is important to note that just as disrupted attachment can lead to vulnerability to depression, secure attachment, and theoretically the cognitive component of it, can also mitigate against the effects of maltreatment. By inference, the cognitive aspect of secure attachment may mitigate the effects of childhood trauma on subsequent psychopathology. In this vein, Toth, Manly, and Cicchetti (1992) studied children's reports of attachment to their parent and maltreatment. Interestingly, maltreated children who were securely attached to their parents were less likely to evidence depressive symptomatology than were maltreated children who were not securely attached to parents. Hence, data showing that insecure attachment is related to depression (presumably via a cognitive route) and that secure attachment can protect against depression suggest clearly that the complex interactions of attachment and maltreatment may ultimately predict the cognitive patterns that predispose toward adult depression.

Summary of Adult Retrospective Studies of Distal Cognitive Vulnerability

The extant data show unquestionably that disrupted interactions with parents pose a risk factor for later depression. Such disruptions may take the form of poor parenting as in lack of care and overcontrol, or may be more malevolent as in the physical, sexual, or emotional abuse of children and adolescents. Theoretical perspectives suggest that the bridge between these parental behaviors and later depression in adulthood is cognitive in nature, whether specified as the operations of schemas or the somewhat more inclusive construct of a cognitive working model. The empirical data on the cognitive effects of these disturbed interactions, however, are sparse and in need of further research. Indeed, research that undertakes examining these presumed cognitive links will be extremely important. Nonetheless, the data in this area thus far are generally supportive of the idea that cognitive variables form mediational pathways between troublesome parent–child/adolescent interactions and depression.

High-Risk Studies of Vulnerability to Depression

Adult-based studies of distal cognitive vulnerability suggest some important conclusions as well as avenues for future research. Such studies, however, leave important gaps and suffer from problems, which do not negate their findings but do certainly limit their utility. We now turn to studies that examine cognitive factors that may create risk for adult depression. Such child-based studies have the advantage of being temporally closer to the assessment of distal factors because such factors are assumed to develop in childhood or adolescence. Nevertheless, as we noted, such studies also, at least for our purposes, generally suffer from some of the same problems as adult-based studies, such as the failure to show that presumed cognitive factors are in fact related to depression in adulthood. Although such empirical relationships have generally not been shown, we do think, however, that these data can provide important clues to the development of the distal cognitive factors that render adults at risk for depression.

Recall from our description in Chapter 8 that high-risk offspring studies assess children of individuals with the disorder of interest, in this case, depression. The underlying assumption of this strategy is that offspring are at increased risk for developing a disorder similar to that of one or both of their parents and thus the offspring of depressed parents should possess the factors that make them vulnerable to depression. Although there are a number of possible avenues of vulnerability transmission that have been proposed by researchers (e.g., genetic, birth or prebirth trauma, etc.), in the case of the type of depression we have operationally defined, the interactional patterns of parents are presumed to be most likely to lead to the developmental of vulnerable cognitive structures.

Parental Depression

Perhaps the most studied vulnerability factor for adult depression has been parental psychopathology. Numerous reviews of the empirical literature indicate that there is no doubt that children of depressed mothers are more vulnerable to a variety of difficulties such as interpersonal and academic problems than are children whose mothers are not depressed. Additionally, children of depressed mothers show both an increased incidence of psychological symptoms as well as increased rates of psychiatric diagnoses, including depression (Beardslee et al., 1983; Blatt & Homann, 1992; Cohn & Campbell, 1992; Downey & Coyne, 1990; Gelfand & Teti, 1990; Hammen, 1991a; Morrison, 1983; M. M. Weissman, 1988). These findings are echoed in the high-risk studies of schizophrenia we mentioned in Chapters 4 and 8, which used depressed mothers as psychiatric controls. Although data on fathers (who may play an important role [Phares, 1996; Phares & Compas, 1992]) are noticeably missing in most of these studies, this line of research nevertheless makes it clear that parental depression is a risk factor for offspring depression.

In a particularly well-done example of the high-risk strategy, Hammen (1991a) examined the offspring of unipolar, bipolar, medically ill control, and normal control mothers. Children were assessed following their mothers' discharge from treatment and then again at 1-, 2-, and

3-year follow-ups. Hammen (1991a) found that children of unipolar mothers were at greater risk for any disorder than were children in any of the other groups. With regard to affective disorders (e.g., major depression, dysthymic disorder), 27% of the offspring of unipolar mothers received a diagnosis of an affective disorder as compared to no children in the bipolar and medically ill groups, and 3% of the normal group. These differences were maintained over the course of the follow-up. For instance, 27%, 16%, and 19% of the children of unipolar mothers received diagnoses of major depression at 1, 2, and 3 years, respectively. The next highest incidence of major depression was in the bipolar group at 1 year and the medical group at 2 years, both with 7% receiving a diagnosis. Thus, not only are the children of depressed mothers at immediate risk, this risk continues over time and perhaps during the course of key developmental periods.

Cognitive Vulnerability Factors

Although data show that the offspring of depressed parents are at increased risk for depression, such data in and of themselves are uninformative about mediational factors, specifically, for our purposes, the role of cognitive factors. Keep in mind in this regard the distinction we have drawn between risk and vulnerability factors. Data showing that the offspring of depressed parents, particularly mothers, are more likely to evidence a number of psychological problems, including depression, are informative only of the probability of offspring experiencing depression (risk) but do not tell us why this is the case (vulnerability). To be sure, such data do provide many important clues about vulnerability, but unless vulnerability mechanisms are specifically assessed, and assessed independently of the increased depression that is seen in the offspring of depressed mothers, the nature of this vulnerability remains speculative.

A small number of studies have examined possible vulnerability factors in the offspring of depressed parents. As we have noted, for instance, one cognitive conceptualization of depression vulnerability concerns attachment processes and cognitions, and hence quality of attachment may constitute a mechanism that renders the children of depressed mothers vulnerable to depression. Specifically, children of depressed parents are particularly likely to be faced with the psychological unavailability of parents for long periods, especially during episodes of depression (Field, 1989).

Indeed, psychological unavailability appears to be a risk factor for development of insecure attachment in children of depressed mothers. Radke-Yarrow, Cummings, Kuczynski, and Chapman (1985) compared patterns of attachment in children of unipolar depressed, bipolar depressed, minorly depressed, and nondepressed mothers. Among children whose caregiver had major depression, 47% had insecure attachments with their primary caregiver and 53% were classified as securely attached. Therefore, depressed mothers may pass on depression to their offspring through factors such as inadequate bonding and subsequent internalization of corresponding models of interpersonal interactions.

In one study that did examine cognitive patterns in conjunction with parental depression, the negative attributional styles of children with mood-disordered mothers were examined. In this study, Radke-Yarrow, Belmont, Nottelmann, and Bottomly (1990) found that children of depressed mothers reported higher negative-toned self-attributions than did children of nondepressed mothers, and their statements were correspondent. That is, the mother who endorsed the statement "I hate myself" was likely to have a child who endorsed the statement "I am bad." The researchers interpreted their findings as a heightened vulnerability for negative self-attributions in offspring of depressed mothers. The potential for this creating cognitive vulnerability to depression in later life seems likely.

In another study assessing possible cognitive vulnerability mechanisms in the children of depressed mothers, Taylor and Ingram (1998) examined information-processing indices of negative self-schemas from a diathesis–stress perspective. As we have previously noted, tests of vulnerability to depression that do not account for the potential activating features of negative events are unlikely to yield much meaningful information, for either adults or children. Participants in the Taylor and Ingram (1997) study were children between the ages of 8 and 12, who had either depressed or nondepressed mothers. Half of the children participated in a mood induction task and the other half participated in a neutral mood induction, and then they all completed the SRET. Results indicated that a negative mood for high-risk children suppressed the endorsement of positive self-descriptors. Moreover, when recall patterns were examined, no differences in the recall of negative words as a function of mood for low-risk children were evidenced, but negative mood enhanced the recall of negative personally relevant stimuli in high-risk children. These results held up even when current levels of depressive symptomatology were controlled for. Hence, these data suggest that depressed mothers may indeed transmit negative cognitive characteristics to their children, which form the basis of a negative self-schema that is activated in response to negative-mood-producing stressful events.

COGNITIVE MECHANISMS IN EARLY DEPRESSION

Another potential way to assess distal cognitive vulnerability factors is to examine the cognitive functioning of depressed children. As we noted at the outset of this chapter, although change in cognitive variables may occur between childhood and adulthood, data on childhood cognitive factors may nonetheless provide important clues about cognitive vulnerability to depression in adults. Indeed, if cognitions can serve as vulnerability factors for adult depression, an important question is whether these same mechanisms appear to function in children and may thus form the basis of distal cognitive vulnerability.

Before attempting to answer this question, it is helpful to consider the issue of negative cognition, specifically self-referent negative cognition, in light of the developmental processes pertaining to children's sense of self. Children's abilities to think about the self (Harter, 1983; Ruble, Parsons, & Ross, 1976) and the causes of events, and to understand the future (Nicholls, 1978) develop with age and begin to stabilize in late adolescence. In this vein, a number of perception researchers have noted a significant change in children's cognition around age 7–8 years. This age shift corresponds to the cognitive transition from preoperational to operational thinking in nonsocial areas and changes in social and self-perceptions (Selman, 1980). Prior to this shift, children view themselves in concrete, physical terms. Following this shift, children view themselves in psychological terms, with characteristics and traits they see as enduring over time. In particular, little doubt exists that by adolescence they have developed the concept of the self (Hammen, 1991a). Also by this time, children shift from viewing themselves in absolute terms to engaging more in social comparisons, and they also think of themselves less in terms of their actions and more in terms of competencies and skills. Hence, evidence for cognitive vulnerability to depression would come from findings that the hypothesized underlying cognitive mechanisms (e.g., dysfunctional thoughts and biased attributional styles) occur in depressed adolescents, whose cognitive structures are relatively developed, as well as adults.

As we noted previously, some cognitive models have been adapted specifically to incorporate key developmental phases into hypothesized vulnerability. In particular, recall that Rose and Abramson (1992) suggest that young children tend to make internal attributions for all events and that, when unpleasant events are encountered that are repetitive and pertain to significant relationships with others, they undermine the developing child's basic need to maintain a positive self-image and hopefulness. Once these basic developmental needs are undermined, the foundation is set for a pattern of hopelessness attributional tendencies.

Empirical Evidence on Cognition in Childhood Depression

What then are the cognitive factors that are characteristic of depression in children? Specifically, do the same kinds of cognitive mechanisms that function in adults also function for children? For early childhood, the answer appears to be no. For example, Nolen-Hoeksema and her colleagues (1992) found that, in early childhood, negative events but not cognitive factors were related to depressive symptoms. However, in later childhood, a pessimistic explanatory style predicted depressive symptoms, both alone and in combination with negative life events (Peterson & Seligman, 1984). Following a depressive episode, children had increased pessimistic explanatory styles. Thus, these older children reported a cognitive vulnerability that was enhanced by the experience of a depressive episode.

A number of studies reported by Garber and colleagues have provided important information about the relationships between cognition and depressive symptomatology in children and adolescents. For instance, in a large scale investigation of children and adolescents in grades 7–12 (an age when depressive disorders can clearly be diagnosed), Garber, Weiss, and Shanley (1993) found a strong association between typical depressogenic cognitions and depressive symptoms in this adolescent age group. In addition, no association between depressogenic thinking and age was found, nor did the strength of the association between cognitions and depression change with age. Further, in a prospective study of adolescent cognitive style and depression, Robinson, Garber, and Hilsman (1995) examined whether depressogenic thinking measured in the sixth grade predicted depression after the stressful transition to seventh grade. Depressogenic thinking directly, and in interaction with stressors, did predict depressive symptoms. However, perceived self-worth appeared to moderate the effect of depressogenic thinking on depressive symptoms. Taken together, these studies clearly support the hypothesis that cognitive vulnerability to depression begins in late childhood and early adolescence. Yet, the extent to which perceived self-worth protects against depression over time is not yet clearly understood.

In the section on the effects of parental depression, we noted a particularly well-done study by Hammen (1991a) that examined the offspring of unipolar, bipolar, medically ill, and normal mothers. This study is also notable for its examination of potentially depressogenic cognitive factors. Such factors can be assessed numerous ways. One particularly useful paradigm for assessing cognition in depressed adults is a self-referent incidental recall task (Rogers, Kuiper, & Kirker, 1977), a task in which the incidental recall of personally relevant adjectives is assessed to make inferences concerning the information-processing schemas and processes that are operative in depression (Ingram & Kendall, 1986). A number of studies have demonstrated that children recall adjectives that are personally descriptive. As with adults, depressed children recall more negative adjectives than do nondepressed children. In the first study to employ this paradigm in children, Hammen and Zupan (1984) found some evidence that negative mood was related to a tendency to recall negative self-descriptive adjectives, suggesting the possible presence of a depressive self-schema.

In an early analysis of data from the Hammen (1991a) study, Zupan, Hammen, and Jaenicke (1987) used this incidental recall paradigm to assess the self-schemas of a subsample of children. They found that children between the ages of 8 and 16 years who had current or prior depression recalled more negative self-descriptive adjectives than did nondepressed children, suggesting that depression is associated with negative self-representations. Thus, similar to adults, depressed children report that they hold more negative views of themselves, even those who are not currently depressed but have been depressed in the past.

Jaenicke et al. (1987) also compared children in Hammen's (1991a) sample on several cognitive measures including the incidental recall task. Recall task results suggested that a lack of positive self-schema information processing was characteristic of the children of both unipolar and bipolar mothers. Children in the unipolar and bipolar groups also reported a less positive self-concept and evidenced a more negative attributional style. Jaenicke et al. (1987) also found that children's positive ratings of their mothers were highly related to their view of themselves, as well as inversely related to attributional style and recall indices of negative self-schemas. Perceptions of maternal criticism were also related to more negative representations of the self as well as to a more negative attributional style. However, because a substantial proportion of these children were also depressed, particularly those with depressed mothers, it is unclear whether these differences were a function of a parental transmission of negative information processing or were related to the presence of depressive symptomatology.

A study reported by Hammen, Adrian, and Hiroto (1988), using this same data set to assess longitudinal cognitive functioning, did not find that attributional style predicted later depression. Specifically, after controlling for initial diagnosis, they found at a 6-month follow-up that attributional style neither alone nor in interaction with stressful events significantly predicted depression (although these variables did predict nonaffective diagnoses). However, they did find that self-concept, independently of stress, predicted depression. Hammen et al. (1987) concluded that a relatively enduring cognitive variable such as self-concept does represent a vulnerability marker for depression in children, at least over a 6-month period of time.

Using a somewhat different recall paradigm, Whitman and Leitenberg (1990) assessed the recall of positive versus negative task feedback in children who were either high or low on depressive symptomatology. Specifically, children were asked to keep track of task responses that had been correct and incorrect, and then later to recall these responses. Results indicated that children higher in depression were less accurate in recalling correct responses but not incorrect responses. These findings were interpreted by Whitman and Leitenberg to indicate deficits in the processing of positive information but not excesses in negative information processing. These results were echoed in a study by Prieto et al. (1992), who also suggested that depressed children may suffer from deficits in the activation of positive self-schemas. In their study of clinic-referred depressed children, they found that these children were less likely to recognize positive self-descriptive words on a recognition task then were nondepressed control groups. Depressed children also remembered fewer positive self-descriptors on an incidental recall task. These results and those of Whitman and Leitenberg find a parallel in the adult literature in a study by Ingram et al. (1983), which found that depressed colleges students had difficulty activating a positive self-schema in response to positive feedback.

Several investigators have also examined children's cognitive distortions such as were proposed by Beck (1967) to be vulnerability factors for depression. In those studies, versions of adult questionnaires adapted for children were used. These studies consistently find that depressed children display more negative cognitive distortions than do nondepressed children (Campbell-Goymer & Allgood, 1984; Haley, Fine, Marriage, Moretti, & Freeman, 1985; Leitenberg, Yost, & Carroll-Wilson, 1986). Similarly, Beck's (1967) cognitive theory suggests that those vulnerable to depression have negative thoughts about the self. Studies of children find that lower self-concept is related to depressive symptoms (Asarnow & Bates, 1988; Garber et al., 1990; Kazdin, Colbus, & Rodgers, 1986; Koenig, 1988). Hammen and Goodman-Brown (1990) divided children into categories of vulnerability in the area of interpersonal relationships or achievement. They then followed children over 6 months and examined whether congruent stressful life events led to depression. Although their sample was small, those youngsters with stressful life events congruent with their vulnerability were more likely to become depressed than those without congruent life events.

As we have previously discussed, attributional style has been shown to predict to depression in adults; stable, global, and internal attributions for negative events are reliably associated with adult depression. Leon, Kendall, and Garber (1980) found that depressed children attribute positive events to external factors and negative events to internal factors. A number of further studies have demonstrated a reasonably consistent relationship between negative explanatory style and depressive symptoms (Garber et al., 1990; Seligman et al., 1984). For example, Nolen-Hoeksema, Girgus, and Seligman (1986) studied children every 3 months for a year and found that attributional style predicted subsequent depression, as well as teacher ratings and achievement behavior.

In an intriguing study examining the cognitive variable of self-complexity in middle childhood, Jordan and Cole (1996) assessed the relationship between this variable and depressive symptoms. Self-complexity represents the organization of self-relevant semantic knowledge into different aspects of the self and had been proposed by Linville (1987) to serve as a buffer between stressful life events and depression. Linville suggests that to the extent that individuals have well-differentiated aspects of the self (i.e., that are relatively compartmentalized), then depression in response to negative events is less likely to occur or, if it does, to be less severe and more short term. The compartmentalization that is function of a heightened degree of self-complexity may thus serve to interrupt the spreading of depressive activation when negative events occur. Jordan and Cole found, however, that reports of depressive symptoms were *positively* related to self-complexity as opposed to the negative association that would be predicted by the buffering hypothesis. Such differences may be due to differences in developmental levels between adults and children in the elaboration of a sufficiently complex sense of self. Correspondingly, it is possible that the occurrence of negative events during the development of self-complexity leads to the generation of negative self-images that become integrated into the overall view of the self and facilitate rather than dampen the spread of activation between affective and cognitive structures.

Summary of Cognitive Functioning in Depressed Children

Hammen (1991a) has summed up nicely the possible relationship between negative cognition and depression in children. While emphasizing the importance of assessing the environmental context for cognitive functioning, Hammen suggests that

> from the point of view of an information-processing perspective on depressive cognitions, the appearance of self-devaluing and pessimistic thoughts in children may merely be the tip of the pernicious psycho-

logical iceberg. Negative cognitions may signal an underlying self-representation that is highly attuned to congruent negative information and resistant to input that does not confirm self-devaluing thoughts. If we find that self-schemas form early and perpetuate themselves, especially if reinforced by difficult life circumstances, we would expect them to exert considerable impact on subsequent development. Negative views of the self and of the future may serve to diminish a child's effort, persistence, and coping in the face of challenges. (p. 104)

Echoing Hammen (1991a), Dodge (1993) has formulated a compelling account of developmental vulnerability to depression that highlights important cognitive features. Accordingly, he postulates that early life experience, coupled with biologically based limits, interact to develop ever-changing knowledge structures or schemas that inform integration of past and future experiences. As such, these schemas organize the processing of new information. Dodge speculates that early life experiences of loss, instability, or excessive pressure to achieve unrealistic goals predisposes children to both negative self-schemas and low self-esteem. Over time, this leads to heightened sensitivity to stressful life events and to negative self-attributions. Because of these depressogenic thinking patterns, these individuals are at heightened risk for depression by the development of a maladaptive and reciprocal cycle of negative information processing and dysfunctional behavior.

SUMMARY AND CONCLUSIONS

We began our discussion of distal cognitive vulnerability factors with a brief overview of the relationship between childhood depression and later depression, and childhood events as distal vulnerability factors, and then discussed both adult- and child-based theories that are relevant to the idea of distal cognitive vulnerability. We also reviewed data stemming from retrospective as well as high-risk studies, and examined the cognitive mechanisms that appear to characterize childhood depression. As we noted, the goal of our discussion was to find clues regarding the relationships between early functioning and later cognitive vulnerability.

As our review indicates, a number of studies have begun to address possible distal factors that may lead to cognitive vulnerability to depression in adulthood. Clearly, those who experience depression in childhood are likely to experience depression in adulthood. Evidence additionally suggests that early depression appears to be related to depression in adulthood. Moreover, a reasonably substantial body of work indicates that depression in adulthood is related to the occurrence of negative events in childhood. These data are generally consistent with theories that predict that aspects of childhood experiences, such as disrupted attachment to adults, should lead to vulnerability to depression; likewise, childhood events such as insecure attachment, childhood physical and/or sexual abuse, and so forth are related to adult depression.

The cognitive characteristics of children who are at risk for depression because of parental depression have also been examined. Data from these studies support the idea that depressed parents transmit negative cognitive characteristics to their children. Furthermore, children at risk for depression appear to have available negative self-schemas that are linked to the appearance of self-devaluing and pessimistic thoughts when accessed. Data further suggest that these kinds of dysfunctional cognitive processes are also detected in vulnerable adults and appear to be linked to experiences with parents during childhood.

What do these data suggest for understanding cognitive vulnerability to depression in general, and distally derived cognitive vulnerability factors in particular? Research specifically examining cognitive distal factors for adult depression vulnerability has been quite limited thus far. Nevertheless, the theory and data that do exist make a strong circumstantial case that negative events in childhood are essential elements in the formation of cognitive structures that eventually predispose adults to the experience of depression; data clearly suggest substantial overlap in the kinds of cognitive processes and mechanisms that appear to characterize depression between childhood and adulthood. No doubt, important differences also exist, but the similarities are striking enough to warrant strong consideration of the idea that developmentally determined cognitive structures in childhood, such as negative self-schemas and dysfunctional information-processing dispositions, create the subsequent cognitive risk for depression in adults. Clearly, drawing lines from childhood experiences to cognitive risk factors for adults requires further study, but, at present, such conclusions are consistent with theory, data, and intuition.

CHAPTER 10

Proximal and Distal Perspectives: An Integrative Approach to Cognitive Vulnerability to Depression

In Chapters 1 through 9 we have dealt with a variety of topics that we believe are important for furthering our understanding of cognitive vulnerability to depression. In Chapter 1 we provided an overview of the cognitive approach to understanding psychopathology, and then in Chapter 2 discussed information relevant to the form of psychopathology in which we are most interested: depression. Chapter 3 tied cognitive constructs and depression together to give an overview of current cognitive theories of depression. Many of these theories include statements about the cognitive antecedents of vulnerability to depression; however, others focus more on the correlates and functioning of depressive cognitive structures and processes. Even though causal statements are commonplace in cognitive theories, few are explicit about vulnerability. Regardless of the focus of extant cognitive theories, a basic understanding of these theories is an essential prerequisite for any exploration of cognitive vulnerability. Chapter 4 discussed the notion of vulnerability in general while Chapter 5 focused on conceptual and definitional issues that pertain not only to vulnerability, but also to depression. Based on these assumptions, in Chapter 6 we assessed methodological issues in the study of proximal cognitive vulnerability, which led to the discussion of theory and data regarding the same in Chapter 7. Following this lead, Chapters 8 and 9 examined the respective methodological issues and data on distal cognitive vulnerability.

Having reviewed theory and data and having thus established a basis for our assumptions concerning cognition, vulnerability, depression, and the study of these interacting variables, we now turn toward an attempt to offer an integrative statement on such variables. We do not claim that we have uncovered all important variables in our exploration of vulnerability to depression. For instance, although our focus is on the cognitive antecedents of vulnerability, this is not intended to diminish the role and contribution of other mediational pathways to depressive vulnerability. Even within the more circumspect cognitive domain that is the focus of our interest we do not intend to suggest that our interpretations, proposals, or understanding are anywhere near complete. Instead, based on the literature as we have interpreted it, we offer several proposals for an integrative understanding of cognitive vulnerability to depression. Such proposals will need empirical verification and, where necessary, revision. Regardless of whether such revision is substantial at some point in the future, or whether subsequent data show that we have missed so much of the conceptual boat that we are left high and dry on the dock, our hope at this point is that we have been able to describe adequately some of the cognitive elements that predispose some people to depression.

To begin our integrative exploration, we start at the most distal point possible in cognitive vulnerability; cognitive propensities as determined by our evolutionary past. We argue that such evolutionarily hard-wired architecture sets the stage for the development of cognitive vulnerability to depression. Moving to somewhat more proximal, but still distal dimensions, we summarize those processes we think may operate when individuals begin to incur cognitive vulnerability through key developmental phases in life. We then proceed to discuss the proximal manifestation of such vulnerability at a later, adult stage of life. Where appropriate we interpret and examine variables that may play a key role in this process, which starts in our ancestry and proceeds onward to the realization of depression in adults.

EVOLUTIONARY ROOTS OF DEPRESSION

The role of evolutionary selection in the development of psychological variables has begun to receive considerable attention (see, e.g., Buss, 1988; Millon, 1990; E. O. Wilson, 1975, 1978). Although a great deal of this attention has been directed to the evolution of personality traits and variables such as aggression (e.g., Buss, 1988), evolutionary theory has a great deal of relevance for understanding vulnerability to depression. In particular, the contribution of the evolutionary forces that have shaped our present psychological functioning as they pertain to depression vulnerability can be understood within the context of attachment theory. Bowlby (1988) argues that, among other things, such forces set the stage for powerful biological urges that have far-reaching implications for a variety of psychological phenomena.

In Chapter 9 we highlighted attachment as providing important insights into distal vulnerability processes. Recall that attachment theory focuses on the processes that are thought to shape the capacity of individuals to form meaningful and enduring emotional bonds with significant others throughout their lives. In a species as inherently social as humans, the capacity to develop attachments to others serves a multitude of important functions, most notably, to maintain bonds between people throughout diverse phases of maturation and life events. From an evolutionary perspective, the development and subsequent propagation of this capacity has most likely played a crucial role in natural selection and thus the survival of the human species. Like several other species (e.g., apes), at birth humans experience a protracted period of helplessness and dependency. Parents possessing an ability to bond emotionally to their children are substantially better able to provide both for their basic survival needs and for protection from danger.

The value of this process in humans is perhaps best illustrated by comparison to other species. For example, many species produce large numbers of offspring that require little or no care from the parents, a reproductive design that has been labeled an *r-reproduction strategy* (Chisholm, 1988; see also Millon, 1990). Animals reproducing by this strategy breed early and frequently, with only a small percentage of the offspring surviving long enough to reproduce. Development is fairly rapid, social and play behavior is limited, and action patterns are relatively fixed. A prototypical example of this strategy is exhibited by the sea turtle, which produces thousands of eggs during its reproductive lifespan. The eggs are buried in sand and left to be hatched; once hatched the offspring must fend for themselves. This strategy requires literally no parental attention to, or investment in, the basic survival needs of offspring because their large numbers produce a high probability that at least some will survive to reproduce.

In contrast, the other end of the spectrum is represented by the *K-reproduction strategy*. Animals that have evolved this strategy mature relatively slowly, play and engage in complex social behavior, exhibit flexible action patterns, and have few offspring. This strategy is typified by several ape species, whose females may produce a single offspring only every few years. For humans, who also embody a K-reproductive strategy, the relatively small number of offspring produced during the mother's fertile years necessitates an intensive commitment of time, energy, and psychological as well as material resources to ensure that some will survive long enough to reproduce and pass on their genes. As we noted in Chapter 9, at a phenomenological level parents can attest to the enormous sense of affective bonding that takes place with their infant children, a phenomenon that is deeply rooted in our evolution and thus has strong genetic and biological foundations (Bowlby, 1988). This bonding helps to assure that caretakers will initiate the necessary commitment to protect the child physically as well as to provide for basic needs.

In the specific context of the evolution of these attachment behaviors, Bowlby (1988) summed up the process and implications in the following way:

> It is . . . more than likely that a human being's powerful propensity to make these deep and long-term relationships is the result of a strong gene-determined bias to do so, a bias that has been selected during the course of evolution. With this frame of reference, a child's strong propensity to attach himself to his mother and father, or to whomever else may be caring for him, can be understood as having the function of reducing the risk of his coming to harm. For to stay in close proximity to, or in easy communication with, someone likely to protect you is the best of all possible insurance policies. Similarly, a parent's concern to care for his or her child plainly has the function of contributing to the child's survival. . . . and thereby the [survival of the] individual's own genes. (pp. 81, 165)

Attachment capacity serves other purposes beyond being a motivational force during the human infant's lengthy period of helplessness and dependency. For example, the learning of increasingly complex sets of skills and abilities that are needed to master progressively more difficult life tasks adequately is facilitated by the mutual ability of caretaker and child to form a significant attachment with one another. Although many tasks in modern life do not have fundamental survival value, from an evolutionary perspective, many tasks that needed to be learned by our ancestors did fulfill basic survival needs (e.g., the ability to recognize and avoid predators, where and how to find food and shelter). It is likely that the learning of these skills was correspondingly dependent on mutual attachment between caretaker and child.

Beyond interactions with caretakers during childhood, attachment capabilities are also essential for the maintenance of proximity between mature members of the same species. Sometimes this maintenance of proximity has survival value in that a group of the members of the same species are better protected than a single individual (i.e., strength in numbers). However, the maintenance of proximity of individuals also serves a much more subtle, but no less important function; that of the ongoing maintenance of affective bonds that play a critical role in our most basic emotional needs, a theme to which we will return shortly. The motivation to bond is thus hard-wired in our history.

It is no evolutionary accident that interpersonal loss is one of the most powerful precipitants of depression; severing attachment bonds with significant others goes to the very core processes of humans. As we have argued, humans are genetically and biologically wired not only to seek out interactions with others in general, but to seek out intimate interactions with at least some people. As some theorists have argued, this social behavior reflects a biologically driven process that eventuates in reproductive success (Gilbert, 1992) and has thus been selected for in the evolutionary process. Indeed, when this social contact seeking is absent it is considered a reflection of psychopathology of another type (e.g., schizoid personality disorder).

But what is the basic survival function of the expression of an affective state that results from the dissolution of a significant relationship? In other arenas of affective expression, survival value and a corresponding evolutionary advantage are obvious. Perhaps the most obvious example is fear; individuals who developed a sense of fear of harmful objects were more likely to avoid such harmful objects and live to reproduce, thus passing on these basic emotional genes to future generations (Buss, 1988). The converse of this example is represented by animals without natural predators, who evolved no sense of fear and who became extinct not long after contact with humans (Quammen, 1996). The transition of fear responses into anxiety states and disorders is also relatively obvious; with fear mechanisms hard-wired, individuals who have inappropriately learned to fear nonharmful situations are likely to develop anxiety states when they perceive that they are, or may be, confronted with a feared situation. This is particularly problematic when the feared object is very general or only vaguely defined (e.g., a heart attack, being alone, fear of rejection, etc.).

The evolutionary survival function of basic sadness and depression is more subtle but no less important than anxiety. Indeed, the capacity to develop and feel profound sadness and depression serves enormous value. If dissolution or loss of a significant interpersonal relationship brings on a profound and aversive state of sadness, this state serves as a powerful motivator to reestablish the relationship where possible or, if not possible, to seek out new relationships. Such a possibility was first advanced in the context of attachment processes by Bowlby in 1969. Thus, we suggest that humans are genetically predisposed to feel an aversive state when losses are suffered, and similarly predisposed to attempt to relieve this aversive state by redeveloping, if possible, preexisting bonds or, if not possible, by developing significant new social bonds. The establishment of these emotional bonds and significant relationships with others helps to ensure the survival of the species. Not only are individuals who are affectively motivated to create interpersonal bonds more likely to reproduce, but if we recall the protracted helplessness experienced by human infants, those who have the benefit of emotionally bonded parents are more likely to survive and pass on attachment-linked sadness genes to their offspring. In turn, these offspring are more likely to survive because the parent possesses the core need to bond to others of the species.

Affective bonding is, indeed, a pervasive phenomenon in humans. Such bonding can even occur to a lesser but still significant degree at an interspecies as well as at an intraspecies level. Pet owners, for instance, report significant emotional bonds with other species and grieve the loss of these companions in a less intense but similar way to the grieving of the loss of a significant human companion (however, replacement is easier for nonhuman animals; human companions can sometimes but not reliably be found at the local animal shelter).

THE DEVELOPMENT OF DISTAL COGNITIVE VULNERABILITY STRUCTURES

Our evolutionary heritage has primed us for the development of a variety of processes that may lead to a predisposition to depression. As we previously noted, the attachment perspective provides an important context in which to understand at least some of these processes. In line with this perspective, we will offer several ideas concerning the development of distal cognitive vulnerability.

When events occur in childhood that affect attachment processes, a variety of effects may occur. Although it is obvious that childhood is a time of enormous and extensive learning, it is important to note that *what* is learned is consolidated in the formation of increasingly intricate and complex neural associations and connections that determine the cognitive and affective development of the child. The occurrence of negative events or situations can thus have a profound effect on the child's developing cognitive–affective networks. The experience of a negative event, however, is hardly an isolated occurrence in childhood. Indeed, occasional negative events are a routine part of growing up.

Rather, to the extent that negative events occur in abundance, occur in the context of multiple and likely interacting domains (e.g., a very dysfunctional family, divorce, high levels of poverty, problematic peer relationships), are chronic or extremely traumatic, cognitive–affective development will be proportionally impacted (for the sake of simplicity we will refer to such significant events of this sort as attachment disruptions). We do not mean to suggest that all such events necessarily have depression vulnerability-producing effects, or that these events are the only effects on the generation of depression-predisposing cognitive networks, but they seem to be likely candidates to affect profoundly the learning structures and processes, and what is learned by the developing child.

In general, several types of interactions with attachment figures are likely to predispose to later depression. For instance, lack of caring or involvement (evidenced in the extreme by abandonment) most likely leaves a vulnerability to depression. This lack of caring can be reflected by neglect in some cases or, in others, by extreme criticism or abuse. Another potential type of cognitive vulnerability-producing interaction is overinvolvement or not allowing the child to achieve age-appropriate levels of independence. Of course, these factors need not be independent. As we have previously noted, caregivers can both lack caring and be overinvolved, a combination known as affectionless control, which is perhaps the most virulent of factors in the genesis of cognitive vulnerability.

Empirical data are sparse on the *precise* predisposing effects that various childhood negative events have on subsequent adult depression. However, in line with our earlier consideration of attachment and the evolution of sadness affective structures, we speculate that the potential long-term effects of negative events are likely to be particularly damaging when they involve key attachment figures. For example, although neglect may have unpleasant effects when experienced as coming from any important figure, when significant and chronic neglect is perceived as coming from the most significant figures (those to whom attachments have been formed, such as parents), then this may produce a particularly negative cognitive self-structure. In this example, the child may not only begin to develop working models that are comprised of cognitive representations of current or future significant others as neglectful or unreliable, but may also develop a cognitive structure that represents the self as unworthy of attention and care (Batagos & Leadbeater, 1995). Similarly, pain is never pleasant, but at the hands of attachment figures it may lead to encoding messages about the nature of others and the self; physically abusive caretakers may produce a cognitive model of others as pain producing and not to be trusted, as well as of an unsafe world in general. Children of abusive caretakers may also develop a cognitive model of themselves as deserving of punishment and pain.

In the developing child, such negative experiences are likely to generate personal themes of derogation and unworthiness that become deeply encoded in self-structures. Also embedded are a variety of concepts linked to the experience of disrupted attachment such as representations about the behavior of significant others and the safety of the world in general. Cognitive structures, however, are not the only neural networks that are developing; affective structures are also in the process of becoming more differentiated and of developing associations to other structures (see Jordan & Cole, 1996). Thus, cognitive self-structures could potentially become closely linked to sadness affective structures through this developmental process. Negative affect, therefore, becomes not only intricately intertwined with unfavorable views of the world and others, but strongly associated with unfavorable conceptions of the self.

The developmental level of the child is also an important consideration. For example, the occurrence of negative affect-invoking events at certain times during key developmental processes may reflect an especially high level of risk for the development of a negative self-structure. For example, early childhood is a time of extensive egocentrism, and children may attribute the occurrence of negative events to themselves, regardless of whether such attributions are accurate (which they rarely are). Such a tendency may have particularly virulent effects when it is activated in the context of developing a consolidated and differentiated self-schema centered around sadness that is (increasingly strongly) being linked to an (increasingly) extensive network of negative representations of the world. Data are not yet clear on precisely when are the most vulnerable times for the development of depressive self-schemas, but, conceptually, those times when the child's sense of self is in the early formative states appear to represent particularly hazardous periods.

If attachment disruption is brief and secure attachment interactions are reestablished, negative cognitive representations are likely to be limited and more weakly linked to affective networks akin to what Bower (1981) has termed "sadness emotion nodes." On the other hand, if the attachment process is more problematic, then such connections between negative self-representations and negative affect should become more extensive and more strongly linked. Thus, to the extent that self-relevant negative emotion-producing events are numerous, traumatic, or chronic, they will have a correspondingly profound effect on the development of, and connections between, representations of the self and others and the experience of negative affective states. Each disruption is likely to strengthen and extend further these connections, thus "pumping up the volume" as these cognitive–affective networks develop. The soon-to-be vulnerable to depression person thus develops a schema of the self as being unlikable and unlovable, which is strongly tied to the experience of negative affect. Hence, self-derogatory cognitive networks are developing and becoming available to be brought online when affective structures are activated in the future. Thus, when individuals with these cognitive–affective links encounter sadness-producing experiences in the future, they not only experience negative emotions, but will also activate a variety of negative cognitions concerning the self.

Numerous events may be associated with sadness and despair for adults. However, within the framework of cognitive vulnerability to depression, once cognitive–affective connections are established during critical developmental periods, future events that occur in adulthood rekindle negative cognitive processes through negative affect. For example, the negative affect surrounding a divorce may evoke powerful negative cognitions established during disruptions in early attachment. Hence, the subsequent loss of key attachment figures will activate a strongly aversive affective state, which will result in sadness (as well as other associated emotions) and the corresponding activation of the now linked dysfunctional self- and other cognitive representation networks. We will discuss this more fully in the section on mature or proximal cognitive vulnerability structures. For now it is important to keep in mind that the reason that this is likely is because we are hard-wired by evolutionary selection for the maintenance of bonds with others, and when these bonds are broken an aversive emotional state is likely to be created that will have profound reverberations for cognitive development.

By emphasizing the collateral development and activation potential of emotional structures and dysfunctional cognitive structures in individuals vulnerable to depression, we do not mean to suggest that these are the only emotional capacities that become fully developed, the only cognitive representations and capacities that are engendered, or the only connections between cognitive and affective structures. In fact, a variety of generalized cognitive capacities as well as other kinds of cognitive self-representations evolve as the child grows. Indeed, examining the development of these other cognitive structures within the context of the evolution of our species, it seems unlikely that vulnerable individuals would survive long enough to reproduce and pass on their genes unless they also developed other competencies. Some of these competencies undoubtedly developed for the purpose of bonding to attachment figures in the future by finding (and holding) these attachments (e.g., the development of procedural knowledge that serves as the basis of social skills). Other basic survival competencies, such as intellectual capabilities, also develop. When operating in states that are quiescent or not emotional, these capacities are likely to guide cognition and behavior, even for those individuals who are vulnerable to depression. Cognitive vulnerabilities thus represent background or latent processes in individuals at risk for depression, which do not become operational in the guidance of the organism until an emotion-producing attachment disruption is experienced.

We have attempted to sketch a broad outline of how certain developmental processes may play a key role in the creation of distal cognitive vulnerability. Similarly, specific theories of depression have incorporated conceptions of these processes into their particular theoretical frameworks. Rose and Abramson's (1992) description of the developmental antecedents of the hopelessness theory of depression is an excellent example (see Chapter 9). They examine the issue of negative and repetitive emotion-eliciting events in children by suggesting that children who experience negative events will attempt to find the causes and significance of these events, which leads to the development of a dysfunctional attributions style for future events. We mention the developmental elaboration of the hopelessness theory not to advocate it or any specific cognitive theory of vulnerability to depression, but rather to suggest that the events and processes that we have described will provide the basic building blocks of distal cognitive vulnerability processes.

PROXIMAL COGNITIVE VULNERABILITY

The processes we have described in key periods in development set the stage for proximal vulnerability. But what do these structures look like in adulthood for vulnerable people? Most likely, they are considerably better differentiated. That is, whereas the link between negative affect and cognition is quite diffuse in children, in adults the links between sadness affective structures and various cognitive networks have become strengthened and firmly established. In this section we speculate on the nature of some of these structures.

Meta-Construct Organization of Proximal Cognitive Vulnerability to Depression

In Chapter 1 we discussed aspects of a meta-construct approach to classifying and organizing various cognitive constructs that have been applied to psychopathology. We employ this framework here to present our speculations concerning the mechanisms that constitute proximal vulnerability variables. As we cautioned earlier when describing this framework, we intend this not as a static or rigid model but rather as a useful organizational heuristic that may aid, in this context, in the understanding of cognitive vulnerability to depression.

Structures

Our assumption is that the basic cognitive vulnerability structures have been established through the sorts of problematic attachment-related learning we discussed earlier. We suspect that in adulthood such vulnerability structures do not look all that different from those proposed by Beck (1967) three decades ago. As we noted earlier, somewhat differing definitions of the very similar constructs of schemas and cognitive networks exist, but nearly all definitions converge on the idea of a stored body of knowledge (declarative and procedural) that is organized, or linked together, in some fashion. As we have suggested, the person vulnerable to depression possesses cognitive self-schemas or structures that have strong associative links to the mechanisms responsible for the activation of sad affect. We view these structures as proximal in the sense that, although they are not fully operational during times of stability or emotionally quiescent functioning for vulnerable individuals, they nevertheless provide the foundation of the cognitive responses to triggering events and thus guide information processing. That is, these cognitive structures that are so closely linked to affective structures are latent but become the first response to events that are appraised as both meaningful and (most likely) interpersonally negative by the person. Hence, an important feature of these structures in individuals who are vulnerable to depression is that they can be activated by various triggering events. We will comment more fully on this activation in the subsequent section on vulnerability cognitive operations and in the section on diathesis–stress interactions.

Propositions

In discussing structural aspects of cognitive vulnerability, our focus has been on the organizational of these variables; specifically, the link between cognitive and affective structures, and how the spread of activation is organized (i.e., direct and indirect activation). Propositions refer to the content of these structures and are thus proximal vulnerability features because they represent the themes and substance of what is activated. It is not possible to detail or catalogue the universe of particular propositions or concepts that vulnerable individuals have encoded in cognitive structures. These will be a function of the specific experiences that each person has encountered as cognitive networks are developing and, once developed, have been encoded through the information-processing guidance of these networks. Cognitive models of depression, however, suggest several generalities or broad themes that tend to be represented within the cognitive structures of vulnerable individuals. As we examined in our discussion of distal structures, and have alluded to several times in this chapter, these propositions are likely to reflect conceptions of (1) the self that are (2) negative, unfavorable, or derogatory in nature. Hence, the general themes of these propositions converge on beliefs of personal inadequacy and worthlessness, perceptions of being unlikable and unlovable, and so forth. These represent the core beliefs or concepts that are activated when the depressive self-schema is brought online in vulnerable people.

The pervasiveness of such self-related propositions may also mediate the frequency with which these propositions are activated. That is, although we have suggested that such networks generally stay dormant until activated, individuals with particularly extensive and well-connected beliefs are likely at great risk for indirect activation. For example, the person who has an extensive self-related network centering around personal inadequacy may be more likely to perceive verification of this inadequacy in interpersonal functioning, whether such verifying data exist or not. If, for instance, the person with such propositions encoded in self-structures is, via a particularly well-elaborated sense of inadequacy, functioning on heightened alert for cues of inadequacy in social situations, then such cues may be found. Thus, in addition to serving to interpret events in a depressogenic manner, these structures may also play a role in the creation of events, or becoming activated when events do not occur. In line with this idea, Hammen (1991b) has argued that depressed individuals contribute to the occurrence of at least some negative life events, a theme to which we will return shortly.

Operations

As we previously reviewed, there is a multitude of data that attest to the fact that, when depressed, individuals attend to, encode, and retrieve information that reflects poorly on the self. Such concepts represent the processing assumptions of cognitive networks or schemas; that is, these constitute some of the mechanisms by which these structures are hypothesized to work. For example, given the role of schemas in guiding information processing, this process takes place partially by determining the sorts of information to which attention will be directed. Similarly, schemas are hypothesized to function by determining or affecting what is encoded for storage or further processing, and by directing what information is, and is not, retrieved from storage. Through these mechanisms, schemas play an important role in structuring virtually all aspects of information processing pertaining to the self.

A central operational construct in our conceptualization of cognitive vulnerability is the idea of activation. Activation of cognitive mechanisms can occur in different ways. Direct activation, for instance, occurs when a cognitive structure is activated by the occurrence of an event whose informational parameters match or closely resemble the parameters represented within the cognitive structure. In Chapter 6 we noted the example of the loss of a spouse that would cognitively resemble the death of a parent. Such an example is prototypically representative of the interpersonal loss that forms the core of attachment disruptions that produce vulnerability.

As we suggested in Chapter 6, there are at least two ways to conceptualize activation of cognitive structures: from the core outward into the network (direct) or from the aspects of the cognitive network into the core (indirect). A key to proximal vulnerability at the structural level is that, when events are cognitively appraised as meaningful and interpersonally unfavorable, they will activate emotional structures (e.g., the core of the structure). Earlier in this chapter we commented on the evolutionary basis for this emotional response, which we view as a core human experience and, as such, a core feature of cognitive networks (i.e., a perception of the disruption of bonding with others is directly linked to the activation of a negative affective state). Thus, one pathway to cognitive vulnerability in this context is that, when certain cognitive networks or schemas have been (1) well developed and elaborated, and (2) strongly linked to this hard-wired negative response to interpersonal disruption, a loss-related event will directly activate these schemas.

Although direct activation of structural mechanisms is an important aspect of proximal vulnerability, the importance of indirect activation should not be underestimated. For example, the individual who possesses an extensive and well-articulated vulnerability structure will perceive and thus perhaps experience a very broad range of events that can be interpreted as negative and meaningful. We will examine the role and functioning of this process in more detail in the section on diathesis–stress interactions, but in the present context this process can be thought of as an indirect activation process. Specifically, the person with an elaborate cognitive structure rendering him or her vulnerable to depression may experience the network being brought fully online by the initial activation of only parts of the network. Recall our earlier example of the vulnerable person being turned down for a date. If this event activates components of a network that generalize beyond such an event to beliefs of personal inadequacy, core emotional structures may become activated. Such a process may be particularly problematic in that it increases the universe of events that may eventually trigger depression.

In discussing the activation patterns of cognitive networks and emotional structures, it is important to emphasize the reciprocal and interacting nature of these patterns. If we assume that both direct and indirect activation are adequate representations of the processes by which networks are brought online, then it follows logically that these processes must interact. For example, a process that feeds activation from a core emotional structure to a cognitive network (direct activation) will eventually have this activation fed back to the core by virtue of the processes that point activation inward toward a core (i.e., indirect activation). Thus, characterizing activation as either direct or indirect may simply reflect the nature of the initial process.

The process we are discussing in the onset (and subsequently the maintenance) of depression is not particularly new. In his seminal 1967 book, Beck suggested the following:

> Let us assume that initially the schema is energized as the result of some psychological trauma. The activation of this cognitive structure leads to the stimulation of the affective structure. The activation of the affective structure produces a burst of energy, which is experienced subjectively as painful emotion. The energy then flows back to the cognitive structure and increases the quantity of energy attached to it. This then produces further innervation of the affective structure. (p. 289)

Although our emphases may differ somewhat, the underlying process is quite similar.

Whether directly or indirectly activated, the functioning of vulnerability networks suggests that network-guided appraisal processes are important aspects of depression onset. In particular, activation of emotional structures is determined by the appraisal of life events. The appraisal construct, as initially discussed by Arnold (1960) and later in more detail by Lazarus (1966, 1968, 1982), refers to the fashion in which life events are linked to existing cognitive structures. More specifically, appraisal is typically seen as the process that gives subjective meaning to external events and is generally thought to be determined by individuals' (1) beliefs about the parameters of a life event and (2) expectancies as to the effects of the event (Averill, 1979). To illustrate, consider the individual who has just experienced a separation from a significant other and believes that the significant other will never been seen again (an event parameter) and that adequate functioning will not be possible without the significant other (a perceived effect of the event).

This event will thus be appraised in a way that will activate sadness emotion structures and the corresponding cognitive networks to which they are linked.

Products

As we noted in Chapter 1, products consist of the cognitions or thoughts that result from the interaction of activated cognitive structures, propositions, and operations, which process the informational parameters and sensory data of events. Products can cover a wide range of constructs, which includes variables such as attributions and self-statements. All people, vulnerable or not, will experience products that are a function of events interpreted and processed via cognitive schemas. For vulnerable people, these will be dysfunctional or depressotypic in the sense that they are self-critical in nature. An attribution of self-blame, for instance, constitutes an example of a depressotypic product. The self-blame part of this has been amplified by the attributional aspects of the hopelessness theory of depression. Thus, to the extent that people who evidence a tendency to blame themselves (internal, stable, and global attributions for the cause of negative events) will be vulnerable to depression because blaming oneself when bad things happen leads to negative affect. Self-statements that are derogatory in nature similarly exacerbate negative affective states. Constructs such as self-blame attributions or negative self-talk are a reflection of cognitive structures; that is, self-talk is the product or surface manifestation of the core beliefs and concepts that are contained in the schemas and activated in response to negative events.

Depressogenesis of Cognitive Mechanisms

In discussing attachment disruptions in childhood, we noted that experiencing negative events is a routine part of growing up and, of course, of being an adult. In all people negative events of sufficient severity lead to negative affective states, and, indeed, the presence of depressive symptoms is not uncommon. In nonvulnerable persons, these negative events are hypothesized to initiate cognitive responses suggesting beliefs about adequacy and the ability to overcome such events. We do not suggest that activating adequacy cognitions is necessarily easy, or that negative events in healthy individuals do not require cognitive and/or behavioral coping. Indeed, with severe negative events, effective coping can be difficult for even the healthiest of people (see Figure 4.2 in Chapter 4). Rather, people who are not vulnerable will have cognitive networks available that will allow and facilitate dealing with such events in ways that do not produce depression.

For vulnerable people, on the other hand, the proximal cognitive response to negative events is the activation of a schema containing themes of inadequacy and a tendency toward self-blame. Cognitively interpreting life stress or negative events in terms of one's own inadequacy and inferiority thus turns a "normal" negative affective state into depression. For example, the person abandoned by a spouse or significant other will experience significant negative affect. The person in this situation who blames him- or herself; sees this as a global and stable phenomenon; engages in negative self-talk and ruminates about the situation, its implications, and his or her perceived inadequacy, inferiority, and ineptitude; and recalls previous failures will experience negative affect that will turn into a depressive state. We are reminded in this context of Freud's (1917) differentiation between mourning and melancholia; in mourning, the person's response to a loss is "This is terrible"; in melancholia, the person's response to this loss is "I am terrible." The vulnerability function or depressogenesis of the cognitive mechanisms we have outlined therefore lies in the transition from normal negative affective states to a depressive psychopathological state.

In sum, there are several depressogenic factors that account for variance in proximal cognitive vulnerability to the onset of depression. The first is simply the possession or availability of well-elaborated negative cognitive self-referent structures, and their various operations and propositions, that are strongly linked with negative affect mechanisms. Secondly, once these structures are available, they will in turn increase the probability that they will be activated by increasing the range of potential triggering events. Theoretically, the possession of negative cognitive–affective self-structures and their influence on information processing increases the chances that nonpathological depressive states will spiral into pathological depression.

Onset and Maintenance

As we noted in Chapter 5, causality can be differentiated according to the onset of depression or the maintenance of the depressed state. Theoretically, different sets of factors may be involved in these two aspects of causality and hence their corresponding vulnerabilities. For instance, a somewhat different set of factors may be implicated in the onset of depression from those factors that are implicated in the maintenance of the depressed state. Although such distinctions are possible, our view of extant theory and data suggests considerable overlap in these vulnerability functions. For instance, to the extent that a schema has become activated, which plays the central role in the onset of depression, the *continuing* activation of this schema serves to maintain depression by guiding both internal and external information processing and by providing access to a negative information flow.

External Information Processing: The Tyrannical Self-Schema

This maintenance process is reminiscent of ideas presented in an article by Greenwald (1980) entitled, "The Totalitarian Ego: Fabrication and Revision of Personal History." Greenwald reviewed evidence from a number of sources suggesting that, through information-processing biases such as selective attention, people have a tendency to revise their personal history in order to protect themselves psychologically; they "rewrite" their experiences to make themselves feel better. Greenwald labeled this behavior "totalitarian" because of the psychological similarity to totalitarian societies that maintain control through information manipulation; history books, for example, are rewritten to serve certain views. But there is another aspect of this analogy that may be particularly germane for depressed people; totalitarian societies maintain control not only through rewriting history, but also through oppression and tyranny. It is in this sense that depressed people might be characterized as operating under the constraints of a totalitarian ego (or perhaps a "tyrannical" self-schema). Such a schema does not serve to protect individuals psychologically but rather "oppresses" individuals' information-processing and meaning systems with access to a steady influx of self-degrading, negative, disheartening, and pessimistic data. This is one manner in which depression is maintained.

Top-Down/Bottom-Up Information Processing. The cognitive maintenance of depression may also be seen in the context of an overreliance on top-down information processing. Recall in Chapter 1 our discussion of the idea that information processing can stem from the top down, indicating the influence of cognitive structures on the data to be processed, or, alternatively, from the bottom up, which suggests that information processing is directed from the data available. Such a distinction has also been characterized as concept-driven versus data-driven information processing. In all likelihood, healthy individuals employ a combination or balance of concept-driven and data-driven information processing, a process that has been long recognized in the basic cognitive theoretical literature (Neisser, 1967). Thus, healthy people employ schemas to help structure and order information-processing operations, but they are also responsive to the data that are processed, which thus influence the operation and content of schemas. Depressed individuals, on the other hand, may have deviated from this healthy balance with an overreliance on concept-driven processing, a fact that may account for the reliable observation that negative affective states are characterized by an imbalance in the ratio of negative to positive thoughts (Schwartz & Garamoni, 1989; Schwartz & Michelson, 1987). Such "cognitive intransigence" (Ingram, 1990) is particularly problematic when the cognitive structures are very dysfunctional in nature, as they are in depression Similarly, and in line with several of our proposals in this book, nondepressed but vulnerable individuals may also evidence this tendency toward more top-down processing, which, when combined with the increased availability of negative self-structures, places them at risk for processing information in a way that will initiate a depressive state. Therefore, one way to view the cognitive functioning of depressed individuals (and those vulnerable to depression) is not only via the operation and content of cognitive self-structures (dysfunctional in this case), but in terms of deviation from the normal balance between top-down and bottom-up processing to a resulting overabundance of top-down to the *relative* exclusion of bottom-up or data-driven processing. Note that this represents a shift in a balance and not a complete abandonment of data processing; functioning even nonadaptively requires some attention to external data, even if depressed individuals insufficiently process it or are cognitively unresponsive to this information (Ingram et al., 1983).

Internal Information Processing: Cognitive Recycling

We previously discussed the reciprocal nature of affective and cognitive processing systems; for instance, direct and indirect activation systems. We noted that these processes can work in concert, and thus activation that spreads outward to cognitive elements is likely to be fed back into the core, presumably at a somewhat degraded strength but still sufficient to re-activate affective structures.

We can apply these principles to the maintenance of depression. When negative affective structures and the dysfunctional cognitive schemas with which they are associated are activated above threshold, activation continues the spread throughout the network. Once started, this process may resemble a "cognitive loop" or "recycling" of activating and re-activating cognitive and emotional structures in which thoughts, memories, and associations consistent with the person's affective state are brought on line (Clark & Isen, 1982; Isen, Shalker, & Clark, 1978). Energy thus continues to spread "out" into the network and then "back" toward affective structures, keeping the cognitive–affective system on-line. Whereas recycling trash is an important activity for preserving a healthy planet, recycling cognitive trash is much less healthy in that it maintains a depressive state. Phenomenologically, this recycling process results in the ruminative cognitions (cognitive products) reported by depressed individuals. For example, it may seem to the individual that negative memories keep coming back, again and again, thus maintaining depressive feelings. Thus, the depression-prone individual who has suffered an interpersonal loss will ruminate on this loss long after such rumination has any functional value.

Continual thinking about a problem is not always a dysfunctional process. A person's rumination on events may lead to new solutions to a problem and thus can serve an important adaptive function. Even in the case of depressive affect, rumination can have similarly positive effects. Through rumination, people may come to new or creative insights into problems. This process most likely has been evolutionarily selected for, to some degree; people who ruminate may be able to evaluate their lives in new ways that lead to adaptive behaviors that were previously unavailable. In the case of the person with a negative self-schema, however, such rumination loses its adaptive function. This may be because there is little flexibility in the rumination process (e.g., the person cannot stop ruminating when it becomes debilitating), and what is ruminated on is negative and unlikely to lead to new or effective solutions to problems (Ingram, 1990).

Decay in the System

Although this recycling process keeps the depressive system online, thus keeping both internal and external information processing dysfunctional, it is not perpetual; energy in any system eventually decays. As activation thus spreads and is ultimately fed back, its gradient gradually decreases over time and this depressogenic process will eventually decay (Ingram, 1984). Thus, affective structures are reactivated at slightly lower levels, and eventually dysfunctional schemas and their associated affective structures will become dormant, as long as there are no additional activating events (such events are discussed in the section on diathesis–stress). Activation and decay functions have not been mapped; thus it is not possible to state how long such decay into dormancy takes place. The fact that most cases of depression do eventually remit, even without treatment, is consistent with the idea of this decay function, but it appears that this process may take place at an extremely slow rate.

Summary of Cognitive Vulnerability Dimensions in Onset and Maintenance

Although vulnerability to onset can differ from vulnerability to maintenance, our conceptualization suggests a great deal of similarity in these vulnerability processes. To some extent this similarity may reflect ambiguity about where to draw the line differentiating the onset of a disorder from its maintenance. For example, DSM-IV specifies that individuals must be depressed for a minimum of 2 weeks before a diagnosis of depression can be made; this in a sense suggests that the disorder must be maintained before its onset can be diagnosed. Our conceptualization of the construct of depression, while not specifying any particular duration, nevertheless suggests that the disorder must persist for a long enough period for it to interfere with adequate functioning. Such ambiguity aside, the most damaging aspect of a disorder such as depression is that it does indeed persist and it is therefore conceptually important to distinguish these facets of the disorder.

In summary, we suggest that people *become* depressed in the face of negative life events because their response to these events is to enter a spiral of schema-driven information processing of self-derogation and blame that interferes with adaptive functioning. They *stay* depressed because the maladaptive structures that have been activated screen information processing in a dysfunctional way, and lead to a ruminative recycling loop that reactivates the negative affective structures and their associated cognitive networks. In many respects, the difference may not be so much in kind or quality as in emphasis; the activation process causes the onset of the depressed state whereas the re-activation process maintains the depressed state.

DIATHESIS–STRESS: COGNITIVE VARIABLES AS THE FINAL COMMON PSYCHOLOGICAL PATHWAY TO DEPRESSION

As is clear from our preceding discussion, depressogenic schemas, the core of cognitive vulnerability, lie dormant until activated by stressful events. Based on speculations from evolutionary psychology, we have also suggested that those stressful events that are interpersonal in nature, particularly those that involve the dissolution of significant relationships, are leading candidates to serve this triggering function. In this section we explore in more detail the nature of this diathesis–stress function in depression.

The Relationship between Stress and Cognition in Depression

In Chapter 4 we suggested that cognitive variables and stress can be conceptually differentiated, and we noted that this separation can be empirically difficult to assess. We also noted that objectively measuring stress is difficult because not only must presumably stressful events be assessed, but contextual factors must be taken into account, and these factors must to some degree be differentiated from individuals' symptom levels and subjective appraisals (Depue & Monroe, 1986; Monroe & Simons, 1991). Aside from the methodological difficulties involved in measuring stress independently of cognition, examination of the conceptual relationship between stress and depression is extremely important for helping to understand the cognitive vulnerability process.

Although our focus is depression, stress is an important factor for understanding a variety of problems. Perspectives adapted from some of the theory and research on these problems may be helpful for conceptualizing some aspects of the relationships among cognition, vulnerability, depression, and stress. For example, in the health psychology arena, particularly that examining Type A or coronary disease-prone behavior, several researchers have examined the interactive functioning of stress and cognition. In this vein, Smith (1986) has outlined two ways in which Type A individuals might create or exacerbate stress levels that appear to serve as a link between hostility and the onset of coronary disease: Type A individuals (1) appraise an overly broad variety of situations as challenging and thus stressful, and (2) actively generate stress by placing themselves in stress-laden situations. In many cases, depressed individuals experience a significant amount of stress in the form of life events, many of which may occur independently of their actions. In a fashion analogous to coronary disease-prone individuals, people prone to either the onset or especially the maintenance of depression may function in ways that increase stress levels.

Depressive Cognition-Linked Appraisal Processes

For purely cognitive reasons, individuals who are prone to depression are apt simply to perceive a greater range of events as stressful, a process, we should note, that is not limited to cognitive vulnerability to depression. Recall in Chapter 4 we discussed Nicholson and Neufeld's (1992) argument that vulnerability to schizophrenia affects the perceptions of stress by affecting the cognitive mechanisms that govern the accuracy with which potentially stressful situations are appraised. Similar perceptual dysfunctions may operate in depression vulnerability in at least two ways.

Lowered Thresholds. Individuals who are experiencing increased levels of stress may also have a lowered threshold for perceiving subsequent events as stressful. As an example, failing to get a raise, which will be stressful for most people, may be perceived as significantly more so for the person experiencing the stress of a dissolving important relationship. Likewise, the normal stress produced by the result of a minor car accident may be perceived as very stressful by the person who has experienced a number of other stressful events and, via the belief that everything is going wrong in his or her life, is on the verge of depression. Even events that are presumably not stressful at all may be appraised as stressful by the vulnerable person afflicted by other stressful events.

Misperception. Stress will similarly be created by the misperception of nonthreatening events as threatening or stressful. In Chapter 4 we noted the example of a person experiencing a significant anxiety state who may misperceive relatively safe events as posing considerable physical or psychological danger. Such misperceptions are governed by the application of affectively linked schemas that guide information processing; in the case of anxiety the predominant affect is one of fear. In the case of depression, schemas (or working models) reflect the depressotypic construal of interpersonal interactions, and hence social events are likely candidates to be misperceived in a manner that increases stress. For instance, the individual vulnerable to depression may perceive social rejection when there is none. A colleague who fails to say hello because he is engrossed in thinking about a problem (or perhaps simply has poor social skills) may be interpreted by the vulnerable person as failing to say hello because of interpersonal dislike. If this vulnerability has been activated by stress in other areas of the individual's social functioning (e.g., relationship difficulties with a significant other), then such a misperceived social rejection will create additional stress.

Stress Generation and Cognition in Depression

In addition to the cognitive processes that may serve to create or exacerbate stress through lowered threshold and misperception, behaviors are also linked to stressful event generation. It is perhaps too simple a dichotomy, but it is clear that stressful events can befall vulnerable individuals (e.g., being rear-ended while sitting at a stoplight) or can be caused by vulnerable people (e.g., rear-ending a car sitting at a stoplight because of not paying attention to traffic and driving cues). Although certainly many stressful events may simply happen to people, several researchers have persuasively argued that other events may constitute the results of a depression-prone person's own actions (Depue & Monroe, 1986; Hammen, 1991b, 1992; Monroe & Simons, 1991; Rutter, 1986a, 1986b). For example, the person with social skills deficits (e.g., inappropriately critical of others) may engender tumultuous relationships with acquaintances, coworkers, and romantic partners that result in the generation of significant levels of stress for the person. As noted previously, Hammen (1991b) found that over the course of a 1-year follow-up, depressed women experienced more interpersonally stressful events, particularly events that involved interpersonal conflict. Hammen (1991b) noted that such events are likely to be the result of the generation of stress by depressed individuals. Vulnerable individuals may therefore play a role in contributing to their own diathesis-activating events. The manner in which this process may function is discussed in the next section.

Final Pathways: The Cognitive–Interpersonal Link in Depression and Vulnerability

Interpersonal and cognitive models have often been seen as competing or incompatible (Gotlib & Hammen, 1992; Safran & Segal, 1990). This division is both unfortunate and artificial in that such approaches are in fact not only complementary, but represent fundamentally related aspects of the same phenomenon (Ingram, 1994). Such a conceptual and empirical partition is no doubt due to the tendency of advocates from one paradigm or the other to pay insufficient attention to other aspects and assumptions in the process of exploring the assumptions of their own paradigms. Although some theorists do represent cognitive and interpersonal approaches as either–or propositions, most acknowledge the validity of a wide variety of contributions from different theoretical perspectives. For example, Beck's 1967 book, which helped launch the cognitive revolution in clinical psychology and established cognitive concepts as important processes in depression, cites a number of examples of the stress that precipitates depression. Virtually every example provided is interpersonal in nature (e.g., a woman losing her family in a car accident, a law professor being relatively unbothered by the lack of a promotion but becoming depressed upon discovering his wife having an affair, a problematic interaction with a woman's son during summer break, etc.). The focus here is clearly on cognition, but the importance of interpersonal events is also plainly recognized.

Similarly, in the cognitive vulnerability model we have described, interpersonal events play several key roles. For example, we have suggested that during key developmental periods distressful interpersonal events activate innate negative affective structures and, correspondingly, begin the process of developing connections between these affective structures and negative self- and other images. Additionally, once these distal vulnerability structures are in place, distressing interpersonal events serve as the triggering agents in the proximal activation of the depressive process. Hence, as with other cognitive models, although the focus is obviously on cognitive factors, interpersonal events account for a considerable amount of theoretical variance.

As we have previously discussed, some cognitive vulnerability theorists have divided cognitively vulnerable individuals into two types (sociotropic–dependent and autonomous–perfectionistic; see Chapters 3 and 7). Accordingly, sociotropic individuals are seen as vulnerable to interpersonal events or the loss of others whereas autonomous types are seen as vulnerable to depression following failure to achieve to the level of their own expectations. Although the high expectations set by autonomous people are internalized (i.e., beliefs they hold themselves), the processes leading to the development of these beliefs are quite likely interpersonal; that is, rigid expectations and demands by caregivers set the stage for the autonomous belief patterns that are encoded in these individuals' self-structures. Furthermore, the sense of failure the autonomous person experiences is generally interpersonal in the sense of feeling that he or she has "let down" others. Therefore, although the focus of autonomous vulnerabilities is not on interpersonal themes per se, we suspect that the context in which they are activated is quite interpersonal in nature.

We have acknowledged that interpersonal events play an important role by serving as potent triggers for the activation of proximal vulnerability, but have not yet commented on the broader relationship between cognitive and interpersonal functioning in depression vulnerability. Although there are any number of psychological models of vulnerability to depression, including interpersonal models, we propose that cognitive factors serve as the *final common pathway* to depression through which these other factors operate. That is, although there are a number of psychological factors that are related to the onset and maintenance of depression, we contend that these all operate via cognitive processes. Similar to Akiskal's (1979; Akiskal & McKinney, 1973, 1975) analysis of depression from a neuroanatomical levels of analysis (the diencephalon as the final neuroanatomical pathway), by final common pathway we mean that cognitive factors mediate all other psychological processes of vulnerability, including interpersonal processes.

In examining the idea that cognitive processes serve as the pathway through which factors such as interpersonal events are linked to depression, consider the ideas that have been advanced about stress generation and depression. As is apparent from our preceding discussion, proximal stressful interpersonal events do not necessarily simply happen to people independent of their actions. By interpreting social information and determining behavioral responses, cognitive structures (such as working models) that provide the template for how other people's actions are interpreted represent the mechanisms that create and mediate stressful interpersonal situations. All social behavior is cognitively mediated in that it has to be processed and interpreted. Indeed, we can think of few interpersonal interactions that are not cognitively mediated. The individual must process and interpret social information and thus respond "accordingly." That is, other people's behaviors, verbalizations, and nonverbal cues are processed and interpreted through the filter of the depressogenic vulnerability schema. Benign interactions thus have the potential to be viewed as nonsupportive or critical, leading to an "appropriate response." Earlier we provided the example of the individual who misinterprets a colleague's benign act of not saying hello as a personal rejection. If the vulnerable individual responds to this perceived slight in kind, interpersonal difficulties would be likely to ensue as a cycle of social rejection is engendered.

There are numerous examples of this central cognitive process. Vulnerable individuals may read social cues in ways that suggest they are being criticized when they are not and to respond accordingly, thus creating negative interpersonal response cycles. Of course, some people are in fact criticized. In line with our earlier discussion, the misperception of stressful events such criticisms, when interpreted via negative cognitive structures, will lead to exacerbated negative responses. The person with a relatively healthy self-concept who hears from a person that he is a "loser" may respond with negative affect but will be unlikely to enter a dysfunctional interpersonal cycle. The person who has incorporated "loser-ness" into personal working models will respond both cognitively and behaviorally in a very different way to such a comment.

Clinical anecdotes may help to illustrate cognitively mediated interpersonal response cycles. Although there are many such examples available, we describe two particularly apt examples. Perhaps the prototypical example of cognitively precipitated dysfunctional interactions comes in the form of paranoid ideation. The paranoid individual interprets even extremely benign cues as evidence of malicious intentions. One depressed patient treated by one of the authors also had strong paranoid features. Prior to the start of the treatment session, the author arrived at the office, greeted the client sitting in the waiting room, and told her he would be with her in just a minute. He then briefly conferred with a colleague sitting behind the receptionist's counter and, at the time scheduled for the appointment, invited the client to the therapy room. She immediately confronted him for talking behind her back and saying unkind things about her. His (true) explanation, that he was merely scheduling a lunch appointment with a colleague, was to no avail. As described by her in therapy sessions, this behavior was quite indicative of her typical perceptions and the negative interactions with others they created. Indeed, after many similar confrontations due to innocuous events being misperceived, people were indeed out to make her life more difficult.

Another patient treated by one of the authors also stands out as a classic example of cognitively mediated dysfunctional interpersonal behavior. As a child, this depressed woman had been sexually abused by several males, thus leading to the cognitive working model of "men are not to be trusted." Even when not in a depressed state, she saw signs of hostility when it was not present, and hostility was consequently "returned." Indeed, before any interaction had taken place, to defend against an impending attack, her strategy was to become aggressive in anticipation of abusiveness by males. This working model led to interpersonal interactions that were exceptionally dysfunctional, particularly in light of her desire to find a satisfying marital relationship (see our discussion of the evolutionarily driven bonding process). Interactions with women were similarly troubled, not so much because she viewed them as threatening or not to be trusted, but because she interpreted the actions of others as evidence that she was unliked (e.g., social gatherings she was not invited to were resented because she believed that people did not like her, and social gatherings she was invited to were declined because she believed that she was only invited because people pitied her). Her interpersonal problems were very real, but were mediated by a depressogenic cognitive style that made it difficult for her to perceive events in ways that allowed her to function effectively in social settings.

This cognitive–interpersonal mediational link can also be shown to be at the heart of some models that argue that interpersonal processes constitute the central feature of depression. There are a variety of interpersonal models, but a particularly prototypical and representative interpersonal model has been proposed by Coyne (1976; Coyne et al., 1990). In brief, this model suggests that with the onset of a depressive state, individuals seek out social support. Such support may have a variety of restorative functions. But, if the individual maintains the depressive state, that is, the support is not particularly effective, supportive individuals may pull back because of the aversiveness of being around people who are depressed (because of the negativity inherent in their perceptions and consequent interactions). Indeed some people have suggested, not completely tongue in cheek, that depression is a contagious disorder for just this reason (i.e., people experience depressed mood if they spend time around depressed people). The disengagement of social support, however, causes the depressed person to intensify support seeking, leading to further disengagement and thus initiating a vicious interpersonal cycle. Although such theories generally do not develop ideas for the remission of depression, such as the cognitive decay functions that we have proposed, they nevertheless capture vitally important components of the depression process.

Clearly such a model places heavy emphasis on the interactional cycles of depressed individuals. Our argument, however, is that cognition is the central pathway to this depressive cycle. The vulnerable individual who seeks out social support in this context is behaving in ways that have been selected for in our evolutionary history and is thus responding quite naturally. In the face of negative interpersonal events, the person who is becoming depressed seeks out such support to cope with the painful feelings. To the extent that other individuals eventually pull back their support, leading to the hypothesized intensification of support seeking, the depressed person is not being appropriately attentive to social cues suggesting that the relationship is starting to tax significant others; the person is *cognitively interpreting* events in a way that will ultimately lead to interpersonal breakdown. Hence, while we find a great deal of validity in such interpersonal models, we suggest that these interpersonal disruptions are cognitively mediated. To get a clear picture of such interpersonal functioning, cognitive mediation must be understood.

Cognitively mediated interpersonal disruptions are not limited to disruptions in existing social relationships, but also impact new relationships. We previously discussed the desire to bond with individuals and, when these bonds are broken, the desire to reestablish bonds or seek out new attachments (when cognitive problems have interfered too much with the existing relationship to repair it). The person who is too cognitively self-focused to attend to social cues so as to establish an adequate relationship with another illustrates such a process. Likewise, the person who cognitively misinterprets social cues (e.g., confesses desperation or neediness on a first date) will have difficulty establishing new bonds. As we noted in Chapter 9, this can colloquially be thought of as the baggage that comes from previous relationships and interferes with the establishment of new relationships. All of which is cognitively mediated and thus is worthy of the term "cognitive depressogenesis."

Stressful events and problematic interpersonal functioning are indeed important elements of the processes that bring about vulnerability. The final common pathway hypothesis suggests that these important factors are dependent on the cognitive processing functions of depressogenic cognitive structures; thus the pathway to the onset or maintenance of depression is through cognitive processes. The idea that cognition serves as the central mediating process is not new. In her discussion of stress generation in depression, for instance, Hammen (1991b) sums this perspective up very nicely when she alludes to this possibility: "Negative cognitions about themselves and events may alter their responses to circumstances or may contribute to an inability to cope with emergent situations and may also determine reactions to personally meaningful events [i.e., stress-generation]. In a sense, therefore, depression causes future depression through the mediation of stressors and cognitions about the self and circumstances" (p. 559). Cognition is the psychological bond that holds the rest of the vulnerability process together.

MEDIATING VARIABLES: COPING AND INTERVENTIONS

Several variables potentially serve to mediate the relations we have specified in our discussion of cognitive vulnerability. Of critical importance is the idea of coping. Coping is typically defined as the instrumental responses, both cognitive and behavioral, that the individual employs to mitigate stressful circumstances (Lazarus, 1966, 1990; Lazarus & Folkman, 1984). To say that the literature on stress and coping is enormous is a profound understatement, and we will thus not attempt a review. However, the relationship between coping and the processes we have described bears some comment.

Psychotherapeutic intervention is another mediational process that can be examined in relationship to cognitive vulnerability. Just as with coping, it is not possible to examine in detail the diversity of psychotherapeutic interventions; nevertheless, several basic therapeutic ideas as they apply to cognitive vulnerability deserve mention.

Coping Processes and Cognitive Vulnerability

Even though our description of many of the key cognitive processes in vulnerability may suggest that they operate in an almost mechanistic fashion, we do not intend to suggest that such processes can not be affected or interrupted. From a functional perspective, we define effective coping within the context of cognitive vulnerability as "any process, whether primarily behavioral or cognitive in nature, that interrupts the activation of the depressogenic cognitive structures and disrupts spreading activation." Such disruptions are hypothesized to prevent, or at least diminish, the transition of "normal" negative affect into a depressive state.

We noted in our discussion of distal vulnerability that children not only develop connections between cognitive self-structures and affect structures, but also other competencies. Even children who are at risk for depression by virtue of developing negative cognitive structures that are closely linked to negative affect, may also develop coping structures that help mitigate against the full-blown activation of depressogenic structures. There are a multitude of possible examples. For example, to the extent that seeking out personal relationships is key to adaptive functioning, vulnerable individuals who have developed a good set of social skills, defined generally as the ability to interact effectively with others, may be a position to prevent or at least diminish the dissolution of emotional bonds with others. Other coping skills might consist of the development of compensatory schemas (Ingram & Hollon, 1986) that serve to guide the individuals to engage in cognitive activities or behavior that help interrupt the depressogenic activation process. Hence, for instance, the individual who activates negative self-referent cognitions following a "failure" may also check out these perceptions with others and thereby be dissuaded from following through on these negative cognitions. We can by no means specify all of the possible coping mechanisms, but these few examples illustrate the functional principle that any process that serves to interrupt the activation of cognitive vulnerability structures will help to diminish the possibility that the individuals will experience significant depression.

No individual will ever avoid periods of negative affect and occasional feelings of sadness when negative events such as the loss of a significant other occurs, but individuals who have developed vulnerability structures might be better able to prevent "normal" depression from spiraling into clinically significant depression if they have also developed coping skills. Sometimes such coping skills can be developed as part of a therapeutic intervention in adulthood, but they are probably most effectively, and thus ideally, established during cognitive development in childhood.

Treatment Implications: Prevention of Relapse and Symptom Return

From the standpoint of intervention, a better understanding of cognitive vulnerabilities for depression could inform treatments in two areas: the prevention of future depression following recovery and the identification of and primary intervention with individuals at increased risk for depression. With respect to the latter, work has been reported in which the goal is to demonstrate the value of the prevention of depressive symptoms in at-risk populations (Munoz, Mrazek, & Haggerty, 1996). For example, studies have been conducted with fifth and sixth grade students (e.g., Gillham, Reivich, Jaycox, & Seligman, 1995) and adolescents (Clarke et al., 1995) that suggest the value of preventive approaches. In fact, the results from at least one randomized controlled trial with patients in a primary care setting are promising

(Munoz & Ying, 1993; Munoz et al., 1995). This work draws upon cognitive and social-learning models to explain the development of depression, although in these accounts cognitive variables cannot be separated from other factors such as behavioral deficits or temperamental differences.

One area in which cognitive variables may be closely linked to treatment strategies is in the prevention of relapse or recurrence of depression following recovery. Although it is true that there are multiple determinants of risk for depressive relapse, including physiological as well as other psychological variables, there are intriguing points of convergence between these domains. Post (1992), for example, has suggested that changes at the level of neuronal function, which follow parameters associated with "kindling" and episode sensitization, underlie episode recurrence. He posits a type of neurobiological "memory trace," which is more sharply defined with each successive depressive episode and which lays a path for new episodes to emerge in response to increasingly minimal cues. "Changes at the level of gene expression and alterations of neuropeptides or the neuronal microstructure" (Post, 1992, p. 1,006) are proposed as mechanisms through which this trace is established. Interestingly, specific changes in the thresholds required to activate the neural structures implicated in depression often depend on such factors as their past frequency of usage and links to mild dysphoric states.

More to the point, several ideas, including the mood dependent accessibility hypothesis model of depression (Teasdale, 1983, 1988), to which we have referred throughout this book, also predict that previous depression puts people at a greater risk for recurrence. Specifically, past usage of negative constructs increases the likelihood of depressive knowledge patterns being activated in the course of future information processing when in periods of mildly depressed mood. In addition, chronic activation patterns enhance generalization of knowledge structure utilization as these structures are deployed in a growing number of contexts over time. This would also explain how smaller magnitude changes in mood would be sufficient to activate them over time. J. M. G. Williams (1992) describes this as "the excessive reactivity of some people, responding to minor fluctuations of mood with large cognitive distortions" (p. 248). This is precisely the implication in the data reported in Chapter 7 when we reviewed empirical studies in which priming is used to study people who had been previously depressed; that is, virtually all of the studies using a priming procedure have demonstrated cognitive reactivity of negative self-structures.

This view also recognizes the possible receding influence of environmental events on the course of depressive disorder over time. Social adversity, for example, is thought to play less of a role in the return of depressive symptoms because the cognitive or biological mechanisms underlying the disorder achieve some degree of functional autonomy from psychosocial triggers. This may be one way that the processes associated with relapse and recurrence differ in important ways from those responsible of the onset and maintenance of the initial episode. Specifically, relapse and recurrence can be viewed as the "retriggering" of the patterns of biological and information-processing activity that characterize the initial episode.

Typically, neither pharmacological nor psychological treatments have been designed to apply this possible distinction between maintenance of the initial episode and the triggering of relapse and recurrence, perhaps because little in known about the intersection between factors that maintain vulnerability to recurrence and those responsible for the initial onset of the disorder. In order to address this possibility, several investigators (Segal, Williams, Teasdale, & Gemar, in press); Teasdale & Barnard, 1993) have suggested that it may be useful to distinguish between (1) the processes responsible for the escalation or "wind-up" of dysphoric states to more intense and persistent states in depressive relapse and recurrence, and (2) the processes responsible for the maintenance of these states, once established.

The possibility of differences between these two aspects of depression implies that it may be helpful to design interventions specifically targeted at preventing the triggering and escalation of depressogenic thinking patterns that seem central to relapse. While not differing in quality, such prophylactic treatments may differ in emphasis from those primarily designed to alleviate established depression (see also Hollon & Cobb, 1993; Hollon et al., 1990). For example, procedures that emphasize training in the volitional allocation and deployment of attention may be sufficient to redirect the processing resources required for the "escalation" of mild depressive states, thus preempting the "wind-up" of depressive relapse. Although insufficient, by itself, as a therapeutic strategy for dealing with an established depression, such attentional redeployment may be invaluable as part of a procedure to nip incipient relapse in the bud (Teasdale, Segal, & Williams, 1995). Such procedures share with existing cognitive therapy techniques the aim of helping patients "decenter" from negative automatic thoughts and feelings and can be combined with training in utilization of basic CBT methods to produce a novel treatment specifically designed for the prevention of future relapse in patients who have already recovered from depression as a result of either pharmacotherapy or cognitive therapy (see Kabat-Zinn, 1990, and Kabat-Zinn et al., 1990, for further details of this approach and its rationale).

One important difference between this approach and currently existing models of CBT delivery after treatment (either in booster sessions or maintenance mode) should be highlighted. In the latter model, patients are encouraged to prepare for future stressful events by rehearsing and augmenting their repertoire of coping behaviors (e.g., performing a situational risk analysis, identifying cognitive triggers, saving records from therapy that can be pulled out and reviewed in response to a stressor). If Post's (1990) analysis is accurate, then the utility of psychosocial stressors as markers of impending episodes will diminish over time, and the patient will be left with an unreliable way of gauging his or her level of risk.

This alternative approach emphasizes acquiring control over a cognitive process that is used on a daily basis (attention) and as such is not so tied to the occurrence of potential distal adversity. Training in attentional deployment can be mastered during periods of euthymia so that patients can be more adept at using it when difficult situations occur. This format is consistent with the needs of a maintenance treatment because the work the patient is expected to do is consistent with recovery and can begin following completion of treatment for more acute problems. In this way it may be possible to redress some of the biasing effects of the increased accessibility of negative structures and patterns of processing that work against the enactment of effective CBT-based strategies in the face of incipient dysphoria. Following this, more standard forms of CBT may be more actively utilized.

COROLLARY ISSUES RELATED TO COGNITIVE VULNERABILITY TO DEPRESSION

Our focus in this volume has been on distal and proximal cognitive vulnerability processes. However, we believe that any attempt to make theoretical statements about a pervasive disorder like depression, no matter what conceptual approach is taken, must at least comment on several issues whose importance is becoming increasingly recognized. In particular, issues of comorbidity, gender differences, and ethnicity demand attention. For example, considering the fact that women are twice as likely to experience and report depression, some discussion is necessary of why and how these differences exist. By the same token, depression is not simply a disorder that afflicts Caucasians, and, given the ethnic and cultural diversity present in North America, particularly in the United States, some theoretical assessment of ethnicity and depression is warranted. We thus believe that it is incumbent on theories of vulnerability and theories of depression, at the very least to comment on these differences. However, data assessing the interactions between these variables and depression are in many respects far less complete than data on cognition and depression. The current lack of data therefore dictates that our suggestions in these arenas are necessarily quite speculative. Our general belief is that, despite individual differences that will affect the expression of vulnerability in some individuals, the processes and mechanisms that we have postulated apply to all potentially vulnerable people.

Comorbidity

We noted early in this book that comorbidity was less of an issue for approaches that, like ours, tend to emphasize a somewhat more dimensional approach to depression. Nevertheless, depressive states frequently coexist with other states, making this construct worthy of comment. Of course, an in-depth exploration of comorbidity is well beyond the scope of this book, and excellent sources are available (Maser & Cloninger, 1990).

Regardless of the occurrence of comorbid states, our basic propositions about the nature of cognitive vulnerability are unchanged. That is, the structures and mechanisms that we postulate to be linked to vulnerability are the same for depression that occurs in relative isolation from other psychopathological states as for that which occurs in conjunction with these other states. Hence, to the extent that individuals evidence well-developed connections between degraded self-schemas and negative affect, depression is likely to occur when events trigger negative affect.

Nevertheless, we also acknowledge that this process does not occur in isolation. That is, factors that affect cognitive vulnerability can be linked to other vulnerabilities as well. For example, a disruption in the attachment process may produce vulnerability to depression *and* anxiety. Indeed, it is certainly possible that the affective structures that control depression and anxiety are closely related, and hence the activation of one may be linked to the activation of another. However, the process that we have outlined should occur if an interpersonal disruption activates sad affect, regardless of whether the person also is feeling anxious affect. In addition, cognitive vulnerability to depression could represent a portion of other cognitive vulnerabilities. As one example, the cognitive vulnerability that underlies borderline personality disorder may also encompass a vulnerability to depression. However, only in an individual who has a well-articulated negative self-structure tied to sad affect will vulnerability to depression be apparent.

Gender Differences

Earlier in this volume, we briefly reviewed the pervasive data showing that women are twice as likely as men to receive a diagnosis of unipolar depression. We also considered several theories aimed at accounting for these differences. We will attempt to offer some ideas as to how the cognitive processes we have outlined are potentially linked to depression vulnerability in both sexes. Before commenting on gender differences, it is important to note a critical yet often overlooked fact in many discussions of these differences, that is, even though it is certainly true that women have a much higher rate of depression, and thus this an undeniably serious problem for women, it is also a reality that many men do get depressed.

Problems in Overemphasizing Sex Differences in Depression

By even the most conservative estimates of the prevalence of depression (see Chapter 2), it is a fact that *millions* of men currently suffer from debilitating and clinically significant depression. Less conservative perspectives also suggest that depression is underestimated in men. For instance, if men employ substance abuse strategies to cope with depression, the resulting higher rates of substance use disorders in men compared with women might mask the true incidence of depression (Hull, 1981; Hull & Reilly, 1986; Ingram et al., 1988). We noted in Chapter 2 the fact that community surveys find different rates of depression in men and women, thus ruling out the possibility of different presentation rates at clinical settings. Yet, even in surveys men may still may be hesitant to admit the occurrence of symptoms that appear to indicate weakness, and these studies might thus still underestimate depression in this group to some degree. By any estimate, depression is a serious problem for a significant number of men as well as for women.

This fact has significant conceptual implications for our efforts to understand gender differences in depression. For example, some theories evidence a tendency to explain gender differences by implying that there are a certain set of factors related to depression that are uniquely associated with women, an implication suggesting that depression does not occur, or is not a problem, for men. In Chapter 2, for instance, we noted biological hypotheses linking neurotransmitter dysregulation to depression, which suggest that women are more vulnerable to depression because of endocrinological differences. We also noted variants to the biological hypotheses proposing that the menstrual cycle, menopause, and postpartum period predispose women to depression. If depression is due to hormonal changes associated with, for example, menopause, then men simply should not experience it.

Certainly not all approaches to gender differences encounter this problem. For example, approaches suggesting that women are more likely to encounter the factors that trigger depression (e.g., certain life events) can more easily account for depression in men by specifying that these events are simply encountered less frequently, but when they are encountered in men depression also results. Although this idea must still be empirically assessed, the assumption itself is conceptually sound. Of course, theories focusing special attention on certain processes in women, such as biological approaches, might also suggest that at least a subset of women might experience different kinds of depression, or different causes of depression than men, thus accounting for gender differences. Few theories specify such relations, however. In general, we argue that any theoretical approach that attempts to account for gender differences must acknowledge that while depression is a particular problem for a great number of women, it is also a significant and serious problem for many men. The focus should thus be on the different *rates* between the genders rather than on why women experience depression.

Cognitive Vulnerability and Gender Differences

Stated briefly, our view of cognitive vulnerability is that the same underlying mechanisms are responsible for vulnerability to depression in both men and women. Thus, for both women and men, we hypothesize that negative experiences in childhood such as attachment disruptions lead to the generation of beliefs of personal derogation and unworthiness, as well as representations about the behavior of others and the safety of the world, that become deeply encoded in cognitive self-structures. As these cognitive structures develop, they also become linked to negative affective structures that result in intricate associations between negative affect and unfavorable views of the world and oneself. Further, once cognitive–affective connections are established during critical developmental periods, the subsequent dissolution of emotional bonds through the loss of an attachment figure constitutes a particularly virulent event for producing the negative affect that is associated with the activation of negative cognitive self-structures.

Where then lie the differences between men and women? Given the universality of cognitive mechanisms that we have proposed, differences may possibly lie in (1) differential rates of developing these mechanisms, (2) differential rates of developing processes that affect these mechanisms, or (3) differences in the events that precipitate the onset of the processes we have specified. We will evaluate each of these possibilities separately although we acknowledge that it is more than likely that if any of these factors are correct, they interact in complex ways to produce a higher rate of depression in women than in men.

Differential Rates of Vulnerability Mechanism Development. If the basic mechanisms of cognitive vulnerability lie in the development of schemas or working models that contain dysfunctional information about the self and others, there is little reason to suggest that differential development underlies gender differences in depression. The biological urge to bond to caretakers, while perhaps differentially expressed by males and females, nevertheless occurs in both sexes. Hence, we see little reason to believe that the ability to experience disruptions in this bonding are not equally distributed across both genders; thus, the negative cognitive effects of these experiences should be similar.

Some specific types of disruptions, however, are more likely to occur in girls as opposed to boys. For example, some estimates of childhood sexual abuse have found higher rates for girls than boys. Finkelhor, Hotaling, Lewis, and Smith (1990) found that 27% of women as compared to 16% of men reported a history of sexual abuse. This experience, particularly when perpetrated by adult caretakers may indeed serve as the type of attachment disruption that creates cognitive vulnerability to depression. Clearly, those with a history of sexual assault are more likely to experience depression (Bifulco, Brown, & Adler, 1991; Burnam, Stein, & Golding, 1992), with some research finding more then double the rates of life time major depressive disorder in those women reporting a history of sexual assault (13%) when compared with those not reporting assault (6%) (Winfield, George, Swartz, & Blazer, 1990). In considering these data, it is important to keep in mind, however, that women (and men) who are not sexually abused do experience depression, and thus although differences in sexual abuse may account for some of the sex-difference variance, they do not account for all of it.

Differential Rates of Developing Processes That Affect These Mechanisms. Although we do not posit basic differences in the acquisition of negative cognitive self- and other structures, we do speculate that boys and girls learn and incorporate information differently, which may have a significant effect on how these processes are expressed. There are relatively well-known differences in the socialization experiences of boys and girls. Boys, for example, are more inclined to be socialized to suppress emotion and to value achievement goals. Girls, on the other hand, are more readily socialized to express emotion and to value interpersonal relationships. Connections may thus be stronger between interpersonal events and negative affect in females. Hence, valuing and nurturing interpersonal relationships, and the facilitated expression of emotion, are linked to a greater vulnerability to depression when disruptions in these relationships occur and trigger negative affect.

We believe that it is important to point out at this juncture, however, that these differences are not absolute. Indeed, in line with our comments about explaining differences, we suggest in this vein that (1) some boys are socialized more to express emotion and value interpersonal relationships than might be "typical," (2) some girls may socialized to suppress emotion and devalue interpersonal relationships. Hence, although these socialization differences may set the stage for affecting cognitive vulnerability mechanisms, the fact that they overlap accounts for different rates of depression and not for why women become depressed.

Conceptually, one way that these differences can be thought of is as coping differences. Recall that we defined effective coping as any process that interrupts the activation of the depressogenic cognitive structures and/or interrupts spreading activation. It is important, however, not to confound coping with outcome; some forms of coping may not only be ineffective, they may exacerbate problems. Recall also that we pointed to the importance of the cognitive recycling process in the genesis of depression. Several theoretical proposals have suggested that women are more inclined to self-focus (Ingram et al., 1988) or ruminate (Nolen-Hoeksema, 1987) than are men. In fact, recent research has found that sex differences in self-focusing are apparent at as early as 13 years of age, with girls being more self- and relationship focused whereas boys are more externally focused. These differences occur at an age when sex-differences in depression are just beginning to emerge (Nolen-Hoeksema, 1987).

If, as we suggested earlier, rumination can be seen as a coping-linked process, then gender differences in the propensity to engage in this process can help to explain gender differences in depression. Thus, to the extent that (1) individuals have developed negative self-referent cognitive networks that are linked to negative affect, (2) ruminative processes help fuel the cycling of activation between negative and affective structures, and (3) women are more inclined to engage in this process, then depression should be more prevalent in women. To the extent that these processes occur in some men, they will be equally at risk, and to the extent that these processes do not occur in some women, they will be less at risk.

Ruminative cognitive processes are but one variable that can be considered within a coping framework. Although we think it is a very central process, other differences in coping may also be linked to sex differences in rates of depression. An active, problem-solving orientation, for instance, may differentiate men and women. Hence, to the extent that adult attachment dissolutions are linked to depressive onset, if men are more likely to engage in active behaviors to cope with or to try to replace attachment bonds, they are less likely to become depressed. On the other hand, not all coping is effective and some coping attempts may lead to more depression or increased rates of other problems (e.g., higher rates of substance abuse, antisocial disorders, etc.), in men.

Differences in the Events That Precipitate the Onset of Depressogenic Processes. Life events are a critical aspect of the diathesis–stress relationship. An equal number of people with the diathesis will experience unequal rates of depression if negative events occur at different rates. An in-depth discussion of cultural inequities is beyond the scope of this book; however, to the extent that women are more likely to encounter stress, they will be more likely to experience depression. Thus, difficulties women have encountered in reaching equity with men (e.g., unequal pay, unequal employment opportunities, glass ceilings, etc.) are likely to be linked to different levels of stress and thus linked to a greater likelihood of encountering stressful events. Similarly, women are more likely experience some kinds of trauma (e.g., rape) than are men (Kessler, Sonnega, Bromet, Hughes, & Nelson, 1995). Again, men are far from immune from negative events, but women may simply encounter more of them.

There is a particular type of stress that may play a key role in gender difference in depression. Even as women have made gains in opportunities for equity, the increased demands that have come with these gains have generally not been accompanied by decreased interpersonal demands. Thus, women still bear a disproportionate level of responsibility for childrearing and maintaining interpersonal connectedness in relationships. These demands make fertile breeding grounds for encountering the stress that triggers cognitive vulnerability mechanisms.

Ethnicity

Ethnicity may be related to psychopathology through a number of interacting variables including cultural factors, minority status, socioeconomic status, acculturation, and immigration experiences (Alvedrez, Azocar, & Miranda, 1996). Before discussing ethnicity, however, it is necessary to note important distinctions between race and ethnicity. Characteristics linked to various racial groups do not hold up to scientific inquiry. In fact, racial traits are not concordant, in that sorting people by "racial" traits leads to different groups depending on which trait is studied. Clearly, defining people according to geographical and social ethnicity makes more sense than racial groupings. Identifying ethnic group composition, however, is anything but straightforward; there is increasing mingling of groups and subsequent mixing of ethnicities in offspring. To make matters even more complicated, there are literally dozens of "officially recognized" ethnic groups represented in North America.

Even if "pure" ethnic individuals can be identified, ethnicity constitutes much more than simply belonging to one ethnic group or the other, or checking one box or the other. According to Malcarne, Chavira, and Liu (1996), for example, ethnicity can be thought of as comprising variables such as how identified and affiliated people are with their ethnic group, how much they feel a part of the ethnic mainstream, and how much discrimination they have perceived. All of these factors may have an effect on depression. The influence of ethnicity is thus not group membership but rather a constellation of cultural differences. When considering all of these factors together, it is clear that the issues involved in understanding the relationship between cognitive vulnerability, depression, and ethnicity are bewilderingly complex.

Compelling data on the link between sex differences and depression are quite limited, and unfortunately there are even fewer data examining the relationship between ethnicity and depression. Nevertheless, as with socialization-linked sex differences, we argue that the same basic structure and mechanisms that operate across sexes also operate across ethnicities. Thus, we posit no basic differences in the structure of cognitive vulnerability for any ethic group. Our reasoning is based on the assumption that the hard-wiring that produces attachment urges, as well as the development of cognitive and affective structures, characterizes all humans. This is not to say that vulnerability and depression may not be expressed in somewhat different ways. Thus, for example, cultural differences may contribute to differences in the content and expression of underlying cognitive structures, in that the latter may be influenced by the cultural context in which learning and psychological development take place.

Different ethnic groups, as with differences in men or women, may also encounter different incidences of triggering negative life events. Certainly differential rates of poverty should be related to differential rates of disorder onset. Even this relationship, however, is extremely complex. Just as we noted reasons why depression may be masked in men (e.g., underreporting, substance abuse), the effects of poverty may also be masked by similar factors.

As should be clear from our brief and very speculative comments on ethnicity and depression, few data have addressed this important area. We believe that the basic cognitive vulnerability to depression propensities are hard-wired and this guides our overall assumptions concerning ethnicity. However, this topic deserves much more attention than our brief comment can do justice to. Perhaps more importantly, empirical data are severely needed to begin to examine the relationship between cognition, depression, and ethnicity.

FINAL COMMENT

As we noted at the outset of this book, depression is a problem that has not only affected untold numbers of people, but affected them at least since, and no doubt considerably before, the beginning of recorded time. The manifestations of this disorder are complex, as are its causes and correlates. Among the multitude of factors that contribute to the cause and course of depression, we believe that cognitive factors play a significant role in many of the forms that a depressive disorder can take. Cognition does not determine reality but it does shape those aspects of reality that we process to make sense out of our world, and unfortunately there is no disputing that reality for many people will be the experience of a profoundly painful state that will be labeled "depression."

There are many ways to examine the interaction between cognitive variables and depression. In an effort to do so, numerous books have been published, hundreds of research findings have been reported, and thousands of people have been studied. Relying on this previous work, we have attempted in this book to capture some of the essential elements of the interaction between cognition and depression as it applies to vulnerability. To do so, we have discussed the nature of depression and have reviewed both research and methodology that apply to the study of depression, ranging from its earliest origins to adulthood. We have attempted to synthesize this information to develop a picture of how certain forms of cognitive functioning render some people at risk for depression. One potentially important and debated issue concerns whether the cognitions that depressed people experience organize their sense of the world in a way that reflects a relatively distorted or a relatively accurate view of reality. Only time and research will tell if our views on this subject have reflected some important reality of the disorder of depression.

References

Abramson, L. Y., & Alloy, L. B. (1990). Search for the "negative cognition" subtype of depression. In D. C. McCann & N. Endler (Eds.), *Depression: New directions in theory, research, and practice.* Toronto: Wall & Thompson.

Abramson, L. Y., Alloy, L. B., & Metalsky, G. I. (1988). The cognitive diathesis–stress theories of depression: Toward an adequate evaluation of the theories' validities. In L. B. Alloy (Ed.), *Cognitive processes in depression.* New York: Guilford Press.

Abramson, L. Y., Metalsky, G. I., & Alloy, L. B. (1989). Hopelessness depression: A theory-based subtype of depression. *Psychological Review, 96,* 358–372.

Abramson, L. Y., Seligman, M. E. P., & Teasdale, J. (1978). Learned helplessness in humans: Critique and reformulation. *Journal of Abnormal Psychology, 87,* 49–74.

Ainsworth, M. D. S. (1989). Attachments beyond infancy. *American Psychologist, 44,* 709–716.

Ainsworth, M. D. S., Blehar, M. C., Waters, E., & Wall, S. (1978). *Patterns of attachment: A psychological study of the Strange Situation.* Hillsdale, NJ: Erlbaum.

Akiskal, H. S. (1979). A biobehavioral approach to depression. In R. A. Depue (Ed.), *The psychobiology of depressive disorders.* New York: Academic Press.

Akiskal, H. S. (1987). Overview of biobehavioral factors in the prevention of mood disorders. In R. F. Munoz (Ed.), *Depression prevention: Research directions.* Washington, DC: Hemisphere.

Akiskal, H. S., & McKinney, W. T. (1973). Depressive disorders: Toward a unified hypothesis. *Science, 182,* 20–29.

Akiskal, H. S., & McKinney, W. T. (1975). Overview of recent research in depression: Integration of ten conceptual models into a comprehensive clinical frame. *Archives of General Psychiatry, 32,* 285–305.

Alba, J. W., & Hasher, L. (1983). Is memory schematic? *Psychological Bulletin,* *93*, 207–231.

Alloy, L. B., & Abramson, L. Y. (1979). Judgment of contingency in depressed and nondepressed students: Sadder but wiser? *Journal of Experimental Psychology: General, 108,* 441–485.

Alloy, L. B., & Abramson, L. Y. (1982). Learned helplessness, depression, and the illusion of control. *Journal of Personality and Social Psychology, 42,* 1114–1126.

Alloy, L. B., & Abramson, L. Y. (1990). *The Temple–Wisconsin Cognitive Vulnerability to Depression Project.* NIMH grant.

Alloy, L. B., Abramson, L. Y., Murray, L. A., Whitehouse, W. G., & Hogan, M. E. (1997). Self-referent information processing in individuals at high and low risk for depression. *Cognition and Emotion, 11,* 539–568.

Alloy, L. B., Hartlage, S., & Abramson, L. Y. (1988). Testing the cognitive diathesis–stress theories of depression: Issues of research design, conceptualization, and assessment. In L. B. Alloy (Ed.), *Cognitive processes in depression.* New York: Guilford Press.

Alloy, L. B., Lipman, A. J., & Abramson, L. Y. (1992). Attributional style as a vulnerability factor for depression: Validation by past history of mood disorders. *Cognitive Therapy and Research, 16,* 391–407.

Alvedrez, J., Azocar, F., & Miranda, J. (1996). Demystifying the concept of ethnicity for psychotherapy researchers. *Journal of Consulting and Clinical Psychology, 64,* 903–908.

Amenson, C. S., & Lewinsohn, P. M. (1981). An investigation into the observed sex difference in prevalence of unipolar depression. *Journal of Abnormal Psychology, 90,* 1–13.

American Psychiatric Association. (1994). *Diagnostic and statistical manual of mental disorders* (4th ed.). Washington, DC: Author.

Andersen, S. M., Spielman, L. A., & Bargh, J. A. (1992). Future-event schemas and certainty about the future: Automaticity in depressives' future-event predictions. *Journal of Personality and Social Psychology, 63,* 711–723.

Anderson, C. A., & Hammen, C. L. (1993). Psychosocial outcomes of children of unipolar depressed, bipolar, medically ill, and normal women: A longitudinal study. *Journal of Consulting and Clinical Psychology, 61,* 448–454.

Anderson, J. R. (1985). *Cognitive psychology and its implications* (2nd ed.). New York: Freeman.

Andreasen, N. C. (1982). Concepts, diagnosis, and classification. In E. S. Paykel (Ed.), *Handbook of affective disorders.* New York: Guilford Press.

Andreasen, N. C., Rice, J., Endicott, J., & Coryell, W. (1987). Familial rates of affective disorder: A report from the National Institute of Mental Health Collaborative Study. *Archives of General Psychiatry, 44,* 461–469.

Andrews, B., & Brewin, C. R. (1990). Attributions of blame for marital violence: A study of antecedents and consequences. *Journal of Marriage and the Family, 52,* 757–767.

Andrews, G., Neilson, M., Hunt, C., & Stewart, G. (1990). Diagnosis, personality and the long-term outcome of depression. *British Journal of Psychiatry, 157,* 13–18.

Aneshensel, C. S. (1985). The natural history of depressive symptoms: Implications for psychiatric epidemiology. *Research in Community and Mental Health, 5*, 45–75.

Aneshensel, C. S., & Frerichs, R. R. (1982). Stress, support, and depression: A longitudinal causal model. *Journal of Community Psychology, 10*, 363–376.

Arnkoff, D. (1980). Psychotherapy from the perspective of cognitive theory. In M. J. Mahoney (Ed.), *Psychotherapy process: Current issues and future directions*. New York: Plenum Press.

Arnold, M. B. (1960). *Emotion and personality.* New York: Columbia University Press.

Asarnow, J. R., & Bates, S. (1988). Depression in child psychiatric inpatients: Cognitive and attributional patterns. *Journal of Abnormal Child Psychology, 16*, 601–615.

Asarnow, J. R., Goldstein, M. J., Thompson, M., & Guthrie, D. (1993). One year outcome of depressive disorders in child psychiatric outpatients: Evaluation of the prognostic power of a brief measure of emotion. *Journal of Child Psychology and Psychiatry, 34*, 129–136.

Averill, J. R. (1979). A selective review of cognitive and behavioral factors involved in the regulation of stress. In R. A. Depue (Ed.), *The psychobiology of the depressive disorders: Implications for the effects of stress*. New York: Academic Press.

Averill, J. R. (1983). Studies on anger and aggression: Implications for theories of emotion. *American Psychologist, 38*, 1145–1160.

Baldessarini, R. J., Finklestein, S., & Arana, G. W. (1983). The predictive power of diagnostic tests and the effect of prevalence of illness. *Archives of General Psychiatry, 40*, 569–573.

Baldwin, M. W. (1992). Relational schemas and the processing of social information. *Psychological Bulletin, 112*, 461–484.

Bandura, A. (1969). *Principles of behavior modification.* New York: Holt, Rinehart & Winston.

Banks, S. M., & Kerns, R. D. (1996). Explaining high rates of depression in chronic pain: A diathesis–stress framework. *Psychological Bulletin, 119*, 95–110.

Bannister, D. (1968). The logical requirements of research into schizophrenia. *British Journal of Psychiatry, 114*, 181–188.

Barerra, M. (1986). Distinctions between social support concepts, measures, and models. *American Journal of Community Psychology, 14*, 413–436.

Barnard, P. J., & Teasdale, J. D. (1991). Interacting cognitive subsystems: A systemic approach to cognitive–affective interaction and change. *Cognition and Emotion, 5*, 1–39.

Barnett, P. A., & Gotlib, I. H. (1988). Psychosocial functioning in depression: Distinguishing among antecedents, concomitants, and consequences. *Psychological Bulletin, 104*, 97–126.

Baron, M., Gruen, R., Asnis, L., & Kane, J. M. (1982). Schizoaffective illness, schizophrenia and affective disorders: Morbidity risk and genetic transmission. *Acta Psychiatrica Scandinavica, 65*, 253–262.

Barraclough, B., Bunch, J., Nelson, B., & Sainsbury, P. (1974). A hundred cases of suicide: Clinical aspects. *British Journal of Psychiatry, 125,* 355–373.

Bartholomew, K., & Horowitz, L. M. (1991). Attachment styles among young adults: A test of a four-category model. *Journal of Personality and Social Psychology, 61,* 226–244.

Batagos, J., & Leadbeater, B. J. (1995). Parental attachment, peer relations, and dysphoria in adolescence. In S. Goldberg, R. Muir, & J. Kerr (Eds.), *Attachment theory: Social, developmental, and clinical perspectives.* Hillsdale, NJ: Analytic Press.

Baxter, L. R., Schwartz, J. M., & Bergman, K. S. (1992). Caudate glucose metabolic rate changes with both drug behaviour therapy for obsessive–compulsive disorder. *Archives of General Psychiatry, 49,* 681–689.

Beardslee, W. R., Bemporad, J., Keller, M. B., & Klerman, G. L. (1983). Children of parents with major affective disorder: A review. *American Journal of Psychiatry, 140,* 825–832.

Beck, A. T. (1963). Thinking and depression: I. Idiosyncratic content and cognitive distortions. *Archives of General Psychiatry, 9,* 324–333.

Beck, A. T. (1967). *Depression: Causes and treatment.* Philadelphia: University of Pennsylvania Press.

Beck, A. T. (1976). *Cognitive therapy and the emotional disorders.* New York: International Universities Press.

Beck, A. T. (1983). Cognitive therapy of depression: New perspectives. In P. J. Clayton & J. E. Barret (Eds.), *Treatment of depression: Old controversies and new approaches.* New York: Raven Press.

Beck, A. T. (1987). Cognitive model of depression. *Journal of Cognitive Psychotherapy, 1,* 2–27.

Beck, A. T., & Emery, G. (1985). *Anxiety disorders and phobias: A cognitive perspective.* New York: Basic Books.

Beck, A. T., Rush, A. J., Shaw, B. F., & Emery, G. (1979). *Cognitive therapy of depression.* New York: Guilford Press.

Beckham, E. E., Leber, W. R., & Youll, L. K. (1995). The diagnostic classification of depression. In E. E. Beckham & W. R. Leber (Eds.), *Handbook of depression* (2nd ed.). New York: Guilford Press.

Beutler, L. E., Scogin, F., Kirkish, P., & Schretlen, D. (1987). Group cognitive therapy and alprazolam in the treatment of depression in older adults. *Journal of Consulting and Clinical Psychology, 55,* 550–556.

Bemporad, J. R., & Romano, S. J. (1992). Childhood maltreatment and adult depression: A review of research. In D. Cicchetti & S. L. Toth (Eds.), *Developmental perspectives on depression.* Rochester, NY: University of Rochester Press.

Bifulco, A., Brown, G. W., & Adler, Z. (1991). Early sexual abuse and clinical depression in adult life. *British Journal of Psychiatry, 159,* 115–122.

Billings, A. G., Cronkite, R. C., & Moos, R. H. (1983). Social-environmental factors in unipolar depression: Comparisons of depressed patients and nondepressed controls. *Journal of Abnormal Psychology, 92,* 119–133.

Billings, A. G., & Moos, R. H. (1982a). Social support and functioning among community and clinical groups: A panel model. *Journal of Behavioral Medicine, 5,* 295–311.

Billings, A. G., & Moos, R. H. (1982b). Work stress and the stress-buffering roles of work and family resources. *Journal of Occupational Behavior, 3,* 215–232.

Billings, A. G., & Moos, R. H. (1983). Comparisons of children of depressed and nondepressed parents: A social-environmental perspective. *Journal of Abnormal Child Psychology, 11,* 463–485.

Billings, A. G., & Moos, R. H. (1985). Life stressors and social resources affect posttreatment outcomes among depressed patients. *Journal of Abnormal Psychology, 94,* 140–153.

Blackburn, I. M., Jones, S., & Lewin, R. J. P. (1986). Cognitive style in depression. *British Journal of Clinical Psychology, 25,* 241–251.

Blackburn, I. M., & Smyth, P. (1985). A test of cognitive vulnerability in individuals prone to depression. *British Journal of Clinical Psychology, 24,* 61–62.

Blackburn, I. M., Whalley, L. J., & Christie, J. E. (1987). Mood, cognition and cortisol: Their temporal relationships during recovery from depressive illness. *Journal of Affective Disorders, 13,* 31–43.

Bland, R. C., Newman, S. C., & Orn, H. (1986). Recurrent and nonrecurrent depression: A family study. *Archives of General Psychiatry, 43,* 1085–1089.

Blaney, P. H. (1986). Affect and memory: A review. *Psychological Bulletin, 99,* 229–246.

Blaney, P. H., Behar, V., & Head, R. (1980). Two measures of depressive cognitions: Their association with depression and with each other. *Journal of Abnormal Psychology, 89,* 678–682.

Blatt, S. J. (1974). Level of object representation in anaclitic and introjective depression. *Psychoanalytic Study of the Child, 29,* 107–157.

Blatt, S. J., & Bers, S. A. (1993). The sense of self in depression: A psychody-namic perspective. In Z. V. Segal & S. J. Blatt (Eds.), *The self in emotional distress: Cognitive and psychodynamic perspectives.* New York: Guilford Press.

Blatt, S. J., D'Afflitti, J. P., & Quinlan, D. M. (1976). Experiences of depression in young adults. *Journal of Abnormal Psychology, 85,* 383–389.

Blatt, S. J., & Homann, E. (1992). Parent–child interaction in the etiology of dependent and self-critical depression. *Clinical Psychology Review, 12,* 47–91.

Blatt, S. J., Quinlan, D., Chevron, E., McDonald, C., & Zuroff, D. (1982). Dependency and self-criticism: Psychological dimensions of depression. *Journal of Consulting and Clinical Psychology, 50,* 113–124.

Blatt, S. J., Wein, S. J., Chevron, E., & Quinlan, D. M. (1979). Parental representations and depression in normal young adults. *Journal of Abnormal Psychology, 88,* 388–397.

Blatt, S. J., & Zuroff, D. C. (1992). Interpersonal relatedness and self-definition: Two prototypes for depression. *Clinical Psychology Review, 12,* 527–562.

Bouchard, T. J., Lykken, D. T., McGue, M., Segal, N. L., & Tellegen, A. (1990).

Sources of human psychological differences: The Minnesota study of twins reared apart. *Science, 250,* 223–250.

Bower, G. H. (1981). Mood and memory. *American Psychologist, 36,* 129–148.

Bower, G. H., & Clapper, J. P. (1989). Experimental methods in cognitive science. In M. L. Posner (Ed.), *Foundations of cognitive science.* Cambridge, MA: MIT Press.

Bowers, W. A. (1990). Treatment of depressed inpatients: Cognitive therapy plus medication, relaxation plus medication, and medication alone. *British Journal of Psychiatry, 156,* 73–78.

Bowlby, J. (1969). *Attachment and loss: Vol. 1. Attachment.* New York: Basic Books.

Bowlby, J. (1973). *Attachment and loss: Vol. 2. Separation, anxiety, and anger.* New York: Basic Books.

Bowlby, J. (1980). *Attachment and loss: Vol. 3. Loss: Sadness and depression.* New York: Basic Books.

Bowlby, J. (1988). *A secure base: Parent–child attachment and healthy human development.* New York: Basic Books.

Boyd, J. H., Burke, J. D., Gruenberg, E., Holzer, C. E. III, Rae, D. S., George, L. K., Karno, M., Stoltzman, R., McEvoy, L., & Nestadt, G. (1984). Exclusion criteria of DSM-III: A study of co-occurrence of hierarchy-free syndromes. *Archives of General Psychiatry, 41,* 983–959.

Brady, E. U., & Kendall, P. C. (1992). Comorbidity of anxiety and depression in children and adolescents. *Psychological Bulletin, 111,* 244–256.

Braff, D. L. (1985). Attention, habituation, and information processing in psychiatric disorders. *Psychiatry, 3,* 1–12.

Brewin, C. R. (1985a). Cognitive change processes in psychotherapy. *Psychological Review, 96,* 379–394.

Brewin, C. R. (1985b). Depression and causal attributions: What is their relation? *Psychological Bulletin, 98,* 297–309.

Brewin, C. R. (1988). *Cognitive foundations of clinical psychology.* Hillsdale, NJ: Erlbaum.

Brewin, C. R., Andrews, B., & Gotlib, I. (1993). Psychopathology and early experience: A reappraisal of retrospective reports. *Psychological Bulletin, 113,* 82–98.

Brewin, C. R., Firth-Cozens, J., Furnham, A., & McManus, C. (1992). Self-criticism in adulthood and recalled childhood experience. *Journal of Abnormal Psychology, 101,* 561–566.

Briere, J. (1992). *Child abuse trauma: Theory and treatment of lasting effects.* Newbury Park, CA: Sage.

Broadhead, W. E., Blazer, D. G., & George, L. K. (1990). Depression, disability days, and days lost from work in a prospective epidemiologic survey. *Journal of the American Medical Association, 264,* 2524–2528.

Brown, G. W., & Harris, T. O. (1978). *Social origins of depression. A study of psychiatric disorder in women.* London: Tavistock.

Brown, G. W., & Harris, T. O. (1989a). Depression. In G. W. Brown & T. O. Harris (Eds.), *Life events and illness.* New York: Guilford Press.

Brown, G. W., & Harris, T. O. (Eds.). (1989b). *Life events and illness.* New York: Guilford Press.

Browne, A., & Finkelhor, D. (1986). Impact of child sexual abuse: A review of the research. *Psychological Bulletin, 99,* 66–77.

Bruner, J. S. (1957). On perceptual readiness. *Psychological Review, 64,* 123–152.

Burbach, D. J., & Borduin, C. M. (1986). Parent–child relations and the etiology of depression. *Clinical Psychology Review, 6,* 133–153.

Burgess, I. S., Jones, L. M., Robertson, S. A., Radcliffe, W. N., & Emerson, E. (1981). The degree of control exerted by phobic and non-phobic verbal stimuli over the recognition behaviour of phobic and non-phobic subjects. *Behaviour Research and Therapy, 19,* 233–242.

Burke, K. C., Burke, J. D., Regier, D. A., & Rae, D. S. (1990). Age at onset of selected disorders in five community populations. *Archives of General Psychiatry, 47,* 511–518.

Burnam, M., Stein, J. A., Golding, J. M., & Siegel, J. M. (1988). Sexual assault and mental disorders in a community population. *Journal of Consulting and Clinical Psychology, 56,* 843–850.

Buss, A. H. (1988). *Personality: Evolutionary heritage and human distinctiveness.* Hillsdale, NJ: Erlbaum.

Calfas, K. J., Ingram, R. E., & Kaplan, R. M. (1997). Information processing and affective distress in osteoarthritis patients. *Journal of Consulting and Clinical Psychology, 65,* 576–581.

Campbell-Goymer, N. R., & Allgood, W. C. (1984). *Cognitive correlates of childhood depression.* Paper presented at the annual meeting of the Southeastern Psychological Association, New Orleans, LA.

Carlson, R., & Levy, N. (1973). Studies of Jungian typology: I. Memory, social perception, and social action. *Journal of Personality, 41,* 559–576.

Carrol, B. J., Feinberg, M., Greden, J. F., Tarika, J., Albala, A. A., Haskett, R. F., James, N., Kronfol, Z., Lohr, N., Steiner, M., deVigne, J. P., & Young, E. (1981). A specific laboratory test for the diagnosis of melancholia. *Archives of General Psychiatry, 38,* 15–22.

Carver, C. S. (1979). A cybernetic model of self-attention processes. *Journal of Personality and Social Psychology, 37,* 1186–1195.

Casper, F., Rothenfluh, T., & Segal, Z. (1992). The appeal of connectionism for clinical psychology. *Clinical Psychology Review, 12,* 719–762.

Cautela, J. R. (1970). Covert negative reinforcement. *Journal of Behavior Therapy and Experimental Psychiatry, 1,* 273–278.

Chassin, L., Curran, P., Hussong, A. M., & Colder, C. R. (1996). The relation of parent alcoholism to adolescent substance use: A longitudinal follow-up study. *Journal of Abnormal Psychology, 105,* 70–80.

Chisholm, J. S. (1988). Toward a developmental evolutionary ecology of humans. In K. M. McDonald (Ed.), *Sociobiological perspectives on human development.* New York: Springer-Verlag.

Clark, D. A. (1986). Cognitive–affective interaction: A test of the "specificity" and "generality" hypotheses. *Cognitive Therapy and Research, 10,* 607–623.

Clark, D. A., Beck, A. T., & Brown, G. (1989). Cognitive mediation in general psychiatric outpatients: A test of the content-specificity hypothesis. *Journal of Personality and Social Psychology, 56,* 958–964.

Clark, L. A., & Watson, D. (1991). Tripartite model of anxiety and depression: Psychometric evidence and taxonomic implications. *Journal of Abnormal Psychology, 100,* 316–336.

Clark, L. A., & Watson, D. (1994). Distinguishing functional from dysfunctional affective responses. In P. Ekman & R. J. Davison (Eds.), *The nature of emotions: Fundamental questions.* New York: Oxford University Press.

Clark, M. S., & Isen, A. M. (1982). Feeling states and social behavior. In A. Hastorf & A. M. Isen (Eds.), *Cognitive social psychology.* Amsterdam: Elsevier.

Clarke, G., Hawkins, W., Murphy, M., Sheeber, L., Lewinsohn, P., & Seeley, J. (1995). Target prevention of unipolar depressive disorder in an at risk sample of high school adolescents: A randomized trial of a group cognitive intervention. *Academy of Child and Adolescent Psychiatry, 34,* 312–321.

Cohen, L. (Ed.). (1988). *Research on stressful life events: Theoretical and methodological issues.* Newbury Park, CA: Sage.

Cohn, J. F., & Campbell, S. B. (1992). Influence of maternal depression on infant affect regulation. In D. Cicchetti & S. L. Toth (Eds.), *Developmental perspectives on depression.* Rochester, NY: University of Rochester Press.

Cole, P. M., & Zahn-Waxler, C. (1992). Emotional dysregulation in disruptive behavior disorders. In D. Cicchetti & S. L. Toth (Eds.), *Developmental perspectives on depression.* Rochester, NY: University of Rochester Press.

Collins, N. L., & Read, S. J. (1990). Adult attachment, working models, and relationship quality in dating couples. *Journal of Personality and Social Psychology, 58,* 644–663.

Compas, B. E., Ey, S., & Grant, K. E. (1993). Taxonomy, assessment, and diagnosis of depression during adolescence. *Psychological Bulletin, 114,* 323–344.

Costello, C. G. (1993a). The advantages of the symptom approach to depression. In C. G. Costello (Ed.), *Symptoms of depression.* New York: Wiley.

Costello, C. G. (1993b). Cognitive causes of psychopathology. In C. G. Costello (Ed.), *Basic issues in psychopathology.* New York: Guilford Press.

Coyne, J. C. (1976). Toward an interactional description of depression. *Psychiatry, 39,* 28–40.

Coyne, J. C. (1982). A critique of cognitions as causal entities with particular reference to depression. *Cognitive Therapy and Research, 6,* 3–13.

Coyne, J. C. (1992). Cognition in depression: A paradigm in crisis. *Psychological Inquiry, 3,* 232–235.

Coyne, J. C. (1994). Self-reported distress: Analog or ersatz depression? *Psychological Bulletin, 116,* 29–45.

Coyne, J. C., Aldwin, C., & Lazarus, R. S. (1981). Depression and coping in stressful episodes. *Journal of Abnormal Psychology, 90,* 439–447.

Coyne, J. C., Burchill, S. A. L., & Styles, W. B. (1990). An interactional perspective on depression. In C. R. Snyder & D. O. Forsyth (Eds.),

Handbook of social and clinical psychology: The health perspective. New York: Pergamon Press.

Coyne, J. C., & Gotlib, I. H. (1983). The role of cognition in depression: A critical appraisal. *Psychological Bulletin, 94,* 472–505.

Coyne, J. C., & Gotlib, I. H. (1986). Studying the role of cognition in depression. Well-trodden paths and cul-de-sacs. *Cognitive Therapy and Research, 10,* 794–812.

Coyne, J. C., Kessler, R. C., Tal, M., Turnbull, J., Wortman, C. B., & Greden, J. F. (1987). Living with a depressed person. *Journal of Consulting and Clinical Psychology, 55,* 347–352.

Coyne, J. C., & Whiffen, V. E. (1995). Issues in personality as diathesis for depression: The case of sociotropy–dependency and autonomy self criticism. *Psychological Bulletin, 118,* 358–378.

Craighead, W. E. (1980). Away from a unitary model of depression. *Behavior Therapy, 11,* 122–128.

Craik, F., & Lockhart, R. (1972). Levels of processing: A framework for memory research. *Journal of Verbal Learning and Verbal Behavior, 11,* 671–684.

Cromwell, R. L. (1975). Assessment of schizophrenia. In M. R. Rosenzweig & L. W. Porter (Eds.), *Annual review of psychology* (Vol. 26). Palo Alto, CA: Annual Reviews.

Culbertson, F. M. (1997). Depression and gender: An international review. *American Psychologist, 52,* 25–31.

Cummings, E. M., & Cicchetti, D. (1990). Toward a transactional model of relations between attachment and depression. In M. Greenberg & D. Cicchetti (Eds.), *Attachment in the preschool years: Theory research, and intervention.* Chicago: University of Chicago Press.

Cutler, S. E., & Nolen-Hoeksema, S. (1991). Accounting for sex differences in depression through female victimization: Childhood sexual abuse. *Sex Roles, 24,* 425–438.

Danion, J., Willard-Schroeder, D., Zimmermann, M., Grange, D., Schlienger, J., & Singer, L. (1991). Explicit memory and repetition priming in depression. *Archives of General Psychiatry, 48,* 707–711.

DeMonbreun, B. G., & Craighead, W. E. (1977). Distortion of perception and recall of positive and neutral feedback in depression. *Cognitive Therapy and Research, 1,* 311–329.

Dent, J., & Teasdale, J. D. (1988). Negative cognition and the persistence of depression. *Journal of Abnormal Psychology, 97,* 29–34.

Depression Guideline Panel. (1993). *Depression in primary care: Vol. 2. Treatment of major depression* (Clinical practice guideline, No. 5; AHCPR Pub. No. 93-0551). Rockville, MD: U.S. Department of Health and Human Services, Public Health Service, Agency for Health Care Policy and Research.

Depue, R. A., & Iacono, W. G. (1989). Neurobehavioral aspects of affective disorders. *Annual Review of Psychology, 40,* 457–492.

Depue, R. A., & Kleiman, R. M. (1979). Free cortisol as a peripheral index of central vulnerability to major forms of unipolar depressive disorders:

Examining stress–biology interactions in subsyndromal high risk persons. In R. A. Depue (Ed.), *The psychobiology of depressive disorders*. New York: Academic Press.

Depue, R. A., Kleiman, R. M., Davis, P., Hutchinson, M., & Krauss, S. (1985). The behavioral high-risk paradigm and bipolar affective disorder: VIII. Serum free cortisol in nonpatient cyclothymic subjects selected by the General Behavior Inventory. *American Journal of Psychiatry, 142,* 175–181.

Depue, R. A., Krauss, S., Spoont, M., & Arbisi, P. (1989). Identification of unipolar and bipolar affective conditions in a university population with the General Behavior Inventory. *Journal of Abnormal Psychology, 98,* 117–126.

Depue, R. A., & Monroe, S. M. (1978a). Learned helplessness in the perspective of the depressive disorders. *Journal of Abnormal Psychology, 87,* 3–20.

Depue, R. A., & Monroe, S. M. (1978b). The unipolar–bipolar distinction in the depressive disorders. *Psychological Bulletin, 85,* 1001–1029.

Depue, R. A., & Monroe, S. M. (1986). Conceptualization and measurement of human disorder and life stress research: The problem of chronic disturbance. *Psychological Bulletin, 99,* 36–51.

Depue, R. A., Slater, J. F., Wolfstetter-Kausch, H., Klein, D., Goplerud, E., & Farr, D. (1981). A behavioral paradigm for identifying persons at risk for bipolar depressive disorder: A conceptual framework and five validation studies [Monograph]. *Journal of Abnormal Psychology, 90,* 381–437.

Derry, P. A., & Kuiper, N. A. (1981). Schematic processing and self-reference in clinical depression. *Journal of Abnormal Psychology, 90,* 286–297.

DeRubeis, R. J., Evans, M. D., & Hollon, S. D. (1990). How does cognitive therapy work? Cognitive change and symptom change in cognitive therapy and pharmacotherapy for depression. *Journal of Consulting and Clinical Psychology, 6,* 862–869.

DiMascio, A., Weissman, M. M., Prusoff, B. A., Neu, C., Zwilling, M., & Klerman, G. L. (1979). Differential symptom reduction by drugs and psychotherapy in acute depression. *Archives of General Psychiatry, 36,* 1450–1456.

Doane, J. A., & Diamond, D. (1994). *Affect and attachment in the family: A family based treatment of major psychiatric disorder.* New York: Basic Books.

Dobson, K. (1985). The relationship between anxiety and depression. *Clinical Psychology Review, 5,* 307–324.

Dobson, K. S. (1989). A meta-analysis of the efficacy of cognitive therapy for depression. *Journal of Consulting and Clinical Psychology, 57,* 414–419.

Dobson, K. S., & Block, L. (1988). Historical and philosophical bases of the cognitive-behavioral therapies. In K. S. Dobson (Ed.), *Handbook of cognitive-behavioral therapies.* New York: Guilford Press.

Dobson, K. S., & Kendall, P. C. (1993). *Psychopathology and cognition.* San Diego: Academic Press.

Dobson, K., & Shaw, B. (1986). Cognitive assessment with major depressive disorders. *Cognitive Therapy and Research, 10,* 13–29.

Dobson, K., & Shaw, B. (1987). Specificity and stability of self-referent encoding in clinical depression. *Journal of Abnormal Psychology, 96,* 34–40.

Dodge, K. A. (1993). Social-cognitive mechanisms in the development of conduct disorder and depression. *Annual Review of Psychology, 44,* 559–584.

Dohr, K. B., Rush, A. J., & Bernstein, I. H. (1989). Cognitive biases in depression. *Journal of Abnormal Psychology, 98,* 263–267.

Dohrenwend, B. S., & Dohrenwend, B. P. (1974). A brief historical introduction to research on stressful life events. In B. P. Dohrenwend & B. S. Dohrenwend (Eds.), *Stressful life events: Their nature and effects.* New York: Wiley.

Dohrenwend, B. P., & Shrout, P. E. (1985). "Hassles" in the conceptualization and measurement of life stress variables. *American Psychologist, 40,* 780–785.

Donders, F. C. (1868–1869). Over de snelheid van psychische processen. Onderzoekingen gedaan in het Physiologisch Laboratorium der Utrechtsche Hoogeschool, 1868–1869, Tweede reeks II, 92–120. [Translated by W. G. Koster in W. G. Koster (Ed.), *Attention and performance: II. Acta Psychologica, 30,* 412–431, 1969.]

Dorzab, J., Baker, M., Winokur, G., & Cadoret, R. J. (1971). Depressive disease: Clinical course. *Diseases of the Nervous System, 32,* 269–273.

Downey, G., & Coyne, J. C. (1990). Children of depressed parents: An integrative review. *Psychological Bulletin, 108,* 50–75.

Dryman, A., & Eaton, W. W. (1991). Affective symptoms associated with the onset of major depression in the community: Findings from the U.S. National Institute of Mental Health Epidemiological Catchment Area program. *Acta Psychiatrica Scandinavica, 84,* 1–5.

Duval, S., & Wicklund, R. (1972). *A theory of objective self-awareness.* New York: Academic Press.

D'Zurilla, T. J. (1986). *Problem-solving therapy: A social competence approach to clinical intervention.* New York: Springer.

Eaton, W. W., Holzer, A., & Von Korff. (1984). The design of the Epidemiologic Catchment Area surveys: The control and measurement of error. *Archives of General Psychiatry, 41,* 942–948.

Eaton, W. W., & Kessler, L. G. (Eds.). (1985). *Epidemiologic field methods in psychiatry: The NIMH Epidemiologic Catchment Area program.* New York: Academic Press.

Eaves, G., & Rush, A. J. (1984). Cognitive patterns in symptomatic and remitted unipolar major depression. *Journal of Abnormal Psychology, 93,* 31–40.

Ebbinghaus, H. (1885). *Uber das Gedachtnis.* [Reprinted as *Memory* (H. A. Ruger & C. E. Busenius, Trans.). New York: Teachers College, 1913.]

Elliot, C. L. & Greene, R. L. (1992). Clinical depression and implicit memory. *Journal of Abnormal Psychology, 101,* 572–574.

Ellis, A. (1962). *Reason and emotion in psychotherapy.* New York: Lyle Stuart.

Ellis, A. (1994). *Reason and emotion in psychotherapy* (2nd ed.). Secausus, NJ: Carol Publishing Group.

Ellis, A. (1996). *Better, deeper and more enduring brief therapy: The rational emotive behavior therapy approach.* New York: Brunner/Mazel.

Ellis, H. C., & Ashbrook, P. A. (1988). The state of mood and memory research: A selective review. *Journal of Social Behavior and Personality, 4,* 1–21.

Engel, R. A., & DeRubeis, R. J. (1993). The role of cognition in depression. In K. S. Dobson & P. C. Kendall (Eds.), *Psychopathology and cognition.* San Diego: Academic Press.

Ensel, W. M. (1982). The role of age in the relationship of gender and marital status to depression. *Journal of Nervous and Mental Disease, 170,* 536–543.

Erdley, C. A., & D'Agostino, P. R. (1988). Cognitive and affective components of automatic priming effects. *Journal of Personality and Social Psychology, 54,* 741–747.

Evans, M. D., & Hollon, S. D. (1988). Patterns of personal and causal inference: Implications for cognitive therapy of depression. In L. B. Alloy (Ed.), *Cognitive processes in depression.* New York: Guilford Press.

Feinstein, A. R. (1970). The pre-therapeutic classification of co-morbidity in chronic disease. *Journal of Chronic Diseases, 23,* 455–468.

Felner, R. D. (1984). Vulnerability in childhood: A preventive framework for understanding children's efforts to cope with life stress and transition. In M. Roberts & L. Peterson (Eds.), *Prevention of problems in childhood: Psychological research and applications.* New York: Wiley.

Fenell, M. J. V., & Campbell, E. A. (1984). The Cognitions Questionnaire: Specific thinking errors in depression. *British Journal of Clinical Psychology, 23,* 81–92.

Field, T. (1989). Maternal depression effects on infant interaction and attachment behavior. In D. Cicchetti (Ed.), *Rochester symposium on developmental psychopathology* (Vol. 1). Hillsdale, NJ: Erlbaum.

Finkelhor, D., Hotaling, G., Lewis, I. A., & Smith, C. (1990). Sexual abuse in a national survey of adult men and women: Prevalence, characteristics, and risk factors. *Child Abuse and Neglect, 14,* 19–28.

First, M. B., Spitzer, R. L., & Williams, J. B. W. (1990). Exclusionary principles and the comorbidity of psychiatric diagnoses: A historical review and implications for the future. In J. D. Maser & C. R. Cloninger (Eds.), *Comorbidity of mood and anxiety disorders.* Washington, DC: American Psychiatric Press.

Flett, G. L., Vredenburg, K., & Krames, L. (1997). The continuity of depression in clinical and nonclinical samples. *Psychological Bulletin, 121,* 395–416.

Foa, E. B., & McNally, R. J. (1986). Sensitivity to feared stimuli in obsessive–compulsives: A dichotic listening analysis. *Cognitive Therapy and Research, 10,* 477–485.

Fogarty, S. J., & Hemsley, D. R. (1983). Depression and the accessibility of memories: A longitudinal study. *British Journal of Psychiatry, 142,* 232–237.

Foulds, G. A. (1973). The relationship between the depressive illnesses. *British Journal of Psychiatry, 123,* 531–533.

Foulds, G. A., & Bedford, B. (1975). Hierarchy of personal illness. *Psychological Medicine, 5,* 181–192.

Frances, A. J., Widiger, T., & Fryer, M. R. (1990). The influence of classification methods on comorbidity. In J. D. Maser & C. R. Cloninger (Eds.), *Comorbidity of mood and anxiety disorders.* Washington, DC: American Psychiatric Press.

Frank, E., Kupfer, D. J., Jacob, M., & Jarrett, D. (1987). Personality features and response to acute treatment in recurrent depression. *Journal of Personality Disorders, 1,* 14–26.

Frank, E., Prien, R. F., Jarret, R. B., Keller, M. B., Kupfer, D. J., Lavori, P. W., Rush, A. J., & Weissman, M. M. (1991). Conceptualization and rationale for consensus definitions of terms in major depressive disorder: Remission, recovery, relapse, and recurrence. *Archives of General Psychiatry, 48,* 851–855.

Fredman, L., Weissman, M. M., Leaf, P. J., & Bruce, M. L. (1988). Social functioning in community residents with depression and other psychiatric disorders: Results of the New Haven Epidemiologic Catchment Area study. *Journal of Affective Disorders, 15,* 103–112.

Freud, S. (1917). Mourning and melancholia. In *Completed psychological works* (Vol. 14). Translated by J. Strachey. London: Hogarth Press.

Friedman, R. C., Aronoff, M. S., Clarkin, J. F., Corn, R., & Hurt, S. W. (1983). History of suicidal behavior in depressed borderline inpatients. *American Journal of Psychiatry, 140,* 1023–1026.

Gabbard, G. O. (1992). Psychodynamic psychiatry in the "decade of the brain." *American Journal of Psychiatry, 149,* 991–998.

Garber, J., & Hollon, S. D. (1991). What can specificity designs say about causality in psychopathology research? *Psychological Bulletin, 110,* 129–136.

Garber, J., Quiggle, N., & Shanley, N. (1990). Cognition and depression in children and adolescents. In R. E. Ingram (Ed.), *Contemporary psychological approaches to depression.* New York: Plenum Press.

Garber, J., Weiss, B., & Shanley, N. (1993). Cognitions, depressive symptoms, and development in adolescents. *Journal of Abnormal Psychology, 102,* 47–57.

Gardner, H. (1985). *The mind's new science.* New York: Basic Books.

Garmezy, N., & Devine, V. (1984). Project competence: The Minnesota studies of children vulnerable to psychopathology. In N. Watt, E. J. Anthony, L. Wynne, & J. Rolf (Eds.), *Children at risk for schizophrenia.* New York: Cambridge University Press.

Garrett, L. (1994). *The coming plague: Newly emerging diseases in a world out of balance.* New York: Farrar, Straus & Giroux.

Garrison, C. Z., Addy, C. L., Jackson, K. L., McKeown, R. E., & Waller, J. L. (1991). The CES-D as a screen for depression and other psychiatric disorders in adolescents. *Journal of the American Academy of Child and Adolescent Psychiatry, 30,* 636–641.

Garrison, C. Z., Addy, C. L., Jackson, K. L., McKeown, R. E., & Waller, J. L. (1992). Major depressive disorder and dysthymia in young adolescents. *American Journal of Epidemiology, 135,* 792–802.

Gaston, L., Marmar, C. R., Thompson, L. W., & Gallagher, D. (1988). Relation of patient pretreatment characteristics to the therapeutic alliance in diverse psychotherapies. *Journal of Consulting and Clinical Psychology, 56,* 483–489.

Gelfand, D. M., & Teti, D. M. (1990). The effects of maternal depression on children. *Clinical Psychology Review, 10,* 329–353.

Gerlsma, C., Emmelkamp, P. M. G., & Arrindell, W. A. (1990). Anxiety, depression, and perception of early parenting: A meta-analysis. *Clinical Psychology Review, 10,* 251–277.

Gershon, E. S., Nurnberger, J. I. (1982). Inheritance of major psychiatric disorders. *Trends in Neurosciences, 5,* 241–242.

Gibbons, F. X., Smith, T. W., Ingram, R. E., Pearce, K., Brehm, S. S., & Schroeder, D. J. (1985). Self-awareness and self-confrontation: Effects of self-focused attention on members of a clinical population. *Journal of Personality and Social Psychology, 78,* 662–675.

Gilbert, P. (1992). *Depression: The evolution of powerlessness.* New York: Guilford Press.

Giles, D. E., Biggs, M. M., Rush, A. J., & Roffwarg, H. P. (1988). Risk factors in families of unipolar depression: I. Psychiatric illness and reduced REM latency. *Journal of Affective Disorders, 14,* 51–59.

Gillham, J. E., Reivich, K., Jaycox, L., & Seligman, M. E. P. (1995). Prevention of depressive symptoms in schoolchildren: A two year follow up. *Psychological Science, 6,* 343–351.

Goldberg, L. R. (1993). The structure of phenotypic personality traits. *American Psychologist, 48,* 26–34.

Goldfried, M. R., & Robins, C. (1983). Self-schemas, cognitive bias, and the processing of therapeutic experiences. In P. C. Kendall (Ed.), *Advances in cognitive-behavioral research and therapy.* New York: Academic Press.

Goldman, N., & Ravid, R. (1980). Community surveys: Sex differences in mental illness. In M. Guttentag, S. Salasin, & D. Bell (Eds.), *The mental health of women.* New York: Academic Press.

Goodwin, F. K., & Jamison, K. R. (1990). *Manic–depressive illness.* New York: Oxford University Press.

Gorenstein, E. E. (1992). Debating mental illness: Implications for science, medicine, and social policy. *American Psychologist, 39,* 50–56.

Gotlib, I. H. (1983). Perception and recall of interpersonal feedback. *Cognitive Therapy and Research, 7,* 399–412.

Gotlib, I. H., & Cane, C. B. (1987). Construct accessibility and clinical depression: A longitudinal investigation. *Journal of Abnormal Psychology, 96,* 199–204.

Gotlib, I. H., & Hammen, C. L. (1992). *Psychological aspects of depression: Toward a cognitive–interpersonal integration.* Chichester, UK: Wiley.

Gotlib, I. H., & Lewinsohn, P. M. (1992). Cognitive models of depression: Critique and directions for future research. *Psychological Inquiry, 3,* 241–244.

Gotlib, I. H., Mount, J. H., Cordy, N. I., & Whiffen, V. E. (1988). Depression and perceptions of early parenting: A longitudinal investigation. *British Journal of Psychiatry, 152,* 24–27.

Gottesman, I. I., & Shields, J. (1972). *Schizophrenia and genetics.* New York: Academic Press.

Greenberg, M. S., & Beck, A. (1989). Depression versus anxiety: A test of the content specificity hypothesis. *Journal of Abnormal Psychology, 98*, 9–13.

Greenberg, P. E., Stiglin, L. E., Finkelstein, S. N., & Berndt, E. R. (1993). The economic burden of depression in 1990. *Journal of Clinical Psychiatry, 54*, 405–418.

Greene, J. G. (1980). Life stress and symptoms at the climacterium. *British Journal of Psychiatry, 136*, 486–491.

Greenwald, A. (1980). The totalitarian ego: Fabrication and revision of personal history. *American Psychologist, 35*, 603–618.

Grunhaus, L., & Greden, J. F. (1994). *Severe depressive disorders.* Washington, DC: American Psychiatric Press.

Guhtrie, E. R. (1935). *Psychology of learning.* New York: Harper.

Guze, S. B., & Robins, E. (1970). Suicide and primary affective disorders. *British Journal of Psychiatry, 117*, 437–438.

Haaga, D. A. F., & Davison, G. C. (1993). An appraisal of rational-emotive therapy. Special section: Recent developments in cognitive and constructivist psychotherapies. *Journal of Consulting and Clinical Psychology, 61*, 215–220.

Haaga, D. A. F., Dyck, M. J., & Ernst, D. (1991). Empirical status of cognitive theory of depression. *Psychological Bulletin, 110*, 215–236.

Haaga, D. A. F., & Solomon, A. (1993). Impact of Kendall, Hollon, Beck, Hammen, and Ingram (1987) on treatment of the continuity issue in "depression" research. *Cognitive Therapy and Research, 17*, 313–324.

Hagnell, O., Lanke, J., Rorsman, B., & Ojesjo, L. (1982). Are we entering an age of melancholy? Depressive illnesses in a prospective epidemiological study over 25 years: The Lundby Study, Sweden. *Psychological Medicine, 12*, 279–289.

Halsam, J. (1809). *Observations on madness and melancholy.* London: G. Hayden.

Haley, G. M., Fine, S., Marriage, K., Moretti, M. M., & Freeman, R. J. (1985). Cognitive bias and depression in psychiatrically disturbed children and adolescents. *Journal of Consulting and Clinical Psychology, 53*, 535–537.

Hamilton, E. W., & Abramson, L. Y. (1983). Cognitive patterns and major depressive disorder: A longitudinal study in a hospital setting. *Journal of Abnormal Psychology, 92*, 173–184.

Hammen, C. (1991a). *Depression runs in families: The social context of risk and resilience in children of depressed mothers.* New York: Springer-Verlag.

Hammen, C. (1991b). The generation of stress in the course of unipolar depression. *Journal of Abnormal Psychology, 100*, 555–561.

Hammen, C. (1992). Life events and depression: The plot thickens. *American Journal of Community Psychology, 20*, 179–193.

Hammen, C. (1995). The social context of risk for depression. In K. D. Craig & K. S. Dobson (Eds.), *Anxiety and depression in adults and children.* Thousand Oaks, CA: Sage.

Hammen, C., Adrian, C., & Hiroto, D. (1988). A longitudinal test of the attributional vulnerability model in children at risk for depression. *British Journal of Clinical Psychology, 27*, 37–46.

Hammen, C., Burge, D., Daley, S., Davila, J., Paley, B., & Rudolph, D. (1995). Interpersonal attachment cognitions and prediction of symptomatic responses to interpersonal stress. *Journal of Abnormal Psychology, 104,* 436–443.

Hammen, C., Ellicott, A., Gitlin, M., & Jamison, K. R. (1989). Sociotropy/autonomy and vulnerability to specific life events in patients with unipolar depression and bipolar disorders. *Journal of Abnormal Psychology, 98,* 154–160.

Hammen, C., & Goodman-Brown, T. (1990). Self-schemas and vulnerability to specific life stress in children at risk for depression. *Cognitive Therapy and Research, 14,* 215–227.

Hammen, C., Gordon, G., Burge, D., Adrian, C., Jaenicke, C., & Hiroto, G. (1987). Maternal affective disorders, illness, and stress: Risk for children's psychopathology. *American Journal of Psychiatry, 144,* 736–741.

Hammen, C., Marks, T., Mayol, A., & deMayo, R. (1985). Depressive self-schemas, life stress, and vulnerability to depression. *Journal of Abnormal Psychology, 94,* 308–319.

Hammen, C., Miklowitz, D., & Dyck, D. (1986). Stability and severity parameters of depressive self-schema responding. *Journal of Social and Clinical Psychology, 4,* 23–45.

Hammen, C., & Zupan, B. A. (1984). Self-schemas and the processing of personal information in children. *Journal of Experimental Child Psychology, 37,* 598–608.

Harrington, R., Fudge, H., Rutter, M., Pickels, A., & Hill, J. (1991). Adult outcomes of childhood and adolescent depression: II. Links with antisocial disorders. *Journal of the American Academy of Child and Adolescent Psychiatry, 30,* 434–439.

Harter, S. (1982). The Perceived Competence Scale for Children. *Child Development, 53,* 87–97.

Hartlage, S. (1990). *Automatic processing of attributional inferences in depressed and cognitively depression-prone individuals.* Unpublished doctoral dissertation, Northwestern University, Evanston, IL.

Hartlage, S., Alloy, L. B., Vazquez, C., & Dykman, B. (1993). Automatic and effortful processing in depression. *Psychological Bulletin, 113,* 247–278.

Hasher, L., & Zacks, R. T. (1979). Automatic and effortful processes in memory. *Journal of Experimental Psychology: General, 108,* 356–388.

Haynes, S. N. (1992). *Models of causality in psychopathology.* New York: Macmillan.

Hazan, C., & Shaver, P. (1987). Conceptualizing romantic love as an attachment process. *Journal of Personality and Social Psychology, 52,* 511–524.

Hedlund, S., & Rude, S. S. (1995). Evidence of latent depressive schemas in formerly depressed individuals. *Journal of Abnormal Psychology, 104,* 517–525.

Hendren, R. I. (1983). Depression in anorexia nervosa. *Journal of the American Academy of Child Psychiatry, 22,* 59–62.

Higgins, E. T. (1989). Knowledge accessibility and activation: Subjectivity and suffering from unconscious sources. In J. S. Uleman & J. A. Bargh (Eds.), *Unintended thought*. New York: Guilford Press.

Higgins, E. T., & King, G. A. (1981). Accessibility of social constructs: Information processing consequences of individual and contextual variability. In N. Cantor & J. F. Kihlstrom (Eds.), *Personality, cognition, and social interaction*. Hillsdale, NJ: Erlbaum.

Higgins, E. T., King, G. A., & Mavin, G. H. (1982). Individual construct accessibility and subjective impressions and recall. *Journal of Personality and Social Psychology, 43*, 35–47.

Hollon, S. D. (1992). Cognitive models of depression from a psychobiological perspective. *Psychological Inquiry, 3*, 250–253.

Hollon, S. D., & Cobb, R. (1993). Relapse and recurrence in psychopathological disorders. In C. G. Costello (Ed.), *Basic issues in psychopathology*. New York: Guilford Press.

Hollon, S. D., Evans, M. D., & DeRubeis, R. J. (1990). Cognitive mediation of relapse prevention following treatment for depression: Implications of differential risk. In R. E. Ingram (Ed.), *Contemporary psychological approaches to depression: Theory, research, and treatment*. New York: Plenum Press.

Hollon, S. D., & Kendall, P. C. (1980). Cognitive self-statements in depression: Development of an automatic thoughts questionnaire. *Cognitive Therapy and Research, 4*, 383–395.

Hollon, S. D., Kendall, P. C., & Lumry, A. (1986). Specificity of depressotypic cognitions in clinical depression. *Journal of Abnormal Psychology, 95*, 52–59.

Hollon, S. D., & Kriss, M. (1984). Cognitive factors in clinical research and practice. *Clinical Psychology Review, 4*, 35–76.

Hooley, J. M. (1985). Expressed emotion: A review of the critical literature. *Clinical Psychology Review, 5*, 119–139.

Hooley, J. M., & Teasdale, J. D. (1989). Predictors of relapse in unipolar depressives: Expressed emotion. *Journal of Abnormal Psychology, 98*, 229–237.

Horowitz, L. M., & Malle, B. F. (1993). Fuzzy concepts in psychotherapy research. *Psychotherapy Research, 3*, 131–148.

Horowitz, M. J. (1988). *Introduction to psychodynamics: A synthesis*. New York: Basic Books.

Hull, J. G. (1981). A self-awareness model of the causes and effects of alcohol consumption. *Journal of Abnormal Psychology, 90*, 585–600.

Hull, J. G., & Reilly, N. P. (1986). An information processing approach to alcohol use and its consequence. In R. E. Ingram (Ed.), *Information processing approaches to clinical psychology*. Orlando, FL: Academic Press.

Imber, S. D., Pilkonis, P. A., Sotsky, S. M., Elkin, I., Watkins, J. T., Collins, J. F., Shea, M. T., Leber, W. R., & Glass, D. R. (1990). Mode-specific effects among three treatments for depression. *Journal of Consulting and Clinical Psychology, 58*, 352–359.

Ingram, R. E. (1984). Toward an information processing analysis of depression. *Cognitive Therapy and Research, 8,* 443–478.

Ingram, R. E. (Ed.). (1986). *Information processing approaches to clinical psychology.* Orlando, FL: Academic Press.

Ingram, R. E. (1989). Affective confounds in social–cognitive research. *Journal of Personality and Social Psychology, 57,* 715–722.

Ingram, R. E. (1990). Self-focused attention in clinical disorders: Review and a conceptual model. *Psychological Bulletin, 107,* 156–176.

Ingram, R. E. (1991a, August). *Cognitive constructs, information processing, and depression.* Invited address at the annual meeting of the American Psychological Association, San Francisco.

Ingram, R. E. (1991b). *Systematic cognitive assessment in dysfunctional states.* NIMH grant.

Ingram, R. E. (1991c). Tilting at windmills: A Response to Pyszczynski, Greenberg, Hamilton, and Nix. *Psychological Bulletin, 110,* 544–550.

Ingram, R. E. (1994). The integration of cognitive and interpersonal aspects of depression: Strained, symbiotic, or synergistic? *Contemporary Psychology, 39,* 403–404.

Ingram, R. E., Bailey, K., & Siegle, G. (1997, August). *Depressotypic information processing in individuals with disrupted parental attachment.* Paper presented at the annual meeting of the American Psychological Association, Chicago.

Ingram, R. E., Bernet, C. Z., & McLaughlin, S. C. (1994). Attentional allocation processes in individuals at risk for depression. *Cognitive Therapy and Research, 18,* 317–332.

Ingram, R. E., Cruet, D., Johnson, B., & Wisnicki, K. S. (1988). Self-focused attention, gender, gender role, and vulnerability to negative affect. *Journal of Personality and Social Psychology, 55,* 967–978.

Ingram, R. E., & Holle, C. (1992). The cognitive science of depression. In D. J. Stein & J. E. Young (Eds.), *Cognitive science and clinical disorders.* Orlando, FL: Academic Press.

Ingram, R. E., & Hollon, S. D. (1986). Cognitive therapy of depression from an information processing perspective. In R. E. Ingram (Ed.), *Information processing approaches to clinical psychology.* Orlando: Academic Press.

Ingram, R. E., Johnson, B. R., Bernet, C. Z., Dombeck, M., & Rowe, M. K. (1992). Cognitive and emotional reactivity in chronically self-focused individuals. *Cognitive Therapy and Research, 16,* 451–472.

Ingram, R. E., & Kendall, P. C. (1986). Cognitive clinical psychology: Implications of an information processing perspective. In R. E. Ingram (Ed.), *Information processing approaches to clinical psychology.* Orlando, FL: Academic Press.

Ingram, R. E., & Kendall, P. C. (1987). The cognitive side of anxiety. *Cognitive Therapy and Research, 11,* 523–536.

Ingram, R. E., Kendall, P. C., & Chen, A. H. (1991). Cognitive-behavioral interventions. In C. R. Snyder & D. R. Forsyth (Eds.), *Handbook of social and clinical psychology: The health perspective.* New York: Pergamon Press.

Ingram, R. E., Kendall, P. C., Smith, T. W., Donnell, C., & Ronan, K. (1987). Cognitive specificity in emotional distress. *Journal of Personality and Social Psychology, 53,* 734–742.

Ingram, R. E., & Ritter, J. (1997). *Cognitive reactivity and parental bonding dimensions of vulnerability to depression.* Manuscript submitted for publication.

Ingram, R. E., Lumry, A. E., Cruet, D., & Sieber, W. (1987). Attentional processes in depressive disorders. *Cognitive Therapy and Research, 11,* 351.

Ingram, R. E., & Reed, M. J. (1986). Information encoding and retrieval in depression: Findings, issues, and future directions. In R. E. Ingram (Ed.), *Information processing approaches to clinical psychology.* Orlando, FL: Academic Press.

Ingram, R. E., & Ritter, J. (1998). *Cognitive reactivity and parental bonding dimensions of vulnerability to depression.* Manuscript submitted for publication.

Ingram, R. E., & Scott, W. (1990). Foundations of cognitive-behavioral approaches to treatment. In A. S. Bellack, M. Hersen, & A. E. Kazdin (Eds.), *International handbook of behavior modification and therapy* (2nd ed.). New York: Plenum Press.

Ingram, R. E., Scott, W., & Siegle, G. (in press). Affective disorders: Cognitive and social aspects. In T. Millon, P. Blaney, & R. Davis (Eds.), *Oxford textbook of psychopathology.* Oxford, UK: Oxford University Press.

Ingram, R. E., & Smith, T. W. (1984). Depression and internal versus external focus of attention. *Cognitive Therapy and Research, 8,* 139–152.

Ingram, R. E., Smith, T. W., & Brehm, S. S. (1983). Depression and information processing: Self-schemata and the encoding of self-relevant information. *Journal of Personality and Social Psychology, 45,* 412–420.

Ingram, R. E., & Wisnicki, K. S. (1991). Cognition in depression. In P. A. Magaro (Ed.), *Annual review of psychopathology.* Newbury Park, CA: Sage.

Isen, A. M., Shalker, T. T., Clark, M., & Karp, L. (1978). Affect, accessibility of material in memory, and behavior: A cognitive loop? *Journal of Personality and Social Psychology, 36,* 1–12.

Izard, C. E. (1993). Four systems for emotion activation: Cognitive and noncognitive processes. *Psychological Review, 100,* 68–90.

Jacobson, N. S., & Anderson, E. A. (1982). Interpersonal skill and depression in college students: An analysis of the timing of self-disclosures. *Behavior Therapy, 13,* 271–282.

Jaenicke, C., Hammen, C. L., Zupan, B., Hiroto, D., Gordon, D., Adrain, C., & Burge, D. (1987). Cognitive vulnerability in children at risk for depression. *Journal of Abnormal Child Psychology, 15,* 559–572.

Jackson, S. W. (1986). *Melancholia and depression: From Hippocratic times to modern times.* New Haven, CT: Yale University Press.

Jacobson, E. (1964). *The self and the object world.* Madison, CT: International Universities Press.

Jacobson, S., Fasman, J., & DiMascio, A. (1975). Deprivation in the childhood of depressed women. *Journal of Nervous and Mental Disease, 160,* 5–14.

Joffe, R., Segal, Z., & Singer, W. (1996). Change in thyroid hormone levels following response to cognitive therapy for major depression. *American Journal of Psychiatry, 153,* 411–413.

Jones, R. (1968). *A factored measure of Ellis's irrational belief system.* Unpublished doctoral dissertation, Texas Technological College, Lubbock, TX.

Jordan, A., & Cole, D. A. (1996). Relation of depressive symptoms to the structure of self-knowledge in childhood. *Journal of Abnormal Psychology, 105,* 530–540.

Just, N., Alloy, L. B., & Abramson, L. Y. (1998). *Remitted depression studies as tests of the cognitive vulnerability hypothesis of depression onset: A critique and conceptual analysis.* Unpublished manuscript.

Jung, C. G. (1910). The association method. *American Journal of Psychology, 21,* 219–269.

Juola, J. F. (1986). Cognitive psychology and information processing: Content and process analysis for a psychology of mind. In R. E. Ingram (Ed.), *Information processing approaches to clinical psychology.* Orlando, FL: Academic Press.

Kabat-Zinn, J. (1990). *Full catastrophe living.* New York: Delacorte.

Kabat-Zinn, J., Massion, A. O., Kristeller, J., Peterson, L. G., Fletcher, K. E., Pbert, L., Lenderking, W. R., & Santorelli, S. F. (1992). Effectiveness of a mediation-based stress reduction program in the treatment of anxiety disorders. *American Journal of Psychiatry, 149,* 936–943.

Kaelber, C. T., Moul, D. E., & Farmer, M. E. (1995). Epidemiology of depression. In E. E. Beckham & W. R. Leber (Eds.), *Handbook of depression* (2nd ed.). New York: Guilford Press.

Kahneman, D. (1973). *Attention and effort.* Englewood Cliffs, NJ: Prentice-Hall.

Kandel, D. B., & Davies, M. (1982). Epidemiology of depressive mood in adolescents: An empirical study. *Archives of General Psychiatry, 39,* 1205–1212.

Kandel, E. R. (1983). From metapsychology to molecular biology: Explorations into the nature of anxiety. *American Journal of Psychiatry, 140,* 1277–1293.

Kandel, E., Mednick, S. A., Kirkegaard-Sorensen, L., Hutchings, B., Knop, J., Rosenberg, R., & Schulsinger, F. (1988). IQ as a protective factor for subjects at high risk for antisocial behavior. *Journal of Consulting and Clinical Psychology, 56,* 224–226.

Kanfer, F. H., & Hagerman, S. M. (1985). Behavior therapy and the information processing paradigm. In S. Reiss & R. R. Bootzin (Eds.), *Theoretical issues in behavior therapy.* New York: Academic Press.

Kanner, A. D., Coyne, J. C., Schaefer, C., & Lazarus, R. S. (1981). Comparison of two modes of stress measurement: Daily hassles and uplifts versus major life events. *Journal of Behavioral Medicine, 4,* 1–39.

Kasl, S. V. (1983). Pursuing the link between stressful life experiences and disease: A time for reappraisal. In C. L. Cooper (Ed.), *Stress research.* New York: Wiley.

Katon, W., & Sullivan, M. D. (1990). Depression and chronic medical illness. *Journal of Clinical Psychiatry, 51,* 3–11.

Katz, R., & McGuffin, P. (1993). The genetics of affective disorders. In L. J. Chapman, J. Chapman, & D. Fowles (Eds.), *Progress in experimental personality and psychopathology research* (Vol. 16). New York: Springer.

Kazdin, A. E. (1983). Psychiatric diagnosis, dimensions of behavior therapy, and child behavior therapy. *Behavior Therapy, 14*, 73–99.

Kazdin, A. E. (1984). Therapy analogues and clinical trials in psychotherapy research. In M. Hersen, L. Michelson, & A. Bellack (Eds.), *Issues in psychotherapy research*. New York: Plenum Press.

Kazdin, A. E. (1992). *Research design in clinical psychology*. Boston: Allyn & Bacon.

Kazdin, A. E., Colbus, D., & Rodgers, A. (1986). Assessment of depression and diagnosis of depressive disorders among psychiatrically disturbed children. *Journal of Abnormal Child Psychology, 14*, 499–515.

Keller, M. B. (1985). Chronic and recurrent affective disorders: Incidence, course, and influencing factors. In D. Kemali & G. Recagni (Eds.), *Chronic treatments in neuropsychiatry*. New York: Raven Press.

Keller, M. B., Shapiro, R. W., Lavori, P. W., & Wolfe, N. (1982). Relapse in RDC major depressive disorders: Analysis with the life table. *Archives of General Psychiatry, 39*, 911–915.

Kendall, P. C. (1985). Cognitive processes and procedures in behavior therapy. In G. T. Wilson, C. M. Franks, P. C. Kendall, & J. P. Foreyt, *Review of behavior therapy: Theory and practice* (Vol. 11). New York: Guilford Press.

Kendall, P. C., & Bemis, K. M. (1983). Thought and action in psychotherapy: The cognitive-behavioral approaches. In M. Hersen, A. E. Kazdin, & A. S. Bellack (Eds.), *The clinical psychology handbook*. Elmsford, NY: Pergamon Press.

Kendall, P. C., & Brady, T. (1995). Comorbidity in the anxiety disorders of childhood: Implications for validity and clinical significance. In K. D. Craig & K. S. Dobson (Eds.), *Anxiety and depression in adults and children*. Thousand Oaks, CA: Sage.

Kendall, P. C., & Butcher, J. N. (Eds.). (1982). *Handbook of research methods in clinical psychology*. New York: Wiley.

Kendall, P. C., & Flannery-Schroeder, E. C. (1995). Rigor, but not rigor mortis, in depression research. *Journal of Personality and Social Psychology, 68*, 892–894.

Kendall, P. C., & Hollon, S. D. (1979). *Cognitive-behavioral interventions: Theory, research, and procedures*. New York: Academic Press.

Kendall, P. C., & Hollon, S. D. (1981). *Assessment strategies for cognitive-behavioral interventions*. New York: Academic Press.

Kendall, P. C., Hollon, S. D., Beck, A. T., Hammen, C. L., & Ingram, R. E. (1987). Issues and recommendations regarding use of the Beck Depression Inventory. *Cognitive Therapy and Research, 11*, 289–299.

Kendall, P. C., & Ingram, R. E. (1987). The future for cognitive assessment of anxiety: Let's get specific. In L. Michelson & M. Ascher (Eds.), *Anxiety and stress disorders: Cognitive-behavioral assessment and treatment*. New York: Guilford Press.

Kendall, P. C., & Ingram, R. E. (1989). Cognitive-behavioral perspectives:

Theory and research on negative affective states. In P. C. Kendall & D. Watson, (Eds.), *Anxiety and depression: Distinctive and overlapping features*. San Diego: Academic Press.

Kendall, P. C., Stark, K. D., & Adam, R. (1990). Cognitive deficit or cognitive distortion in childhood depression. *Journal of Abnormal Child Psychology, 18,* 255–270.

Kendall, P. C., & Watson, D. (Eds.). (1989). *Negative affective conditions*. San Diego: Academic Press.

Kendall-Tackett, K. A., Williams, L. M., & Finkelhor, D. (1993). Impact of sexual abuse on children: A review and synthesis of recent empirical studies. *Psychological Bulletin, 113,* 164–180.

Kendell, R. E. (1968). *The classification of depressive illness*. London: Oxford University Press.

Kendell, R. E. (1975). *The role of diagnosis in psychiatry*. Oxford, UK: Blackwell.

Kendler, K. S., Kessler, R. C., & Neale, M. C. (1993). The prediction of major depression in women: Toward an integrated etiologic model. *American Journal of Psychiatry, 150,* 1139–1148.

Kendler, K. S., Neale, M. C., Kessler, R. C., & Heath, A. C. (1992). Familial influences on the clinical characteristics of major depression: A twin study. *Acta Psychiatrica Scandinavica, 86,* 371–378.

Kernberg, O. (1976). *Object-relations theory and clinical psychoanalysis*. Northvale, NJ: Aronson.

Kessler, R. C., McGonagle, K. A., Swartz, M., Blazer, D. G., & Nelson, C. B. (1993). Sex and depression in the National Comorbidity Survey: I. Lifetime prevalence, chronicity and recurrence. *Journal of Affective Disorders, 29,* 85–96.

Kessler, R. C., McGonagle, K. A., Zhao, S., Nelson, C. B., Hughes, M., Eshleman, S., Wittchen, H. U., & Kendler, K. S. (1994). Lifetime and 12-month prevalence of results from the National Comorbidity Survey. *Archives of General Psychiatry, 51,* 8–19.

Kessler, R. C., Sonnega, A., Bromet, E., Hughes, M., & Nelson, C. B. (1995). Posttraumatic stress disorder in the National Comorbidity Survey. *Archives of General Psychiatry, 52,* 1048–1060.

Kety, S. S., Rosenthal, D., Wender, P. H., & Schulsinger, F. (1968). The types and prevalence of mental illness in the biological and adoptive families of adopted schizophrenics. In D. Rosenthal & S. S. Kety (Eds.), *Transmission of schizophrenia*. Oxford, UK: Pergamon Press.

Khantzian, E. J. (1985). The self-medication hypothesis of addictive disorders: Focus on heroin and cocaine dependence. *American Journal of Psychiatry, 142,* 1259–1264.

Kihlstrom, J. F., & Cantor, N. (1984). Mental representations of the self. In L. Berkowitz (Ed.), *Advances in experimental social psychology* (Vol. 15). New York: Academic Press.

Kihlstrom, J. F., & Nasby, W. (1981). Cognitive tasks in clinical assessment: An exercise in applied psychology. In P. C. Kendall & S. D. Hollon (Eds.), *Assessment strategies for cognitive-behavioral interventions*. New York: Academic Press.

Klein, D., Depue, R. A., & Krauss, S. P. (1986). Social adjustment in the offspring of parents with bipolar affective disorder. *Journal of Psychopathology and Behavioral Assessment, 8*, 355–366.

Klein, D., Harding, K., Taylor, E. B., & Dickstein, S. (1988). Dependency and self-criticism in depression: Evaluation in a clinical population. *Journal of Abnormal Psychology, 97*, 399–404.

Klein, D., & Riso, L. P. (1993). Psychiatric disorders: Problems of boundaries and comorbidity. In C. G. Costello (Ed.), *Basic issues in psychopathology.* New York: Guilford Press.

Klein, M. H., Kupfer, D. J., & Shea, M. T. (1993). *Personality and depression.* New York: Guilford Press.

Klerman, G. L., Lavori, P. W., Rice, J., Reich, T., Endicott, J., Andreasen, N. C., Keller, M. B., & Hirschfeld, R. M. A. (1985). Birth-cohort trends in rates of major depressive disorder among relatives of patients with affective disorder. *Archives of General Psychiatry, 42*, 689–693.

Klerman, G. L., & Weissman, M. M. (1992). The course, morbidity, and costs of depression. *Archives of General Psychiatry, 49*, 831–834.

Klerman, G. L., Weissman, M. M., Rounsaville, B. J., & Chevron, E. (1984). *Interpersonal psychotherapy of depression.* New York: Basic Books.

Koenig, L. J. (1988). Self-image of emotionally disturbed adolescents. *Journal of Abnormal Child Psychology, 16*, 111–126.

Kovacs, M., Feinberg, T. L., Crouse-Novak, M. A., Paulauskas, S. L., Pollock, M., & Finkelstein, R. (1984). Depressive disorders in childhood: II. A longitudinal study of the risk for a subsequent major depression. *Archives of General Psychiatry, 41*, 643–649.

Kraemer, H., Kazdin, A., Offord, D., Kessler, R., Jensen, P., & Kupfer, D. (1997). Coming to terms with the terms of risk. *Archives of General Psychiatry, 54*, 337–343.

Krantz, S., & Hammen, C. (1979). Assessment of cognitive bias in depression. *Journal of Abnormal Psychology, 50*, 169–174.

Krantz, S., & Moos, R. H. (1988). Risk factors at intake predict nonremission among depressed patients. *Journal of Consulting and Clinical Psychology, 56*, 863–869.

Kroger, R. O., & Wood, L. A. (1993). Reification, "faking," and the big five. *American Psychologist, 48*, 1297–1298.

Kuiper, N. A., & Olinger, L. J. (1986). Dysfunctional attitudes and a self-worth contingency model of depression. In P. C. Kendall (Ed.), *Advances in cognitive-behavioral research and therapy* (Vol. 5). New York: Academic Press.

Kuiper, N. A., Olinger, L. J., & MacDonald, M. (1988). Vulnerability and episodic cognitions in a self-worth contingency model of depression. In L. B. Alloy (Ed.), *Cognitive processes in depression.* New York: Guilford Press.

Kuyken, W., & Brewin, C. R. (1995). Autobiographical memory functioning in depression and reports of early abuse. *Journal of Abnormal Psychology, 104*, 585–591.

Labarge, A. S., Cash, T. F., & Brown, T. A. (1995). *The use of a modified Stroop task to examine appearance-schematic information processing in college women.* Unpublished manuscript.

Lachman, R., & Lachman, J. (1986). Information processing psychology: Origins and extensions. In R. E. Ingram (Ed.), *Information processing approaches to clinical psychology.* Orlando, FL: Academic Press.

Lang, P. J. (1977). Fear imagery: An information-processing analysis. *Behaviour Research and Therapy, 8,* 495–512.

Lavori, P. W., Kessler, M. B., & Klerman, G. L. (1984). Relapse in affective disorders: A reanalysis of the literature using life table methods. *Journal of Psychiatric Research, 18,* 13–25.

Lazarus, R. S. (1966). *Psychological stress and the coping process.* New York: McGraw-Hill.

Lazarus, R. S. (1968). Emotions and adaptation: Conceptual and empirical relations. In W. Arnold (Ed.), *Nebraska symposium on motivation* (Vol. 16). Lincoln, NE: University of Nebraska Press.

Lazarus, R. S. (1982). Thoughts on the relations between emotion and cognition. *American Psychologist, 37,* 1019–1024.

Lazarus, R. S. (1990). Theory-based stress management. *Psychological Inquiry, 1,* 3–13.

Lazarus, R. S., & Folkman, S. (1984). *Stress, appraisal, and coping.* New York: Springer.

Lefebve, M. (1981). Cognitive distortions and cognitive errors in depressed psychiatric and low back pain patients. *Journal of Consulting and Clinical Psychology, 49,* 517–525.

Lehmann, H. J. (1959). Psychiatric concepts of depression: Nomenclature and classification. *Canadian Psychiatric Association Journal Supplement, 4,* 1–12.

Leitenberg, H., Yost, L. W., & Carroll-Wilson, M. (1986). Negative cognitive errors in children: Questionnaire development, normative data, and comparisons between children with and without self-reported symptoms of depression, low self-esteem, and evaluation anxiety. *Journal of Consulting and Clinical Psychology, 54,* 528–536.

Leon, G. R., Kendall, P. C., & Garber, J. (1980). Depression in children: Parent, teacher, and child perspectives. *Journal of Abnormal Child Psychology, 8,* 221–235.

Lewinsohn, P. (1985). A behavioral approach to depression. In J. C. Coyne (Ed.), *Essential papers in depression.* New York: New York University Press.

Lewinsohn, P. M., Duncan, E. M., Stanton, A. K., & Fischer, S. A. (1993). Age at first onset for nonbipolar depression. *Journal of Abnormal Psychology, 102,* 110–120.

Lewinsohn, P. M., Hoberman, H. M., Teri, L., & Hautzinger, M. (1985). An integrative theory of depression. In S. Reiss & R. R. Bootzin (Eds.), *Theoretical issues in behavior therapy.* Orlando, FL: Academic Press.

Lewinsohn, P. M., Hops, H., Roberts, R. E., Seeley, J. R., & Andrews, B. (1993). Adolescent psychopathology: I. Prevalence and incidence of depression and other DSM-III-R disorders in high school students. *Journal of Abnormal Psychology, 102,* 133–144.

Lewinsohn, P. M., & Rosenbaum, M. (1987). Recall of parental behavior by acute depressives, remitted depressives, and nondepressives. *Journal of Personality and Social Psychology, 52,* 611–619.

Lewinsohn, P. M., Steinmetz, L., Larson, D. W., & Franklin, J. (1981). Depression-related cognitions: Antecedent or consequence? *Journal of Abnormal Psychology, 90,* 213–219.

Lilienfeld, S. O., & Marino, L. (1995). Mental disorder as a Roschian concept: A critique of Wakefield's "harmful dysfunction" analysis. *Journal of Abnormal Psychology, 104,* 411–420.

Lilienfeld, S. O., Waldman, I. D., & Israel, A. C. (1994). A critical examination of the use and the concept of comorbidity in psychopathology research. *Clinical Psychology: Science and Practice, 1,* 71–83.

Linville, P. W. (1987). Self-complexity as a cognitive buffer against stress-related illness and depression. *Journal of Personality and Social Psychology, 52,* 663–676.

Luthar, S. S., & Zigler, E. (1991). Vulnerability and competence: A review of research on resilience in childhood. *American Journal of Orthopsychiatry, 61,* 6–22.

MacDonald, M. R., & Kuiper, N. A. (1982). Self and other in mild depression. *Cognitive Therapy and Research, 1,* 223–239.

MacLeod, C., Mathews, A., & Tata, P. (1986). Attentional bias in emotional disorders. *Journal of Abnormal Psychology, 95,* 15–20.

Magaro, P. A (1991). *Annual Review of Psychopathology: Cognitive bases of mental disorders..* Newbury Park, CA: Sage.

Maher, B. (1970). *Introduction to research in psychopathology.* New York: McGraw-Hill.

Mahoney, M. J. (1990). *Human change processes.* New York: Basic Books.

Mahoney, M. J., & Arnkoff, D. (1978). Cognitive and self-control therapies. In S. Garfield & A. E. Bergin (Eds.), *Handbook of therapy and behavior change: An empirical analysis* (2nd ed.). New York: Wiley.

Main, M., Kaplan, N., & Cassidy, J. (1985). Security in infancy, childhood, and adulthood: A move to the level of representation. In I. Bretherton & E. Waters (Eds.), Growing points in attachment theory and research. *Monographs of the Society for Research in Child Development, 50*(1–2, Serial No. 209), 66–106.

Malcarne, V. L., Chavira, D. A., & Liu, P. (1996). *The scale of ethnic experience: A measure for use across groups.* Presented at the meeting of the American Psychological Association, Toronto.

Malcarne, V. L., & Ingram, R. E. (1994). Cognition and negative affectivity. In T. H Ollendick & R. J. Prinz (Eds.), *Advances in clinical child psychology* (Vol. 16). New York: Plenum Press.

Mandler, G. (1967). Organization and memory. In K. W. Spence & J. T. Spence (Eds.), *The psychology of learning and motivation: Advances in research and theory* (Vol. 1). New York: Academic Press.

Marcus, M. D., Wing, R. R., Guare, J., Blair, E. H., & Jawad, A. (1992). Lifetime prevalence of major depression and its effect on treatment outcome in obese type II diabetic patients. *Diabetes Care, 15,* 253–255.

Markowitz, J. C., & Weissman, M. M. (1995). Interpersonal psychotherapy. In E. E. Beckham & W. R. Leber (Eds.), *Handbook of depression* (2nd ed.). New York: Guilford Press.

Marsella, A. J., Sartorius, M., Jablensky, A., & Fenton, F. R. (1985). Cross-cultural studies of depressive disorders: An overview. In A. Kleinman & B. Good (Eds.), *Culture and depression: Studies in the anthropology and cross-cultural psychiatry of affect and disorder.* Berkeley: University of California Press.

Maser, J. D., & Cloninger, R. (Eds.). (1990). *Comorbidity of mood and anxiety disorders.* Washington, DC: American Psychiatric Association Press.

Maser, J. D., Weise, R., & Gwirtsman, H. (1995). Depression and its boundaries with selected Axis I disorders. In E. E. Beckham & W. R. Leber (Eds.), *Handbook of depression* (2nd ed.). New York: Guilford Press.

Massie, M. J., & Holland, J. C. (1987). The cancer patient with pain: Psychiatric complications and their management. *Medical Clinics of North America, 71,* 243–258.

Mayou, R. A., Peveler, R., Davies, B., Mann, J., & Fairburn, C. (1991). Psychiatric comorbidity in young adults with insulin-dependent diabetes mellitus. *Psychological Medicine, 21,* 639–645.

Mathews, A., & MacLeod, C. (1985). Selective processing of threat cues in anxiety states. *Journal of Abnormal Psychology, 95,* 131–138.

Matthews, G. (in press). *Cognitive science perspectives on personality and emotion.* New York: Elsevier Science.

McCabe, S. B., & Gotlib, I. H. (1993). Attentional processing in clinically depressed subjects: A longitudinal investigation. *Cognitive Therapy and Research, 17,* 359–377.

McCauley, E., Mitchell, J., Burke, P., & Moss, S. (1988). Cognitive attributes of depression in children and adolescents. *Journal of Consulting and Clinical Psychology, 56,* 903–908.

McCranie, E. W., & Bass, J. D. (1984). Childhood family antecedents of dependency and self-criticism: Implications for depression. *Journal of Abnormal Psychology, 93,* 3–8.

McFarlane, A. H., Norman, G. R., Streiner, D. L., Roy, R., & Scott, D. J. (1980). A longitudinal study of the influence of the psychosocial environment on health status: A preliminary report. *Journal of Health and Social Behavior, 21,* 124–133.

McGue, M., & Gottesman, I. I. (1989). Genetic linkage in schizophrenia: Perspectives from genetic epidemiology. *Schizophrenia Bulletin, 15,* 453–464.

McGuffin, P., Katz, R., Aldrich, J., & Bebbington, P. E. (1988). The Camberwell Collaborative Depression Study: II. Investigation of family members. *British Journal of Psychiatry, 152,* 766–774.

McGuffin, P., Katz, R., & Rutherford, J. (1991). Nature, nurture and depression: A twin study. *Psychological Medicine, 21,* 329–335.

McKnight, D. L., Nelson-Gray, R. O., & Barnhill, J. (1992). Dexamethasone suppression test and response to cognitive therapy and antidepressant medication. *Behavior Therapy, 23,* 99–111.

Mednick, S. A., & Schulsinger, F. (1968). Some premorbid characteristics related to breakdown in children of with schizophrenic mothers. In D. Rosenthal & S. S. Kety (Eds.), *Transmission of schizophrenia*. Oxford, UK: Pergamon Press.

Meehl, P. E. (1962). Schizotaxia, schizotypy, schizophrenia. *American Psychologist, 17*, 827–838.

Meehl, P. E. (1986). Diagnostic taxia as open concepts: Meta-theoretical and statistical questions about reliability and construct validity in the grand strategy of nosological revision. In T. Millon & G. L. Klerman (Eds.), *Contemporary directions in psychopathology: Toward the DSM-IV*. New York: Guilford Press.

Metalsky, G. I., Abramson, L. Y., Seligman, M. E. P., Semmel, A., & Peterson, C. R. (1982). Attributional styles and life events in the classroom: Vulnerability and invulnerability to depressive mood reactions. *Journal of Personality and Social Psychology, 43*, 612–617.

Metalsky, G. I., Halberstadt, L. J., & Abramson, L. Y. (1987). Vulnerability to depressive mood reactions: Toward a more powerful test of the diathesis–stress and causal mediation components of the reformulated theory of depression. *Journal of Personality and Social Psychology, 52*, 386–393.

Metalsky, G. I., Joiner, T. E., Hardin, T. S., & Abramson, L. Y. (1993). Depressive reactions to failure in a naturalistic setting: A test of the hopelessness and self-esteem theories of depression. *Journal of Abnormal Psychology, 102*, 101–109.

Meyer, D. E., & Schvaneveldt, R. W. (1971). Facilitation in recognizing pairs of words: Evidence of a dependence between retrieval operations. *Journal of Experimental Psychology, 90*, 227–234.

Miller, A. (1983). *For your own good: The roots of violence in child-rearing*. New York: Farrar, Straus, & Giroux.

Millon, T. (1969). *Modern psychopathology*. Philadelphia: Saunders.

Millon, T. (1990). *Toward a new personology: An evolutionary model*. New York: Wiley.

Miranda, J., Gross, J., Persons, J., & Hahn, J. (in press). Mood matters: Negative mood induction activates dysfunctional attitudes in women vulnerable to depression. *Cognitive Therapy and Research*.

Miranda, J., & Persons, J. B. (1988). Dysfunctional attitudes are mood-state dependent. *Journal of Abnormal Psychology, 97*, 76–79.

Miranda, J., Persons, J. B., & Byers, C. (1990). Endorsement of dysfunctional beliefs depends on current mood state. *Journal of Abnormal Psychology, 99*, 237–241.

Mogg, K., Bradley, B., Williams, R., & Mathews, A. (1993). Subliminal processing of emotional information in anxiety and depression. *Journal of Abnormal Psychology, 102*, 304–311

Monroe, S. M. (1989). Stress and social support: Assessment issues. In N. Schneiderman, S. M. Weiss, & P. G. Kaufman (Eds.), *Handbook of research in cardiovascular behavioral medicine*. New York: Plenum Press.

Monroe, S. M., & Peterman, A. M. (1988). Life stress and psychopathology. In

L. Cohen (Ed.), *Research on stressful life events: Theoretical and methodological issues.* Newbury Park, CA: Sage.

Monroe, S. M., Kupfer, D. J., & Frank, E. (1992). Life stress and treatment course of recurrent depression: I. Response during index episode. *Journal of Consulting and Clinical Psychology, 60,* 718–724.

Monroe, S. M., & Simons, A. D. (1991). Diathesis–stress theories in the context of life stress research: Implications for the depressive disorders. *Psychological Bulletin, 110,* 406–425.

Moos, R. H., Fenn, C., Billings, A., & Moos, B. (1989). Assessing life stressors and social resources: Applications to alcoholic patients. *Journal of Substance Abuse, 1,* 135–152.

Moos, R. H., & Moos, B. (1992). *Life Stressors and Social Resources Inventory—Adult Form Manual.* Palo Alto, CA: Stanford University Medical Center, Center for Health Care Evaluation/Department of Veterans Affairs Medical Center.

Moretti, M. M., Segal, Z. V., McCann, C. D., Shaw, B. F., Vella, D., & Miller, D. T. (1996). Self-referent versus other-referent information processing in mildly depressed, clinically depressed and remitted depressed subjects. *Personality and Social Psychology Bulletin, 22,* 68–80.

Morrison, H. L. (Ed.). (1983). *Children of depressed parents: Risk, identification, and intervention.* New York: Grune & Stratton.

Munoz, R. F., Mrazek, P. J., & Haggerty, R. J. (1996). Institute of Medicine report on prevention of mental disorders: Summary and commentary. *American Psychologist, 51,* 1116–1122.

Munoz, R. F., Ying, Y., Perez-Stable, E. J., & Miranda, J. (1993). *The prevention of depression. Research and practice.* Baltimore: Johns Hopkins University Press.

Murphy, H., Wittkower, E., & Chance, N. (1964). Cross-cultural inquiry into the symptomatology of depression. *Transcultural Psychiatric Research Review, 1,* 5–21.

Musson, R. F., & Alloy, L. B. (1988). Depression and self-directed attention. In L. B. Alloy (Ed.), *Cognitive processes in depression.* New York: Guilford Press.

Nasby, W., & Kihlstrom, J. F. (1986). Cognitive assessment of personality and psychopathology. In R. E. Ingram (Ed.), *Information processing approaches to clinical psychology.* Orlando, FL: Academic Press.

Neisser, U. (1967). *Cognitive psychology.* New York: Appleton.

Neisser, U. (1976). *Cognition and reality.* San Francisco: Freeman.

Newell, A., & Simon, H. A. (1972). *Human problem solving.* Englewood Cliffs, NJ: Prentice Hall.

Nicholls, J. G. (1978). Development of causal attributions and evaluative responses to success and failure in Maori and Pakeha children. *Developmental Psychology, 14,* 687–688.

Nicholson, I. R., & Neufeld, R. W. J. (1992). A dynamic vulnerability perspective on stress and schizophrenia. *American Journal of Orthopsychiatry, 62,* 117–130.

Nietzel, M. T., & Harris, M. J. (1990). Relationship of dependency and achievement/autonomy to depression. *Clinical Psychology Review, 10,* 279–297.

Nisbett, R. E., & Wilson, T. D. (1977). Telling more than we can know: Verbal reports on mental processes. *Psychological Review, 84,* 231–259.

Nolen-Hoeksema, S. (1987). Sex differences in unipolar depression: Evidence and theory. *Psychological Bulletin, 101,* 259–282.

Nolen-Hoeksema, S. (1991). Responses to depression and their effects on the duration of depressive episodes. *Journal of Abnormal Psychology, 100,* 569–582.

Nolen-Hoeksema, S., Girgus, J. S., & Seligman, M. E. P. (1986). Learned helplessness in children: A longitudinal study of depression, achievement, and explanatory style. *Journal of Personality and Social Psychology, 51,* 435–442.

Nolen-Hoeksema, S., Girgus, J. S., & Seligman, M. E. P. (1992). Predictors and consequences of childhood depressive symptoms: A 5-year longitudinal study. *Journal of Abnormal Psychology, 101,* 405–422.

Norman, D. A. (1969). *Memory and attention.* Chichester, UK: Wiley.

Norman, D. A. (1986). Toward a theory of memory and attention. *Psychological Review, 75,* 522–536.

Nurcombe, B. (1992). The evolution and validity of the diagnosis of major depression in childhood and adolescence. In D. Cicchetti & S. L. Toth (Eds.), *Developmental perspectives on depression.* Rochester, NY: University of Rochester Press.

O'Hara, M. W., Zekoski, E. M., Phillips, L. H., & Wright, E. J. (1990). Controlled prospective study of postpartum mood disorders: Comparison of childbearing and nonchildbearing women. *Journal of Abnormal Psychology, 99,* 3–15.

Pardo, J. V., Pardo, P. J., & Raichle, M. E. (1993). Neural correlates of self-induced dysphoria. *American Journal of Psychiatry, 150,* 713–719.

Parker, G. (1979). Parental characteristics in relation to depressive disorders. *British Journal of Psychiatry, 134,* 138–147.

Parker, G. (1983). Parental "affectionless control" as an antecedent to adult depression: A risk factor delineated. *Archives of General Psychiatry, 40,* 956–960.

Parker, G., Tupling, H., & Brown, L. B. (1979). A parental bonding instrument. *British Journal of Medical Psychology, 52,* 1010.

Paykel, E. S. (1974). Life stress and psychiatric disorder: Applications of the clinical approach. In B. S. Dohrenwend & B. P. Dohrenwend (Eds.), *Stressful life events: Their nature and effects.* New York: Wiley.

Paykel, E. S. (1979). Causal relationships between clinical depression and life events. In J. E. Barrett (Ed.), *Stress and mental disorder.* New York: Raven Press.

Pearlin, L. I., & Schooler, C. (1978). The structure of coping. *Journal of Health and Social Behavior, 19,* 2–21.

Pearson, J. L., Cohn, D. A., Cowan, P. A., & Cowan, C. P. (1994). Earned- and continuous-security in adult attachment: Relation to depressive symptomatology and parenting style. *Development and Psychopathology, 6, 359–373*.

Peck, J. R., Smith, T. W., Ward, J. R., & Milano, F. (1989). Disability and depression in rheumatoid arthritis. A multitrait–multimethod investigation. *Arthritis and Rheumatism, 29,* 1456–1466.

Persons, J. B. (1986). The advantages of studying psychological phenomena rather than psychiatric diagnoses. *American Psychologist, 41,* 1252–1260.

Persons, J. B., & Miranda, J. (1992). Cognitive theories of depression: Reconciling negative evidence. *Cognitive Therapy and Research, 16,* 485–502.

Persons, J. B., & Rao, P. A. (1985). Longitudinal study of cognitions, life events and depression in psychiatric inpatients. *Journal of Abnormal Psychology, 94,* 51–63.

Petersen, A. C., Compas, B. E., Brooks-Gunn, J., Stemmler, M., Ey, S., & Grant, K. E. (1993). Depression in adolescence. *American Psychologist, 48,* 155–168.

Peterson, C., & Seligman, M. E. (1984). Causal explanations as risk factors for depression: Theory and evidence. *Psychological Review, 91,* 347–374.

Phares, V. (1996). *Fathers and developmental psychopathology.* New York: Wiley.

Phares, V., & Compas, B. E. (1992). The role of fathers in child and adolescent psychopathology: Make room for daddy. *Psychological Bulletin, 111,* 387–412.

Phillips, D., & Segal, B. (1969). Sexual status and psychiatric symptoms. *American Sociological Review, 34,* 58–72.

Pilkonis, P., & Frank, E. (1988). Personality pathology in recurrent depression: Nature, prevalence, and relationship to treatment response. *American Journal of Psychiatry, 145,* 435–441.

Pitt, E. (1982). Depression and childbirth. In E. S. Paykel (Ed.), *Handbook of affective disorders.* New York: Guilford Press.

Popper, K. R. (1959). *The logic of scientific discovery.* New York: Basic Books.

Posner, M. I. (1978). *Chronometric explorations of mind.* Hillsdale, NJ: Erlbaum.

Posner, M. I., & McLeod, P. (1982). Information processing models—In search of elementary operations. In M. R. Rosenzweig & L. W. Porter (Eds.), *Annual review of psychology* (Vol. 33). Palo Alto, CA: Annual Reviews.

Posner, M. I., & Warren, R. E. (1972). Traces, concepts and conscious constructions. In A. W. Melton & E. Martin (Eds.), *Coding processes in human memory.* Washington, DC: Winston & Sons.

Post, R. M. (1992). Transduction of psychsocial stress into the neurobiology of recurrent affective disorder. *American Journal of Psychiatry, 149,* 999–1010.

Pribram, K. H. (1986). The cognitive revolution and mind/brain issues. *American Psychologist, 41,* 507–520.

Prieto, S. L., Cole, D. A., & Tageson, C. W. (1992). Depressive self-schemas in clinic and nonclinic children. *Cognitive Therapy and Research, 16,* 521–534.

Pyszczynski, T., & Greenberg, J. (1987). Self-regulatory perseveration and the depressive self-focusing style: A self-awareness theory of reactive depression. *Psychological Bulletin, 102*, 1–17.

Pyszczynski, T., & Greenberg, J. (1992a). *Hanging on and letting go: Understanding the onset, progression and remission of depression.* New York: Springer-Verlag.

Pyszczynski, T., & Greenberg, J. (1992b). Putting cognitive constructs in their place: Is depression really just a matter of interpretation? *Psychological Inquiry, 3*, 255–258.

Pyszczynski, T., Greenberg, J., Hamilton, J., & Nix, G. (1991). On the relationship between self-focused attention and psychological disorder: A critical reappraisal. *Psychological Bulletin, 110*, 538–543.

Quammen, D. (1996). *The song of the dodo: Island biogeography in an age of extinctions.* New York: Scribners.

Radke-Yarrow, M., Belmont, B., Nottelmann, E., & Bottomly, L. (1990). Young children's self-conceptions: Origins in the natural discourse of depressed and normal mothers and their children. In D. Cicchetti & M. Beeghly (Eds.), *The self in transition.* Chicago: University of Chicago Press.

Radke-Yarrow, M., Cummings, E. M., Kuczynski, L., & Chapman, M. (1985). Patterns of attachment in two- and three-year olds in normal families and families with parental depression. *Child Development, 36*, 884–893.

Radloff, L. (1975). Sex differences in depression: The effects of occupation and marital status. *Sex Roles, 1*, 249–265.

Radloff, L., & Rae, D. S. (1979). Susceptibility and precipitation factors in depression: Sex differences and similarities. *Journal of Abnormal Psychology, 88*, 174–181.

Randolph, J. J., & Dykman, B. M. (in press). Perceptions of parenting and depression-proneness in the Offspring: Dysfunctional attitudes as a mediating mechanism. *Cognitive Therapy and Research.*

Reda, M. A., Carpiniello, B., Secchiaroli, L., & Blanco, S. (1985). Thinking, depression, and antidepressants: Modified and unmodified depressive beliefs during treatment with amitriptyline. *Cognitive Therapy and Research, 9*, 135–143.

Regier, D. A., Boyd, J. H., Burke, J. D., Rae, D. S., Myers, J. K., Kramer, M., Robins, L. N., George, L. K., Karno, M., & Locke, B. Z. (1988). One-month prevalence of mental disorders in the United States: Based on five Epidemiologic Catchment Area sites. *Archives of General Psychiatry, 45*, 977–986.

Regier, D. A., Myers, K. J., & Kramer, M. (1984). The NIMH Epidemiologic Catchment Area program: Historical context, major objectives, and study population characteristics. *Archives of General Psychiatry, 41*, 934–941.

Rehm, L. P. (1977). A self-control model of depression. *Behavior Therapy, 8*, 787–804.

Reid, W. H., & Morrison, H. L. (1983). Risk factors in children of depressed parents. In H. L. Morrison (Ed.), *Children of depressed parents: Risk, identification, and intervention.* New York: Grune & Stratton.

Revicki, D. A., Whitley, T. W., Gallery, M. E., & Allison, E. J., Jr. (1993). Impact of work environment characteristics on work-related stress and depression in emergency medicine residents: A longitudinal study. *Journal of Community and Applied Social Psychology, 3,* 273–284.

Ricks, M. (1985). The social transmission of parental attitudes: Attachment across generations. In I. Bretherton & E. Waters (Eds.), Growing points in attachment theory and research. *Monographs of the Society for Research in Child Development, 50*(1–2, Serial No. 209), 445–466.

Riskind, J. H., & Rholes, W. S. (1984). Cognitive accessibility and the capacity of cognitions to predict future depression. *Cognitive Therapy and Research, 8,* 1–12.

Roberts, J. E., Gotlib, I. H., & Kassel, J. D. (1996). Adult attachment mediates security and symptoms of depression: Mediating roles of dysfunctional attitudes and low self-esteem. *Journal of Personality and Social Psychology, 70,* 310–320.

Roberts, J. E., & Kassel, J. D. (1996). Mood state dependence in cognitive vulnerability to depression: The roles of positive and negative affect. *Cognitive Therapy and Research, 20,* 1–12.

Robins, C. J. (1990). Congruence of personality and life events in depression. *Journal of Abnormal Psychology, 99,* 393–397.

Robins, C. J., & Block, P. (1988). Personal vulnerability, life events, and depressive symptoms: A test of a specific interactional model. *Journal of Personality and Social Psychology, 54,* 847–852.

Robins, C. J., & Luten, A. G. (1991). Sociotropy and autonomy: Differential patterns of clinical presentation in unipolar depression. *Journal of Abnormal Psychology, 100,* 74–77.

Robins, L. N., Helzer, J. E., Croughan, J., & Ratcliff, K. S. (1981). National Institute of Mental Health Diagnostic Interview Schedule: Its history, characteristics, and validity. *Archives of General Psychiatry, 38,* 381–389.

Robinson, N. S., Garber, J., & Hilsman, R. (1995). Cognitions and stress: Direct and moderating effects on depressive versus externalizing symptoms during the junior high school transition. *Journal of Abnormal Psychology, 104,* 453–463.

Rogers, T. B., Kuiper, N. A., & Kirker, W. S. (1977). Self-reference and the encoding of personal information. *Journal of Personality and Social Psychology, 35,* 677–688.

Rohde, P., Lewinsohn, P. M., & Seely, J. R. (1990). Are people changed by the experience of having an episode of depression? A further test of the scar hypothesis. *Journal of Abnormal Psychology, 99,* 264–271.

Rolf, J. (1972). The social and academic competence of children vulnerable to schizophrenia and other behavior pathologies. *Journal of Abnormal Psychology, 80,* 225–243.

Rolf, J., & Garmezy, M. (1974). The school performance of children vulnerable to behavior pathology. In D. F. Ricks & M. Roff (Eds.), *Life history research in psychopathology.* Minneapolis: University of Minnesota Press.

Romano, J. M., & Turner, J. A. (1985). Chronic pain and depression: Does the evidence support a relationship? *Psychological Bulletin, 97,* 18–34.

Rose, D. T., & Abramson, L. Y. (1992). Developmental predictors of depressive cognitive style: Research and theory. In D. Cicchetti & S. L. Toth (Eds.), *Developmental perspectives on depression*. Rochester, NY: University of Rochester Press.

Rose, D. T., & Abramson, L. Y. (1995). *Developmental maltreatment and cognitive vulnerability to hopelessness depression*. Paper presented at the annual meeting of the Association for the Advancement of Behavior Therapy, Washington, DC.

Rose, D. T., Abramson, L. Y., Hodulik, C. J., Halberstadt, L., & Leff, G. (1994). Heterogeneity of cognitive style among depressed inpatients. *Journal of Abnormal Psychology, 103*, 419–429.

Rosenthal, D. (1970). *Genetic theory and abnormal behavior*. New York: McGraw-Hill.

Rosenthal, D., Wender, P. H., Kety, S. S., Schulsinger, F., Welner, J., & Ostergaard, L. (1968). Schizophrenics' offspring reared in adoptive homes. In D. Rosenthal & S. S. Kety (Eds.), *Transmission of schizophrenia*. Oxford, UK: Pergamon Press.

Ruble, N., Parsons, J. E., & Ross, J. (1976). Self-evaluative responses of children in an achievement setting. *Child Development, 47*, 990–997.

Rude, S. S., & Burnham, B. L. (1993). Do interpersonal and achievement vulnerabilities interact with congruent events to predict depression? Comparison of DEQ, SAS, DAS, and combined scales. *Cognitive Therapy and Research, 17*, 531–548.

Rutter, M. (1986a). Meyerian psychobiology, personality development, and the role of life experiences. *American Journal of Psychiatry, 143*, 1077–1087.

Rutter, M. (1986b). The developmental psychopathology of depression: Issues and perspectives. In M. Rutter, C. E. Izard, & P. B. Read (Eds.), *Depression in young people: Developmental and clinical perspectives*. New York: Guilford Press.

Rutter, M. (1987). Psychosocial resilience and protective mechanisms. *American Journal of Orthopsychiatry, 57*, 316–331.

Rutter, M. (1988). Longitudinal data in the study of causal processes: Some uses and some pitfalls. In M. Rutter (Ed.), *Studies of psychosocial risk: The power of longitudinal data*. Cambridge, UK: Cambridge University Press.

Rutter, M., Maughan, B., Mortimore, P., & Ouston, J. (1979). *Fifteen thousand hours: Secondary schools and their effects on children*. London: Open Books.

Sacco, W. P., & Beck, A. T. (1995). Cognitive theory and therapy. In E. E Beckham & W. R. Leber (Eds.), *Handbook of depression* (2nd ed.). New York: Guilford Press.

Safran, J. D. (1990). Towards a refinement of cognitive theory in light of interpersonal theory: I. Theory. *Clinical Psychology Review, 10*, 87–103.

Safran, J. D., & Segal, Z. V. (1990). *Interpersonal process in cognitive therapy*. New York: Basic Books.

Sargeant, J. K., Bruce, M. L., Florio, L. P., & Weissman, M. M. (1990). Factors associated with 1-year outcome of major depression in the community. *Archives of General Psychiatry, 47*, 519–526.

Sartorius, N., Jablensky, A., Gulbinat, W., & Ernberg, G. (1980). WHO collaborative study: Assessment of depressive disorders. *Psychological Medicine, 10,* 743–749.

Sattler, J. (1995). *Assessment of children* (4th ed.). San Diego: Sattler.

Schaefer, C., Coyne, J. C., & Lazarus, R. S. (1981). The health-related functions of social support. *Journal of Behavioral Medicine, 4,* 381–406.

Scher, C., & Ingram, R. E. (1998). *Attachment schemas as a potential vulnerability factor for depression among the adult offspring of depressed parents.* Manuscript in preparation.

Schleifer, S. J., Macari-Hinson, M. M., Coyle, D. A., Slater, W. R., Kahn, M., Gorlin, R., & Zucker, H. D. (1989). The nature and course of depression following myocardial infarction. *Archives of Internal Medicine, 149,* 1785–1789.

Schmidt, P. J., Nieman, L. K., Grover, G. N., Muller, K. L., Merriam, G. R., & Rubinow, D. R. (1991). Lack of effect of induced menses on symptoms in women with premenstrual syndrome. *New England Journal of Medicine, 324,* 1174–1179.

Schwartz, R. M., & Garamoni, G. L. (1989). Cognitive balance and psychopathology: Evaluation of an information processing model of positive and negative states of mind. *Clinical Psychology Review, 9,* 271–294.

Schwartz, R. M., & Michelson, L. (1987). States-of-mind model: Cognitive balance in the treatment of agoraphobia. *Journal of Consulting and Clinical Psychology, 55,* 557–565.

Sears, R. R., Maccoby, E. E., & Leven, H. (1957). *Patterns of childrearing.* Evanston, IL: Row Peterson.

Segal, Z. V. (1988). Appraisal of the self-schema construct in cognitive models of depression. *Psychological Bulletin, 103,* 147–162.

Segal, Z. V., & Dobson, K. S. (1992). Cognitive models of depression: Report from a consensus conference. *Psychological Inquiry, 3,* 225–229.

Segal, Z. V., Gemar, M., & Williams, S. (1998). *Differential cognitive response to a mood induction following successful cognitive therapy or pharmacotherapy for depression.* Manuscript submitted for publication.

Segal, Z. V., & Ingram, R. E. (1994). Mood priming and construct activation in tests of cognitive vulnerability to unipolar depression. *Clinical Psychology Review, 14,* 663–695.

Segal, Z. V., & Shaw, B. F. (1986). Cognition in depression: A reappraisal of Coyne and Gotlib's critique. *Cognitive Therapy and Research, 10,* 671–694.

Segal, Z. V., Shaw, B. F., Vella, D. D., & Katz, R. (1992). Cognitive and life stress predictors of relapse in remitted unipolar depressed patients: Test of the congruency hypothesis. *Journal of Abnormal Psychology, 101,* 26–36.

Segal, Z. V., & Vella, D. D. (1990). Self-schema in major depression: Replication and extension of a priming methodology. *Cognitive Therapy and Research, 14,* 161–176.

Segal, Z. V., Williams, J. M. G., Teasdale, J. D., & Gemar, M. (1996). A cognitive science perspective on kindling and episode sensitization in recurrent affective disorder. *Psychological Medicine, 26,* 371–380.

Seligman, M. E. P. (1975). *Helplessness: On depression, development, and death.* San Francisco: Freeman.

Seligman, M. E. P. (1990). Why is there so much depression today? The waxing of the individual and the waning of the common. In R. E. Ingram (Ed.), *Contemporary psychological approaches to depression*. New York: Plenum Press.

Seligman, M. E. P., & Abramson, L., Semmel, A., & von Baeyer, C. (1979). Depressive attributional style. *Journal of Abnormal Psychology, 88,* 242–248.

Seligman, M. E. P., Castellon, C., Cacciola, J., Schulman, P., Luborsky, L., Ollove, M., & Downing, R. (1988). Explanatory style changes during cognitive therapy for unipolar depression. *Journal of Abnormal Psychology, 97,* 13–18.

Seligman, M. E. P., Peterson, C., Kaslow, N. J., Tenenbaum, R. L., Alloy, L. B., & Abramson, L. Y. (1984). Attributional style and depressive symptoms among children. *Journal of Abnormal Psychology, 93,* 235–241.

Selman, R. (1980). *The growth of interpersonal understanding: Developmental and clinical analyses.* New York: Academic Press.

Selye, H. (1936). A syndrome produced by diverse noxious agents. *Nature, 138,* 32.

Shea, T., Glass, D., Pilkonis, P., Watkins, J., & Docherty, J. (1987). Frequency and implications of personality disorders in a sample of depressed outpatients. *Journal of Personality Disorders, 1,* 27–42.

Shelton, R. C., Hollon, S. D., Purdon, S. E., & Loosen, P. T. (1991). Biological and psychological aspects of depression. *Behavior Therapy, 22,* 201–228.

Sher, K. J., & Trull, T. J. (1996). Methodological issues in psychopathology research. *Annual Review of Psychology, 47,* 371–400.

Shiffrin, R. M., & Schneider, W. (1977). Controlled and automatic human processing: Perceptual learning, automatic attending and a general theory. *Psychological Review, 84,* 127–190.

Shorkey, C. T., & Whiteman, V. L. (1977). Development of the rational behavior inventory: Initial validity and reliability. *Educational and Psychological Measurement, 37,* 527–534.

Siegle, G., & Ingram, R. E. (1997). The big picture. *Contemporary Psychology, 41,* 163–164.

Siegle, G., & Ingram, R. E. (1997). Modeling individual differences in negative information processing biases. In G. Matthews (Ed.), *Cognitive science perspectives on personality and emotion*. New York: Elsevier Science.

Silverman, J. S., Silverman, J. A., & Eardley, D. A. (1984). Do maladaptive attitudes cause depression? *Archives of General Psychiatry, 41,* 28–30.

Simons, A., Garfield, S., & Murphy, G. (1984). The process of change in cognitive therapy and pharmacotherapy: Changes in mood and cognition. *Archives of General Psychiatry, 41,* 45–51.

Simons, A. D., & Thase, M. E. (1992). Biological markers, treatment outcome, and 1-year follow-up in endogenous depression: Electroencephalographic sleep studies and response to cognitive therapy. *Journal of Consulting and Clinical Psychology, 69,* 392–401.

Slife, B. D., Miura, S., Thompson, L. W., Shapiro, J. L., & Gallagher, D. (1984). Differential recall as a function of mood disorder in clinically depressed patients: Between- and within-subject differences. *Journal of Abnormal Psychology, 93,* 391–400.

Smith, K. A., Teasdale, J. D., & Cowen, P. J. (1998). *Effects of pharmacological mood induction on measures of depressive thinking in recovered depressed patients.* Manuscript submitted for publication.

Smith, T. W. (1986). Type A behavior and cardiovascular disease: An information processing approach. In R. E. Ingram (Ed.), *Information processing approaches to clinical psychology.* Orlando, FL: Academic Press.

Smith, T. W. (1989). Assessment in rational-emotive therapy: Empirical access to the ABCD model. In M. E. Bernard & R. DiGiuseppe (Eds.), *Inside rational-emotive therapy: A critical appraisal of the theory and therapy of Albert Ellis.* San Diego: Academic Press.

Smith, T. W., & Greenberg, J. (1981). Depression and self-focused attention. *Motivation and Emotion, 5,* 323–331.

Smith, T. W., Ingram, R. E., & Brehm, S. S. (1983). Social anxiety, self-preoccupation, and recall of self-relevant information. *Journal of Personality and Social Psychology, 44,* 1276–1283.

Smith, T. W., Ingram, R. E., & Roth, D. L. (1985). Self-focused attention and depression: Self-evaluation, affect, and life stress. *Motivation and Emotion, 9,* 381–389.

Smith, T. W., O'Keefe, J. C., & Jenkins, M. (1988). Dependency and self-criticism: Correlates of depression or moderators of the effects of stressful events? *Journal of Personality Disorders, 2,* 160–169.

Smith, T. W., & Rhodewalt, F. T. (1991). Methodological challenges at the social/clinical interface. In C. R. Snyder & D. R. Forsyth (Eds.), *Handbook of social and clinical psychology: The health perspective.* New York: Pergamon Press.

Smith, T. W., Wallston, K. A., & Dwyer, K. A. (1995). On babies and bathwater: Disease impact and negative affectivity in the self-reports of persons with rheumatoid arthritis. *Health Psychology, 14,* 64, 73.

Speier, P. L., Sherak, D. L., Hirsch, S., & Cantwell, D. P. (1995). Depression in children and adolescents. In E. E. Beckham & W. R. Leber (Eds.). *Handbook of depression* (2nd ed.). New York: Guilford Press.

Spitzer, R. L., & Endicott, J. (1978). Medical and mental disorder: Proposed definition and criteria. In R. L. Spitzer & D. F. Klein (Eds.), *Critical issues in psychiatric diagnosis.* New York: Raven Press.

Stancer, H. C., Persad, E., Wagener, D. K., & Jorna, T. (1987). Evidence for homogeneity of major depression and bipolar affective disorder. *Journal of Psychiatric Research, 21,* 37–53.

Stein, D. J., & Young, J. E. (1992). *Cognitive science and clinical disorders.* San Diego: Academic Press.

Sternberg, S. (1969). The discovery of processing stages: Extensions of Donders method. *Acta Psychologia, 30,* 276–315.

Stinson, C. H., & Palmer, S. E. (1991). Parallel distributed processing models of person schemas and psychopathologies. In M. J. Horowitz (Ed.), *Person schemas and maladaptive interpersonal patterns.* Chicago: University of Chicago Press.

Strauman, T. J. (1989). Self-discrepancies in clinical depression and social phobia: Cognitive structures that underlie emotional disorders? *Journal of Abnormal Psychology, 98,* 5–14.

Strickland, B. R. (1988). Sex-related differences in health and illness. Special Issue: Women's health: Our minds, our bodies. *Psychology of Women Quarterly, 12,* 381–399.

Sturt, E., Kumakura, N., & Der, G. (1984). How depressing life is: Life-long morbidity risk for depressive disorder in the general population. *Journal of Affective Disorders, 7,* 109–122.

Sweeney, P. D., Anderson, K., & Bailey, S. (1986). Attributional style in depression: A meta-analytic review. *Journal of Personality and Social Psychology, 50,* 974–991

Szasz, T. S. (1960). The myth of mental illness. *American Psychologist, 15,* 113–118.

Taylor, L., & Ingram, R. E. (1998). *Cognitive reactivity and depressotypic information processing in the children of depressed mothers.* Manuscript submitted for publication.

Teasdale, J. D. (1983). Negative thinking in depression: Cause, effect, or reciprocal relationship? *Advances in Behavior Research and Therapy, 5,* 3–25.

Teasdale, J. D. (1988). Cognitive vulnerability to persistent depression. *Cognition and Emotion, 2,* 247–274.

Teasdale, J. D. (1993). Emotion and two kinds of meaning: Cognitive therapy and applied cognitive science. *Behaviour Research and Therapy, 31,* 339–354.

Teasdale, J. D., & Barnard, P. J. (1993). *Affect, cognition, and change.* Hillsdale, NJ: Erlbaum.

Teasdale, J. D., & Dent, J. (1987). Cognitive vulnerability to depression: An investigation of two hypotheses. *British Journal of Clinical Psychology, 26,* 113–126.

Teasdale, J. D., Segal, Z. V., & Williams, J. M. G. (1995). An information-processing analysis of depressive relapse and its prevention: The theoretical background to Attentional Control Training. *Behaviour Research and Therapy, 33,* 25–39.

Thase, M. E., Simons, A. D., & Cahalane, J. F. (1991). Cognitive behavior therapy of endogenous depression: Part 1: An outpatient clinical replication series. *Behavior Therapy, 22,* 457–467.

Thase, M. E., Simons, A. D., McGeary, J., Cahalane, J. F., Hughes, C., Harden, T., & Friedman, E. (1992). Relapse after cognitive behavior therapy of depression: Potential implications for longer courses of treatment. *American Journal of Psychiatry, 149,* 1046–1052.

Tennen, H., Hall, J. A., & Affleck, G. (1995a). Depression research methodologies in the Journal of Personality and Social Psychology: A review and critique. *Journal of Personality and Social Psychology, 68,* 870–884.

Tennen, H., Hall, J. A., & Affleck, G. (1995b). Rigor, rigor mortis, and conspiratorial views of depression research. *Journal of Personality and Social Psychology, 68,* 895–900.

Thurber, S., Crow, L. A., Thurber, J. A., & Woffington, L. M. (1990). Cognitive distortions and depression in psychiatrically disturbed adolescent inpatients. *Journal of Clinical Psychology, 46,* 57–60.

Tolman, E. C. (1932). *Purposive behavior in animals and man.* New York: Century.

Torgerson, S. (1986). Genetic factors in moderately severe and mild affective disorders. *Archives of General Psychiatry, 43,* 222–226.

Toth, S. L., Manly, J., & Cicchetti, D. (1992). Child maltreatment and vulnerability to depression. *Development and Psychopathology, 4,* 92–112.

Trull, T. J., Widiger, T. A., & Guthrie, P. (1990). Categorical versus dimensional status of borderline personality disorder. *Journal of Abnormal Psychology, 99,* 40–48.

Tversky, A., & Kahneman, D. (1973). Availability: A heuristic for judging frequency and probability. *Cognitive Psychology, 5,* 207–232.

Vasta, R., Haith, M. M., & Miller, S. A. (1992). *Child psychology: The modern science.* New York: Wiley.

Velten, E. (1968). A laboratory task for induction of mood states. *Behaviour Research and Therapy, 6,* 473–482.

Vredenburg, K., Flett, G. L., & Krames, L. (1993). Analogue versus clinical depression: A critical reappraisal. *Psychological Bulletin, 113,* 327–344.

Wachtel, P. (1987). *Action and insight.* New York: Guilford Press.

Wakefield J. C. (1992a). Disorder as harmful dysfunction: A conceptual critique of DSM-III-R's definition of mental disorder. *Psychological Review, 99,* 232–247.

Wakefield J. C. (1992b). The concept of mental disorder: On the boundary between biological facts and social values. *American Psychologist, 47,* 373–388.

Walker, E., & Hoppes, E. (1984). Longitudinal research in schizophrenia: The high risk method. In S. A. Mednick & M. Harway (Eds.), *Handbook of longitudinal research.* New York: Praeger.

Walsh, B. T., Roose, S. P., Glassman, A. H., Gladis, M., & Sadik, C. (1985). Bulimia and depression. *Psychosomatic Medicine, 47,* 123–131.

Watson, D., & Clark, L. A. (1984). Negative affectivity: The disposition to experience negative emotional states. *Psychological Bulletin, 96,* 465–490.

Watson, D., & Kendall, P. C. (1989). *Anxiety and depression: Distinctive and overlapping features.* San Diego: Academic Press.

Weary, G., Edwards, J. A., & Jacobson, J. A. (1995). Depression research methodologies in the Journal of Personality and Social Psychology: A reply. *Journal of Personality and Social Psychology, 68,* 885–891.

Weintraub, S. (1987). Risk factors in schizophrenia: The Stony Brook high-risk project. *Schizophrenia Bulletin, 13,* 439–450.

Weintraub, S., Winters, K. C., & Neale, J. M. (1986). Competence and vulnerability in children with an affectively disordered parent. In M. Rutter, C. E. Izard, & P. B. Read (Eds.), *Depression in young people: Developmental and clinical perspectives.* New York: Guilford Press.

Weissman, M. M. (1988). Psychopathology in the children of depressed parents:

Direct interview studies. In D. L. Dunner, E. S. Gershon, & J. E. Barett (Eds.), *Relatives at risk for mental disorders.* New York: Raven Press.

Weissman, M. M., Gershon, E. S., Kidd, K. K., Prusoff, B. A., & Leckman, J. F. (1984). Psychiatric disorders in the relatives of probands with affective disorders. *Archives of General Psychiatry, 41,* 13–21.

Weissman, M. M., & Klerman, G. L. (1977). Sex differences and the epidemiology of depression. *Archives of General Psychiatry, 34,* 98–111.

Weissman, M. M., & Klerman, G. L. (1985). Gender and depression. *Trends in Neuroscience, 8,* 416–420.

Weissman, M. M., Klerman, G. L., Prusoff, B. A., Sholomskas, D., & Padian, N. (1981). Depressed outpatients: Results one year after treatment with drugs and/or interpersonal psychotherapy. *Archives of General Psychiatry, 38,* 52–55.

Weissman, M. M., Leaf, P. J., Holzer, C. E., Myers, J. K., & Tischler, G. L. (1984). The epidemiology of depression: An update on sex differences in rates. *Journal of Affective Disorders, 7,* 179–188.

Wells, K. B., Golding, J. M., & Burnam, M. A. (1988). Psychiatric disorder and limitations in physical functioning in a sample of the Los Angeles general population. *American Journal of Psychiatry, 145,* 712–717.

Wells, K. B., Stewart, A., Hays, R. D., Burnam, M. A., Rogers, W., Daniels, M., Berry, S., Greenfield, S., & Ware, J. (1989). The functioning and well-being of depressed patients: Results from the Medical Outcomes Study. *Journal of the American Medical Association, 262,* 914-919.

Westen, D. (1991). Social cognition and object relations. *Psychological Bulletin, 109,* 429–455.

Weissman, A., & Beck, A. T. (1978). *Development and validation of the Dysfunctional Attitude Scale: A preliminary investigation.* Paper presented at the annual meeting of the American Educational Research Association, Toronto, Canada.

Whisman, M. A., & Kwon, P. (1992). Parental representations, cognitive distortions, and mild depression. *Cognitive Therapy and Research, 16,* 557–568.

Whisman, M. A., Miller, I. W., Norman, W. H., & Keitner, G. I. (1992). Cognitive therapy with depressed inpatients: Specific effects on dysfunctional cognitions. *Journal of Consulting and Clinical Psychology, 59,* 282–288.

Whitman, P. B., & Leitenberg, H. (1990). Negatively biased recall in children with self-reported symptoms of depression. *Journal of Abnormal Child Psychology, 18,* 15–27.

Widiger, T. A., & Trull, T. J. (1985). The empty debate over the existence of mental illness: Comments on Gorenstein. *American Psychologist, 40,* 468–471.

Widom, C. (1977). A methodology for studying noninstitutionalized psychopaths. *Journal of Consulting and Clinical Psychology, 45,* 674–683.

Wilkinson, I. M., & Blackburn, I. M. (1981). Cognitive style in depressed and recovered depressed patients. *British Journal of Clinical Psychology, 20,* 283–292.

Williams, J. M. G. (1992). *The psychological treatment of depression*. London: Routledge.

Williams, J. M. G. (1997). *Cry of pain*. London: Penguin Books.

Williams, J. M. G., Watts, F. N., MacLeod, C., & Mathews, A. (1997). *Cognitive psychology and emotional disorders*. Chichester, UK: Wiley.

Williams, R. M. (1988). *Individual differences in the effects of mood on cognition*. Unpublished doctoral dissertation, University of Oxford.

Wilson, E. O. (1975). *Sociobiology: The new synthesis*. Cambridge, MA: Harvard University Press.

Wilson, E. O. (1978). *On human nature*. Cambridge, MA: Harvard University Press.

Wilson, J. S., & Costanzo, P. R. (1996). A preliminary study of attachment, attention, and schizotypy in early adulthood. *Journal of Social and Clinical Psychology, 15*, 231–260.

Winfield, I., George, L. K., Swartz, M., & Blazer, D. G. (1990). Sexual assault and psychiatric disorders among a community sample of women. *American Journal of Psychiatry, 147*, 335–341.

Winokur, G., & Clayton, P. J. (1967). Family history studies: II. Sex differences and alcoholism in primary affective illness. *British Journal of Psychiatry, 113*, 973–979.

Winokur, G., Clayton, P., & Reich, T. (1969). *Manic depressive illness*. St. Louis: Mosby.

Winokur, G., Coryell, W., Endicott, J., & Akiskal, H. (1993a). Further distinctions between manic–depressive illness (bipolar disorder) and primary depressive disorder (unipolar depression). *American Journal of Psychiatry, 150*, 1176–1181.

Winokur, G., Tsuang, M., & Crowe, R. (1982). The Iowa 500: Affective disorder in relatives of manic and depressed patients. *American Journal of Psychiatry, 139*, 209–212.

Worland, J., Janes, C., Anthony, E., McGinnis, M., & Cass, L. (1984). St. Louis Risk Research project: Comprehensive progress report of experimental studies. In N. Watt, E. J. Anthony, L. Wynne, & J. Rolf (Eds.), *Children at risk for schizophrenia*. New York: Cambridge University Press.

Worland, J., Weeks, D. G., Janes, C. L., & Strock, B. D. (1984). Intelligence, classroom behavior, and academic achievement in children at high and low risk for psychopathology: A structural equation analysis. *Journal of Abnormal Child Psychology, 12*, 437–454.

World Health Organization. (1992). *The ICD-10 classification of mental and behavioral disorders: Diagnostic criteria for research*. Geneva, Switzerland: Author.

Wundt, W. (1899). Zur Kritik tachistoskosckopischer Versuche. *Philosophische Studien, 15*, 287–317.

Zajonc, R. B. (1980). Feeling and thinking: Preferences need no inferences. *American Psychologist, 35*, 151–175.

Zeiss, A. M., & Lewinsohn, P. M. (1988). Enduring deficits after remission of depression: A test of the scar hypothesis. *Behaviour Research and Therapy, 26*, 151–158.

Zeitlin, H. (1985). *The natural history of psychiatric disorders in children*. New York: Oxford University Press.

Zimmerman, M., Coryell, W., Pfohl, B., Corenthal, C., & Stangl, D. (1986). ECT response in depressed patients with and without a DSM-III personality disorder. *American Journal of Psychiatry, 143*, 1030–1032.

Zubin, J., & Spring, B. (1977). Vulnerability—A new view of schizophrenia. *Journal of Abnormal Psychology, 86*, 103–126.

Zupan, B. A., Hammen, C., & Jaenicke, C. (1987). The effects of current mood and prior depressive history on self-schematic processing in children. *Journal of Experimental Child Psychology, 43*, 149–158.

Zurawski, R. M., & Smith, T. W. (1987). Assessing irrational beliefs and emotional distress: Evidence and implications of limited discriminant validity. *Journal of Counseling Psychology, 34*, 224–227.

Zuroff, D. C., Koestner, R., & Powers, T. A. (1994). Self-criticism at age 12: Longitudinal study of adjustment. *Cognitive Therapy and Research, 18*, 267–386.

Zuroff, D. C., & Mongrain, M. (1987). Dependency and self-criticism: Vulnerability factors for depressive affective states. *Journal of Abnormal Psychology, 96*, 14–22.

Author Index

Subject Index